Register Now for Onl[...] to Your Boo[...]

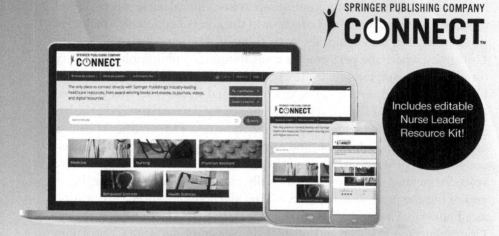

Your print purchase of *Compassion Fatigue and Burnout in Nursing, Second Edition* **includes online access to the contents of your book**— increasing accessibility, portability, and searchability!

Access today at:

http://connect.springerpub.com/content/book/978-0-8261-5521-4 or scan the QR code at the right with your smartphone and enter the access code below.

GUJV5FLH

Scan here for quick access.

SPRINGER PUBLISHING COMPANY

View all our products at springerpub.com

Vidette Todaro-Franceschi, PhD, RN, FT, is a tenured professor of nursing at the College of Staten Island and appointed doctoral nursing faculty at the Graduate Center, both of the City University of New York. A registered nurse for 37 years, she has worked in a variety of roles and settings as staff, head nurse, assistant director, clinical supervisor, clinical nurse specialist, and educator. A nurse scholar and educator in the areas of end-of-life/palliative care, ethics, and leadership, she earned her PhD in nursing at New York University, where she performed a transdisciplinary philosophical inquiry on ideas of energy, for which she earned several awards. She is the author of two books, many articles, chapters, and digital stories. Her first authored book, *The Enigma of Energy*, is based on her initial doctoral research; she has since then performed seminal research in the areas of bereavement healing, end-of-life nursing education, and professional quality of life, and has been consulted by professionals around the world about her work. A passionate voice for nursing, she has presented locally, nationally, and internationally on end of life and professional quality of life. She holds advanced certification as a Fellow in Thanatology from the Association for Death Education and Counseling and has been an End-of-Life Nursing Education Consortium (ELNEC) trainer since the first cohort in 2001.

The first edition of this book, *Compassion Fatigue and Burnout in Nursing: Enhancing Professional Quality of Life*, received critical acclaim from numerous reviewers and was chosen to be listed on the LPN to BSN Online "Ultimate Reading List for Nurses."

Compassion Fatigue and Burnout in Nursing

Enhancing Professional Quality of Life

Second Edition

Vidette Todaro-Franceschi, PhD, RN, FT

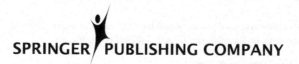

SPRINGER PUBLISHING COMPANY

Copyright © 2019 Springer Publishing Company, LLC

Springer Publishing Company, LLC
11 West 42nd Street
New York, NY 10036
www.springerpub.com
http://connect.springerpub.com/home

Acquisitions Editor: Joseph Morita
Compositor: Exeter Premedia Services Private Ltd.

ISBN: 978-0-8261-5519-1
ebook ISBN: 978-0-8261-5521-4
Nurse Leader Resource Kit ISBN: 978-0-8261-3664-0
DOI: 10.1891/9780826155214

Nurse Leader Resource Kit is available for download from https://www.springerpub.com/cfbn

19 20 21 22 23 / 5 4 3 2 1

The author and the publisher of this Work have made every effort to use sources believed to be reliable to provide information that is accurate and compatible with the standards generally accepted at the time of publication. The author and publisher shall not be liable for any special, consequential, or exemplary damages resulting, in whole or in part, from the readers' use of, or reliance on, the information contained in this book. The publisher has no responsibility for the persistence or accuracy of URLs for external or third-party Internet websites referred to in this publication and does not guarantee that any content on such websites is, or will remain, accurate or appropriate.

Library of Congress Cataloging-in-Publication Data

Names: Todaro-Franceschi, Vidette, author.
Title: Compassion fatigue and burnout in nursing: enhancing professional
   quality of life / Vidette Todaro-Franceschi.
Description: Second edition. | New York, NY: Springer Publishing Company,
   LLC, [2019] | Includes bibliographical references and index.
Identifiers: LCCN 2018052481| ISBN 9780826155191 | ISBN 9780826136640 (Nurse
   Leader Resource Kit) | ISBN 9780826155214 (ebook)
Subjects: | MESH: Nurses—psychology | Philosophy, Nursing | Empathy |
   Burnout, Professional—psychology | Burnout, Professional—prevention &
   control | Quality of Life
Classification: LCC RT86 | NLM WY 87 | DDC 610.73—dc23
LC record available at https://lccn.loc.gov/2018052481

Contact us to receive discount rates on bulk purchases.
We can also customize our books to meet your needs.
For more information please contact: sales@springerpub.com

Publisher's Note: New and used products purchased from third-party sellers are not guaranteed for quality, authenticity, or access to any included digital components.

Printed in the United States of America.

Once again,
I dedicate this book to nurse colleagues everywhere with
the hope that you will go about your work heartfully and
with passion, knowing that what you do is so important and
that each and every day you are making a difference.

Contents

Foreword Mary Koloroutis, MSN, RN   *ix*
Preface   *xiii*

Part I: Professional Quality of Life

1. The Good, Bad, and Ugly of Professional Quality of Life   *3*

2. Transforming Both Health and Care in Healthcare   *15*

Part II: Unity, Purpose, and the Good: An Ethic of Caring

3. Compassion and Contentment: Being Heartful and
    Happy at Work   *33*

4. Values and Excellences in Nursing   *51*

5. The *ART* of Reaffirming Purpose: A Healing Model
    for Carers   *63*

Part III: The Bad: Compassion Fatigue and Moral Distress

6. Compassion Fatigue: A Heavy Heart Hurts   *83*

7. Moral Distress: I Know What I Ought to Do!   *99*

**Part IV: The Ugly, Uglier, and Ugliest: Burnout and
Workplace Violence**

8. Burnout: Feeling Empty-Hearted and Disheartened   *123*

9. Bullying and Incivility in Nursing: An Oxymoron   *147*

Part V: Facing Death

10. Being Prepared to Care for the Dying   *171*

11. Collective Trauma and Healing in Healthcare:
     Aching, Breaking Hearts   *191*

Part VI: Beating the Odds

12. Changing the Mindset in Nursing Education   *207*

13. Cultivating Collective Mindful Awareness in Nursing:
     A Leadership Agenda   *227*

14. Imagining and Actualizing the Power of Nursing   *249*

Appendix A   ProQOL Tool for Self-Assessment of PQOL   263
Appendix B   PPACD Tool for Preparedness and Ability to Care for the Dying   267
Appendix C   Resources   269
Appendix D   Nurse Leader Resource Kit   279
Index   295

Foreword

Although the world is full of suffering, it is full also of the overcoming of it.

—Helen Keller

For the past 20 years, I have had the privilege of sitting with patients, nurses, physicians, therapists, administrators, social workers, environmental service workers, and others in healthcare to talk about the work of human caring and what it means for all of us. Some of the most enlightening conversations have been those in which patients and families join with healthcare professionals and share their lived experiences of illness and vulnerability.

In these conversations, a safe space is created—like the white space on a page, intentionally left blank—in which the meaning and purpose of the work of human caring, in the absence of everything else, is illuminated. These safe spaces serve as a catalyst for healing because they allow us to gain greater self-awareness. We experience acceptance without judgment. Tears are common in these circles—tears of frustration, tears of compassion, tears of joy, tears of revelation, tears of pain and suffering. And what so often follows are apologies for the tears, as the message in our healthcare cultures is that we must put on a brave face, let it go, soldier on, shake it off. People who work so intimately with people going through some of the most difficult things they will ever face should not be expected to figure out, on their own time, how to cope. We must change our paradigm in healthcare, accepting the responsibility, as institutions, to make time available for healthcare workers to connect with their own needs and humanity, and provide knowledge-based support to improve the healthcare environment.

In this second edition of *Compassion Fatigue and Burnout in Nursing*, Dr. Vidette Todaro-Franceschi shares stories of human connection and the intimacy of the caring experience. She helps us see that as we gain understanding about the importance of human connection, and as these connections deepen, the tears of those caring for others are no longer dismissed. In a workplace where caring relationships are valued, emotional responses are understood as natural expressions of human compassion. Tears and other expressions of emotion are seen as a way to become more aware of the power, love, and sorrow that are inherent parts of caring for another human being who is hurting. Professionalism does not require turning away from our lived experience. In fact, it necessitates exactly the opposite. To thrive professionally we need to learn how to turn toward our experience, especially in the face of suffering. We need to learn how to meet it and make sense of it, and know that when we express emotion, we will not be left behind. As Dr. Todaro-Franceschi writes in her chapter on being prepared to care for the dying, "There is nothing wrong with crying and showing human emotion . . . it is the nurse who *doesn't* cry who worries me."

Listening to the voices in her narratives stirs resolve in me to do what I can to inspire more compassionate, relationship-based healthcare cultures—cultures in which human connection is central and human isolation is not tolerated. This will not happen by accident. The ability to meet human suffering with compassion is a skill that requires cultivation. Unless we create safe spaces to make meaning of experience and recognize what we in healthcare are experiencing physically, mentally, and spiritually, we are left with a default way of managing—that is, turning away, distracting ourselves to numb the pain.

I am struck by the paradox that the work of healthcare includes so many painful elements of the human experience and is still, somehow, profoundly beautiful. That contradiction is no small thing, and it's a lot for any one person to hold. How is one person supposed to make sense of it, sort it out, or reconcile the paradox of it. None of us can reconcile the complexity in isolation. We need each other.

When I discovered the first edition of *Compassion Fatigue and Burnout in Nursing*, I immediately reached out to Dr. Todaro-Franceschi. I was touched by how in sync our thoughts are about our beloved profession of nursing and our shared understanding of how important and meaningful the work of human caring is. I particularly appreciated her thinking about the nature of the work of caring when I read her words, "We are connected, *one* with those we care for—and it is this unity and purpose that manifest the potential to heal." I was further struck by her clear assertion, "It is impossible to disengage the quality of care for the patient from the carer's professional quality of life; they are one."

I wanted to let Dr. Todaro-Franceschi know that her work matters. I wanted her to know that I will use her book to guide my own work, and to thank her for her meaningful contribution to our profession. Her response was immediate and gracious. She reinforced how important it is for those of us working to improve healthcare systems throughout the world to stay focused on our shared humanity and the preservation of individual dignity.

Dr. Todaro-Franceschi's scholarly rigor is a gift to her readers. I also appreciate that it does not diminish the exquisite openness and vulnerability with which she writes. She invites her readers in as honored colleagues to share her lived experience in caring for patients and teaching students, as well as her own experiences as a patient and loved one. Dr. Todaro-Franceschi calls us to look with open eyes, open hearts, and open minds at the good, the bad, the ugly, the uglier, and the ugliest in healthcare so that together we can cultivate a healthcare world in which compassion prevails and our shared humanity is embraced.

I am truly inspired by the breadth and depth of this new edition of *Compassion Fatigue and Burnout in Nursing*. There are three areas in particular in which Dr. Todaro-Franceschi gave me new language and expanded awareness: (a) we have an ethical imperative to claim and value our professional quality of life, (b) there is much to be learned about preparing clinicians in all disciplines to care for the dying, and (c) finding meaning in our work is a fundamental way to prevent compassion fatigue and burnout.

In order to understand what leads to compassion fatigue and burnout, Dr. Todaro-Franceschi helps us to understand the difference between the two. Her explanation of this difference, along with the section on the existence of collective trauma in healthcare, can be instrumental in helping to have valuable conversations about the emotional strain of caring. The strong desire to help, coupled with the consistent challenges inherent in our work, set us up to feel isolated in our suffering, at least until we tap into the support of others who are going through the same things. Just as soldiers coming back after combat need to connect with people who have been through similar experiences, people in healthcare must have the support of their own coworkers. Dr. Todaro-Franceschi speaks of the unique plight of healthcare workers this way:

> The idea that healthcare professionals, and particularly nurses, might suffer from "death overload," collective trauma, and possibly PTSD has not been given much attention. . . We [nurses] readily acknowledge when others are traumatized and are suffering. For our own quality of life, both personal and professional, it is perhaps time for us to acknowledge that we have been and continue to be collectively traumatized in our work environments. We can encourage ourselves and each other to make meaning from our collective suffering.

Dr. Todaro-Franceschi describes our society's denial of death, highlighting that death and dying are not topics consistently taught in academic programs for nurses and physicians. Yet, death and dying are central to nursing practice, and if we are not prepared, we likely are not as effective as we want to be and as our patients and their loved ones need us to be. Dr. Todaro-Franceschi reflects on her own experience as a nursing student, which still seems to be the norm in student preparation:

> We were taught basic postmortem care—how to clean and wrap a body after death. We were never taught how to make eye contact with the patient who was dying, or his loved ones who asked, "Is he dying?" We were never taught how to talk, or listen, for that matter, to patients nearing the end of life. And we were certainly never taught how to comfort those who were left behind after their loved ones died.

Making meaning from our experiences with patients and their loved ones who are suffering is a fundamental way to support our professional quality of life. Every word in this superb book can act as a catalyst for courageous conversations about what it means to work in the midst of human suffering and trauma. I hope you will use what you learn here to talk with your colleagues in all healthcare disciplines about what it takes for all of us to be fully present to ourselves, to each other, and to our patients in the midst of all of the hurt and pain we're surrounded with every day. What does it take to prevent ourselves from becoming overwhelmed and disconnected? What does it take to keep from being diminished in our own humanity and subsequently diminishing the humanity of those in our care?

Twentieth-century author, professor, and theologian, Henri Nouwen, wrote, "Anyone who willingly enters into the pain of a stranger is truly a remarkable person." If you work in healthcare, you are surrounded by such remarkable people every day. Perhaps the greatest resources in our healthcare systems are the truly remarkable nurses, physicians, therapists, social workers, service workers, and administrators who show up every day and willingly enter into the pain of strangers. It is up to all of us to hold and safeguard each other in this sacred work. Dr. Todaro-Franceschi helps us in this mission through this extraordinary book.

I hope nurses and all caregivers experience this book as a true validation of the importance and beauty of their work. I hope healthcare leaders and educators turn to this book for insights and guidance in creating compassionate cultures of care, driven by a deep respect for the mission of human caring and all who willingly enter the pain of strangers. I know I will turn to this book often.

Mary Koloroutis, MSN, RN
CEO, Creative Health Care Management
Minneapolis, Minnesota

Preface

In the seminal edition of this book published in 2012, I underscored the need for nurses to focus more on our own well-being, for the benefit of everyone. I am pleased to note that in recent years there has been considerably more emphasis on the importance of our professional quality of life. However, a workforce crisis still exists in nursing, and as I was working on this second edition, I was occasionally seized with a sense of desperation about it. For as both a nurse and a consumer of healthcare, I am scared. The data continue to accrue; the environment where people work plays a part not only in the health and happiness of the workforce but also the quality of the work that they do. People depend on us to *care* in health*care*. They expect us to advocate for and protect them from harm. But how can we do that, if we have lost our zest for nursing?

In the preface to the first edition, I began by sharing how I had woken up one day after years in practice and realized I didn't look forward to work anymore. It was a subtle change that happened over time and then WHAM! It hit me. I hated going to work. In one of my disillusioned moments during my nursing career, I decided to apply for a job outside of nursing. I had been working as a staff nurse in critical care for several years and I wasn't happy. Don't get me wrong; I love nursing. I was just tired of seeing people so sick, often dying. Tired of working every other weekend, every other holiday, knowing full well that we would be short-staffed and I wouldn't be able to take a break or more importantly provide the quality care that I wanted to give to my patients. Tired of getting talked down to by the occasional pompous physician, and well, I was just plain *tired*. So, I applied for a job at Macy's.

Yup, I went in to their personnel department on my day off, while the kids were in school, filled out the paperwork, and took a short test. I didn't mention it to any of my friends or family; I knew they wouldn't understand.

A week later they called me to schedule an interview at which time they offered me a supervisory position. They said I was "overqualified" to be a salesperson. Hmm, I thought. I could easily switch careers and get a great shopping discount to boot. I seriously thought about it, for all of one day. When I sat down to dinner that night and told my husband about my interview and Macy's offer, he said, "Are you crazy? Are you kidding? Why would you leave nursing to work in Macy's?" Of course he was right. How could I consider throwing away my nursing career? So, I didn't. And after 37 years as a nurse, I am still glad I stayed in nursing.

The paramount question for most who will read this book is: How do I remain in a profession I love and continue to love the work I do when it seems like the entire system is working against me? It is my hope that you find the answer to that question in this book. Yet, I also want to emphasize that while readers can use the information provided to enhance their own professional quality of life, my real goal is to reach out to the collective. Change begins with each of us, sure, but at some point, we must make a concerted effort to fix what is broken and transform our work environment. Otherwise, we are just putting a temporary Band-Aid on a wound and it will eventually fall off. We have to heal the *whole*, and that will take courage as well as resilience, compassion, and yes, passion.

Some readers of the first edition may recall a few of the stories I shared in the third person; in this book I disclose that several were personal. They were in fact about a family member's hospitalization experiences in a facility where there was an obvious disconnect between the carers and the *care*. Readers may wonder why I have chosen to disclose this now, and the answer is multifaceted. The simple answer is that in order to be true to myself, to be authentic—as a nurse, an educator, and the wife of a man harmed in a healthcare system—I *had* to share the experiences, and since the first printing of this book, I have done so in various places and forums.

In the wonderful movie *You've Got Mail*, when Tom Hanks, who plays the character that owns a large franchise of bookstores, tells Meg Ryan, playing the part of a small independent bookstore owner, that his having run her out of business wasn't personal, she says something along the lines of "What does that mean? If anything, everything ought to begin with it being personal." I agree. We are human beings, and *how we treat one another*, whether in business or not, whether professional or not, *is personal*. When we are wounded by others it is personal, and when we are cared for by others, whether they are formal carers or not, *it is personal*.

There is nothing *im*personal about nurses caring for people at their most vulnerable. So, herein I share a personal account of our family's experience in a healthcare system. There is no need to point any fingers explicitly here. It could have been anywhere; it could happen anywhere. *It is happening* *everywhere.* This particular story, I think, serves to bring together and make absolutely clear the many issues that coalesce into a crisis of care for all of us. For *no one is safe in a broken healthcare system* where nurses and other carers cannot, for whatever reason, competently and compassionately *care.* And it doesn't matter *who* you know or *what* you know.

Unfortunately, many of the nurses who are living these experiences—working in sometimes quite appalling environments—feel that their voices do not count. Some are fearful for their livelihood, and feel boxed in with nowhere to go. Consequently, they remain in unhealthy work environments where they can only give substandard care, harming themselves because they know full well they are not being true to their calling as carers. They become silent voices and witnesses. What's more, nurses (and other carers) who continue to work in places where less than optimal care is the mainstay know that they are not just hurting themselves, they are hurting innocent people who have put their complete trust in them to *do the right thing.*

Since the writing of the first edition I have met thousands of healthcare professionals at various events, and have taught hundreds more students in different classes. Many individuals have shared atrocious stories about personal and/or professional healthcare experiences and ugly workplace environments. At one of many memorable conferences after I did a keynote, a nurse came up to me with the handout from my talk and asked me if I would sign it. That was a first for me; I have had people ask me to autograph books, but no one had ever asked me to sign one of my presentation handouts before. As I signed it, I asked her why she wanted me to do so, and with tears in her eyes, she said that she had been a silent voice for a long time. She went on to tell me that she was going to hang it on her wall at work to always remind herself that she didn't have to be one. My heart hurt; I was so moved by her words that I started to cry, too.

I am regularly contacted via email, LinkedIn, Twitter, and an occasional phone call, from nurses and other healthcare professionals who have read my work and/or heard me speak. I want you to know that I heard you all, and I continue to hear your voices in my head as I write this now. I also want those of you who, to date, feel that you have been silent voices, to know that I hear you, too. *Your voices ALL count, they matter. Thank you for caring.*

The Nurse Leader Resource Kit is available for download as an editable file from https://www.springerpub.com/cfbn

ACKNOWLEDGMENTS

The seed for the first edition of this book was planted many years ago but really came to fruition while I was on sabbatical in 2009 and up at Hastings

Center as a visiting scholar roaming through its wonderful library, participating in lunch discussions, sharing ideas, and renewing myself on its beautiful grounds in Garrison, New York. Once again, thank you, Dan Callahan, for creating that wondrous space where dialogue and reflection on some of the most important issues related to living–dying have been valued and encouraged. Appreciation also goes to Thomas H. Murray and all the staff at the center for making me feel welcome during that time.

Much appreciation goes to the Springer team for all their efforts on behalf of this work: Joe Morita, Senior Acquisitions Editor at Springer, for inviting me to write a second edition of this text; Rachel Landes, Associate Editor, for regularly checking in with me to ask how things were going, and who answered my email queries along the way; Rose Mary Piscitelli, Senior Production Editor, for her gracious understanding and attentiveness; and the compositor team at Exeter Premedia Services. Lastly, a great big shout out to Ellen Zanolle, the cover designer, for her incredible artistry (and of course, for providing me with my monarch).

Students continue to reaffirm my purpose as a nurse educator. I often hear from old students, sometimes many years after they graduate. They tell me how well I taught them, but as I have said before, they should know that they taught me extraordinarily well, too. My continued appreciation to the multitude of students and nurses who have shared their stories over the years is humbly expressed through this publication and is accompanied by a heartfelt wish for their happiness.

Last, love and gratitude to the family members and friends who have encouraged and supported me over the years; you know who you are. A special thanks to my daughter, Laura, whose substantive background in both social work and teaching made her a great reader for this work. She took time to critique it and also reassured me that I was on the right path when I needed encouragement. An added bonus is that she teaches English; she made editing suggestions, too! As always, Michael, no words can express my gratitude. Once more I took precious time from you to lock myself in the den to work. Thank you, too, for continuing to be my sounding board and inspiring me.

Professional Quality of Life

Professionally speaking, are you alive or just lingering?
Are the people who work with you or for you thriving or
barely surviving? If the quality of your professional life is
questionable, prolonging it may be a grave disservice. There
are worse things than death for a person or a professional.
If you have to make a choice, go for quality.
                                        —Melodie Chenevert

The Good, Bad, and Ugly of Professional Quality of Life

Our prime purpose in this life is to help others. And if you can't help them, at least don't hurt them.

—Dalai Lama

Introduction to positive and negative aspects of professional quality of life:

- Compassion contentment
- Compassion fatigue
- Burnout

INTRODUCTION

Nurses know all about "quality of life." It is the main focus of our profession—we provide care to enhance the quality of our patients' lives. However, many nurses may not know that their *own* quality of life is at stake, depending upon how they go about their work each day. Indeed, a lot of nurses, although familiar with the terms *compassion fatigue* and *burnout*, cannot identify how it manifests or whether they or their coworkers are experiencing it.

Countless individuals have emphasized the potential detriment to self that can arise from the unique work of healthcare professionals. However, psychologist and scholar Beth Stamm (2002, 2010) has paid equal attention to the positive aspects of professional quality of life. In looking at the negative consequences of providing care, she came to realize that not everyone who witnesses suffering when caring for others actually develops compassion fatigue; many people still manage to go about their work in a joyful manner. Thus, she expounds upon three components of professional quality of life: *compassion satisfaction*, *compassion fatigue*, and *burnout* (Stamm, 2002, 2009, 2010).

The positive aspect of professional quality of life, what Stamm (2002, 2010) refers to as compassion satisfaction, is derived from doing caring work and readily manifests itself as happiness, or at the very least, contentment, in the workplace. It is the pleasure that one gets from helping others (Stamm, 2002). I rather like the term *compassion contentment*, for it seems to better allude to a sense of pleasure, something greater than "satisfaction," which to me could be merely passable.

When we can appreciate our work as meaningful, we feel content. Stamm's (2002) approach to professional quality of life can be useful for those who are interested in fostering healthy work environments, particularly in light of all the work being done with appreciative inquiry as a means of enabling and enhancing constructive change in organizations. With appreciative inquiry, one focuses on the positive aspects of things rather than the negative in order to come to understand what can be done to replicate the good and, in so doing, diminish the bad.

Compassion fatigue and burnout are the two most frequently talked about aspects of professional quality of life. Nurse Carla Joinson (1992) first used the term *compassion fatigue* in nursing when writing about the negative feelings that nurses sometimes experience while caring for people who are suffering. She wisely noted that "compassion fatigue is almost impossible to recognize without a heightened awareness of it" (p. 116). And, while 25 years later we know this to be the case, we still do not insist that our nursing workforce and leadership be well-versed in this area. In fact, there is a great deal of conflicting information in the accumulating literature on the subjects of compassion fatigue and burnout; sometimes the terms are used interchangeably, and in the early literature, compassion fatigue was simply a form of burnout specific to carers (nurses, physicians, therapists, etc.). In much of the later writings on the subject, however, the two syndromes have been described as distinct entities, and in this book, I, too, differentiate between them.

Although each may contribute to the other, compassion fatigue and burnout are different in how they come about and manifest in each of us. I will reiterate a disclaimer here that I noted in the first edition: I am not attempting to reconcile any discrepancies in the literature. Instead of getting caught up on terminology, I am even more fervently seeking to get right to what I perceive to be the essence or *heart* of the matter. The nurse's overall professional quality of life is important for both the carers *and* the recipients of care. They are one, so the heart of the matter is *heart*. Heart is a synonym for many pertinent words; if you look at a thesaurus, you will find that it can also mean compassion, empathy, kindness, sensitivity, and spirit, among other love-conjuring terms.

I think of people who love caring for others and are content doing their work as *heartful*, and I cannot help relating it to the spiritual aspects of human nature. For me, spiritual denotes a sense of belonging to everything else in the universe and to each other. It encompasses the scientific but makes subjective aspects (for instance, how we feel and what we think) just as essential, and sometimes even more so, than the objective (what we can see and measure) aspects of existence. People who are *heartful* tend to be more aware of their connection to everything else.

Compassion fatigue is relational in nature, meaning it arises through one's relationships with others. Typically, compassion fatigue manifests suddenly while caring for those who are suffering from any kind of physical or mental anguish or trauma. The suffering rubs off on the carers and can be, as Joinson noted, "emotionally devastating" (1992, p. 116). A social worker who has talked and written about the subject, Karl La Rowe, refers to compassion fatigue as having a *heavy heart* (Perry, 2008, p. 87), a description I find most applicable and one that I use throughout the following pages.

Whereas compassion fatigue is related to our connection to others and our ability to bear witness to the suffering of others, burnout arises out of a more generalized dissatisfaction with one's work life, and it is usually the result of a multitude of things. Of course, one's relationship with others can be a big factor, but workload, environment, salary, benefits, organizational culture—many things can set the stage for burnout. Burnout develops gradually over time with prolonged emotional and physical exhaustion, and it ultimately results in widespread apathy, a disinterest in work and relationships (Maslach, 1982).

People who are burned out and work in healthcare are frequently seen as *dis*passionate because their apathy appears to indicate a lack of caring. In other words, they appear *heartless* (or *empty-hearted*) and usually feel quite hopeless (dis*heart*ened!) to make things better in their work lives. The feelings of discontent that may arise from one's work and which lead to the development of burnout can, and frequently do, spill over into our personal lives. If we are not mindful, it can even snuff the enjoyment out of our daily living (and can also remove the joy from our loved ones' lives in the process!). So when I refer to the good, the bad, and the ugly of professional quality of life, I am referring to *compassion contentment*—heartful (the good); *compassion fatigue*—heavy hearted (the bad); and *burnout*—seemingly heartless or empty-hearted (the ugly).

HEARTFUL, HEAVY HEARTED, AND HEARTLESS

We definitely cannot afford to be ostensibly heartless and yet I repeatedly hear from students and nurses that what they are seeing in their clinical practicums and work environments is a workforce that seems predominantly empty-hearted. The display of dispassionate care can be extremely disturbing, especially to undergraduate students, and it can be challenging to try to put it all in context. At different times in our lives, each of us may be heartful, heart heavy, or seemingly empty-hearted or heartless. The point is, in nursing we really need to be *heartful*, at least most of the time—it is a matter of health and healing for us as well as those we care for.

I often share the story of John Doe, a homeless young man who had been found unresponsive on a street corner, and who quickly went from being simply unresponsive without a known diagnosis into a full-blown multisystem failure (Todaro-Franceschi, 2008, 2011). We had no health history, no name, and consequently no family or friends to call. I was assigned to care for John during the first night tour that he was on our unit. He was a one-to-one patient, his care acuity being high enough to warrant one nurse to work with him for a full shift.

John had tubes for everything: a central line, an arterial line, a Foley catheter, a nasogastric tube for feeding, and he was intubated and on a respirator. He was dirty, really dirty. There was caked muck under his nails and toenails and in his hair. There was dirt between his fingers and toes and even in his eyebrows. That first night I spent a significant amount of time bathing him, trying to remove all the grime; I only partially succeeded.

I wondered about him; he was a fairly nice-looking young man, with dark blonde hair and gray-blue eyes. How did he come to be homeless? Did he have family members somewhere who wanted to know where he was and who would be there right now holding his hand if they did know? What caused him to be so ill? How might we help him? How might I help him? I quickly realized that aside from maintaining the status quo in terms of trying to keep him stabilized, the only thing I could do was acknowledge his humanness by talking to him as I cared for him and trying to ensure that he was as comfortable as possible.

John was assigned to me the following two nights and they were difficult, to say the least. He had not regained consciousness. He was on multiple intravenous (IV) medications, which I was constantly titrating up and down to maintain homeostasis; but that was not the hardest part of caring for John. The most difficult thing was to see unrealized potential, to watch a human being who was clearly dying without loved ones, without us knowing who he was and had been. I continued to talk to him as I cared for him, and each night I took over where the day tour nurse had left off, as we each slowly and painstakingly removed what appeared to be years of dirt and grime from his body.

This was a week when I was scheduled to work four nights in a row and I had difficulty sleeping when I went home. As I drove back to work, I dreaded the thought of caring for John another shift, and when I reported to the unit for my fourth consecutive tour, the charge nurse started to assign me to work with him again. I began to cry and told her I simply could not spend another night in the room with him; it was just too painful. I was fortunate in that our charge nurse was an understanding leader, and she quickly made out a new assignment for me.

That night, John coded and I ended up in his room for much of the shift, helping a coworker who had been assigned to care for him. I felt so terrible, for both the patient and my coworker. John was pronounced dead after several tortuous hours of trying to keep him alive. When we did postmortem care we removed the little remaining dirt; he was finally clean. In a way, his cleanliness had a sad element attached to it too, because by having removed the last vestiges of grime, in a way it erased what was known about who he was and how he had lived.

My coworker and I consoled each other; we had done everything humanly possible to save our John Doe. As I drove home that morning, I was comforted with knowing I had talked to him and cleaned him as best I could. Perhaps, by my having done so, John had, on some level, been aware that he was cared for by another human being. After all, it is said that hearing is the last sense to go. On autopsy they found that he had contracted leptospirosis, a serious disease carried by various animals and spread through contaminated water, food, or soil.

Twenty-five years later, I can still see John ever so clearly in my mind. I recognized years ago that, at that time, I was suffering from compassion fatigue. It is possible that I was experiencing a bit of death overload, too, having been working in critical care and bearing witness to many deaths by that time. I also realize, in retrospect, that John was, in part, the reason for my shift in focus; he was a turning point for me. I went from critical care nursing to a focus on care of the dying. Most notably, I have come to appreciate that cases like John and so many other individuals that I have worked with over the years, by their sustaining memory, continually help to reaffirm a sense of purpose, a sense that there is always a reason why I do the things I do as a carer. I know that if I keep that sense of purpose first and foremost in my mind, it guides me to always do whatever I do with compassion and, I might add, passion.

The story of John is an example of the good, the bad, and what could have turned out to be the ugly. My being able to bear witness to his suffering—cleaning him, touching him, speaking with him—these were actions that get at compassion contentment. My dreading the thought of working with him one more night was indicative of my ability to suffer with, to internalize the anguish of the John Does in this world who die young and alone with strangers; I quickly manifested compassion fatigue. Had my charge nurse been less of a leader, she might not have changed my assignment, creating a bigger wound that could have festered over time, contributing to eventual burnout. The wound would have been bigger, because, without her sincere acknowledgment of my hurting—my humanity—I would have certainly felt worse than I did.

Compassion fatigue can be healed and many times even averted if we are mindfully aware of how we are acting in the workplace (Todaro-Franceschi, 2008). If we can take note of the things that scare us and the ways we are acting—for instance, my dreading going to work to care for John or being overly upset by the suffering of particular patients and/or their loved ones—we can mindfully care for ourselves to ensure our own well-being.

GOING TO THE PLACES THAT SCARE US

We all have sustaining memories that, on occasion, pop into our awareness. It is important to reflect upon them and consider what our past experiences have contributed to who we are today, even if it means reliving difficult times in our lives. Pema Chodron (2001), an American Buddhist nun, explains that we need to *choose* to go to the places that scare us. By learning to be fearless, we can grow and develop more fully our compassionate nature. If we, in nursing, are unwilling to go, or can no longer go, to the places that scare us (or if we always circumvent around those places, for example, we do not like to care for people who are dying or perhaps we choose not to make eye contact with them or their loved ones), then we have work to do in order to heal from and/or prevent compassion fatigue.

That fourth night going into work, I was distressed at the thought that I would have to care for John yet another shift. It was a place that scared me. As a critical care nurse, having had many experiences with patients who were close to death, I was still terribly uncomfortable with dying and death at times. Watching him die was very hard for me.

Most of us in nursing have gotten the impression somewhere along our professional life journey that it is not right to be distressed or to refuse an assignment, when really we should be okay with our discomfort, because after all, we are humans, not robots—we think, we feel, we hurt, we laugh, and we love. We should be more than okay with speaking up and saying, I just *cannot* do this now. Everyone, leaders and educators, as well as staff—all of us—need to keep prominently in mind that we *are* human beings as we go about the many times overwhelmingly difficult job of nursing; we *all* have our limits. Knowing this, then, can help us remain true to ourselves and our intrinsic caring nature.

Recognizing our limitations and our own distress is very important, so even while we may occasionally say, "I cannot do this now," by acknowledging that where we are right now in this moment *is* a place that scares us, we are, in reality, facing it and embracing it as part of our own humanness. That is *always* a good thing, not a bad thing.

TURNING POINTS

Various experiences lead to turning points in our lives. Turning points are occasionally referred to as critical incidents, and these incidents can be positive or negative. Sometimes we are aware of what has led up to a change in our way of thinking and/or being in the world. But, more often than not, the transformation is subtle and we do not take notice. Over time, we subsume our experiences into the core of our being and sometimes we forget who we used to be. It is in looking back that we come to know what has contributed to who we have become. Thus, the goal here is for some of the stories I share to jar *your* memories.

Keep in mind that at the time when many of our most memorable experiences occur, we do not know how important the events will be in the shaping of our careers and lives. For me, it was only through the intentional effort of trying to make sense of things, usually at times when I felt a bit lost, that I recognized some of my important turning points. That really is the way it happens for many of us, most of the time. Looking back helps us to look forward. Hopefully, as you recall some of your own stories, you will reflect upon how your experiences have changed the way you go about being in the world.

WORKING AGAINST THE ODDS

Nurses who bear witness to human suffering on a regular basis are especially at risk of compassion fatigue; however, there are many things that contribute to the development of diminished professional quality of life. Work conditions—the physical environment as well as organizational culture—can enhance or hinder contentment on the job, and nurses who work in certain areas may be more likely to develop compassion fatigue and/or burnout over time. My own observations and studies have led me to believe that how nurses are educated also plays a significant part in their ability (or inability) to be *heartful* while working.

In an especially telling exploration of what nursing is and the difficulties inherent in the profession of nursing, writer Suzanne Gordon (2005) portrayed us as working *against the odds*. In a lot of ways, we are working against the odds. Chaotic changes in healthcare systems, attributed in part to the increasing complexity of healthcare, along with economic constraints, have contributed to the sense that everyone involved in care delivery is working against the odds, and nurses as frontline carers are even more so than any other healthcare professional. Some of these things are not of our choosing or making, but some of the reasons why the odds seem to be against us definitely are of our making, and I think the way we have been, and continue to be, educated is a big part of the problem. We, in nursing, have to some extent *stacked the deck* against ourselves.

We are a *collective* body, and we are faced with a crisis in our profession, unlike any other in the history of nursing. We are not dealing with just a shortage of nurses, which is going to worsen as our aging workforce retires. We have issues with recruitment, retention, productivity, unhealthy work environments (which includes a whole other cadre of problems such as incivility and bullying, lack of resources, heavy workload)—all of these and more are contributing to a crisis that is manifesting in instances of individual and collective compassion fatigue, moral distress, and burnout. However, in this era of unprecedented challenges for us in nursing, there is also a collective opportunity.

In the first edition of this book I had emphasized that I was not pointing an accusatory finger at any one group because no one group owns the current state of affairs in nursing; not staff, educators, or leaders. I especially want to commend the efforts being made by nurses to address some of the issues I had written about. Since 2012, when the book was first published, the American Nurses Association (ANA) has focused extensively on the well-being of our workforce and has championed efforts to address bullying, incivility, staffing, self-care, compassion fatigue, and moral distress. Yet, I am still troubled by the lack of progress in nursing education and leadership areas to address nursing professional quality of life. We can, and we must, reshuffle the deck to bring the odds in our favor. On the following pages, I hope to illuminate how we can do it.

The ultimate goal is for us to individually and collectively bring some of the missing joy back into nursing. I would like to begin here by pointing to what might make one more than capable of working against the odds— whatever those odds might be. To work against the odds takes passion (or if you prefer, enthusiasm), along with resiliency and maybe more than a little sense of one's own importance. We *have* to believe in ourselves and in what we are about. I do not believe that all, or even most, nurses are educated to believe in ourselves and the power we have collectively as a profession.

No matter what leads to compassion fatigue and burnout, it is clear that some kind of purposeful action is necessary in order to heal from these syndromes, and with adequate knowledge of contributing factors, one may be able to evade the occurrence or at least minimize the effects of compassion fatigue and/or burnout. Thus, the first step is to be able to recognize and acknowledge that there is a problem brewing.

Nurses most likely to quickly relate to the topics explored herein will be those with firsthand experience working with the very ill and dying individuals and their loved ones. Staff nurses and advanced practice nurses who work in emergency rooms, ICUs, and those who work on medical–surgical, oncology, and palliative care units will easily relate to these topics; however, I believe that most nurses, at some point or another during the course of their career, will experience a degree of compassion fatigue and/or burnout, whether it is due to their frequent exposure to suffering, or to the chaos of their workplace environment, or even more likely, a combination of the two. Consequently, every nurse should have a knowledge of the factors that play a part in how both syndromes can develop and what steps can be taken to facilitate compassion contentment, thereby enhancing professional quality of life and minimizing the potential purportedly negative consequences of our work.

Nurses who work in leadership positions will also benefit from reading this book. I recall having a discussion with a clinical nurse leader student who worked in nursing administration; she asked me, "During this program, will I learn how to motivate my staff?" The answer to that is complex, because in many places, there is collective compassion fatigue and perhaps collective burnout. I discuss this in further detail later; it suffices to say here that leaders cannot hope to motivate staff who have disconnected with the meaning and purpose of their work, and in essence, that is what eventually happens to many nurses who suffer from compassion fatigue for any length of time. Accordingly, those who would lead others in healthcare today need to know how to identify and address the serious workforce woes that impact professional quality of life in order to preserve the integrity and quality of healthcare, as well as the integrity and quality of life for their staff. It is all one.

Throughout this book, I expound upon the different aspects of professional quality of life, and in various instances, I use storytelling; some of the stories are mine and span across my years of nursing practice. Some are narratives that have been imparted by students and friends. Still others are anecdotes about experiences I had as a recipient of care or while witnessing a loved one who was receiving care. All are shared as part of a whole, to get at what it means to be a nurse and to do the actions of nursing.

In the next chapter, I discuss the integral relationship between the cared for and the carers, with an emphasis on an ethic of care, which I perceive to be inherent in our discipline. In Part II, I discuss the positive aspects of our professional quality of life, focusing on compassion contentment and its relationship to our ethical foundation—the values and excellences identified and solidified in our code of ethics. I introduce a healing model ($ART^{©}$) specifically designed to address the enhancement of professional quality of life (Todaro-Franceschi, 2008, 2013, 2015). For the remainder of the book, in each chapter addressing different aspects of professional quality of life (compassion fatigue, moral distress, burnout, workplace violence, facing death, posttraumatic stress disorder [PTSD], leadership), I describe how ART can be applied.

Part III covers the bad—both compassion fatigue and moral distress. Part IV delineates the ugly, uglier, and ugliest aspects of professional quality of life. In a discussion of burnout, I again make no attempt to reconcile what is out there in the literature. Rather, I draw from the literature, along with my own experiences and observations to put forward ideas related to how burnout manifests and how it can negatively transform our lives along with the lives of our coworkers, patients, and loved ones.

Some readers familiar with the first edition will note that I have shifted things around and added two new chapters (Chapters 9 and 13) to expand upon topics I felt needed to be more prominent and deserved their own space. Incivility and bullying now has its own chapter and has been placed accordingly in Part IV because it is definitely the *uglier* side of nursing.

In Part V, I discuss how facing death can negatively affect us and, conversely, how it can positively transform the way we go about being in the world and how we go about caring for the dying and their loved ones. I include a discussion on collective trauma and death overload, from both natural and man-made disasters, along with posttraumatic stress. In Part VI, the discussion is expanded to include the collective healing of our profession through nursing education and leadership efforts and how, through knowing participation, we can work toward transforming the workplace and enhancing our professional quality of life.

KEY POINTS

- The quality of our professional life is important for us—nurse carers—and equally important for those entrusted to our care.

- Our work contributes to how we go about being in the world, personally and professionally.

- When we are content with our work, it is good and we feel heartful.

- When we internalize suffering, it is bad; we become compassion fatigued and heart heavy.

- When we are discontent and become disconnected from our work, distancing ourselves from others, it is ugly; we are suffering from burnout and are seemingly empty-hearted or heartless.

- How we go about our work is important and can provide clues as to what we need to do for ourselves and for others to transform health and healing for all.

REFERENCES

Chodron, P. (2001). *The places that scare you: A guide to fearlessness in difficult times.* Boston, MA: Shambala.

Gordon, S. (2005). *Nursing against the odds: How health care cost cutting, media stereotypes, and medical hubris undermine nurses and patient care.* Ithaca, NY: ILR Press (an imprint of Cornell University Press).

Joinson, C. (1992). Coping with compassion fatigue. *Nursing, 22,* 116–121. doi:10.1097/00152193-199204000-00035

Maslach, C. (1982). *Burnout: The cost of caring.* Englewood Cliffs, NJ: Prentice-Hall.

Perry, B. (2008). Why exemplary oncology nurses seem to avoid compassion fatigue. *Canadian Oncology Nursing Journal, 18*(2), 87–92. doi:10.5737/1181912x1828792

Stamm, B. H. (2002). Measuring compassion satisfaction as well as fatigue: Developmental history of the compassion fatigue and satisfaction test. In C. R. Figley (Ed.), *Treating compassion fatigue* (pp. 107–119). New York, NY: Brunner Mazel.

Stamm, B. H. (2009). *Research Information on the ProQOL.* Retrieved from http://www.compassionfatigue.org

Stamm, B. H. (2010). *The ProQOL (Professional Quality of Life Scale: Compassion Satisfaction and Compassion Fatigue).* Pocatello, ID: ProQOL.org. Retrieved from www.proqol.org

Todaro-Franceschi, V. (2008). Preventing compassion fatigue and reaffirming purpose in nursing. *Proceedings on the 3rd European Federation of Critical Care Nursing Congress and 27th Aniarti Conference, Influencing Critical Care Nursing in Europe,* Florence, Italy (October).

Todaro-Franceschi, V. (2011). *Vestiges [A digital story].* Jackson, NJ: Author.

Todaro-Franceschi, V. (2013). *Compassion fatigue and burnout in nursing: Enhancing professional quality of life.* New York, NY: Springer Publishing.

Todaro-Franceschi, V. (2015). The ART of maintaining the "care" in healthcare. *Nursing Management, 46*(6), 53–55. doi:10.1097/01.numa.0000465407.76450.ab

2

Transforming Both Health and Care in Healthcare

It is a beautiful and mysterious power that one human being can have on another through the mere act of caring. . . . A great truth, the act of caring is the first step in the power to heal.

—Phillip Moffitt

KEY TOPICS

- What is a nurse?
- Ideas of energy, health, and healing
- Unity and purposeful change
- Subtle influences and butterfly power
- Caring in nursing

INTRODUCTION

Very often we talk about cure of illness, prevention, and promotion of health as the main aspects of healthcare, but in actuality, it is all about transforming the quality of living and dying. Nurses are instrumental in this transformation. The following story, shared by a student in focused group discussions on end-of-life care, depicts the wholeness of our caring work:

> *I lost my mom during the summer of 1991, right before my 21st birthday. Her death was a shock to my family and me. She had a severe vomiting episode and fell unconscious after having lunch. For six days she was in a vegetative state, hooked up to a ventilator from a ruptured cerebral aneurysm. She had hemorrhaged badly and the physicians couldn't do anything to help her. My dad had to make the most difficult decision by signing the "Do Not Resuscitate" (DNR) papers. My mom was only 59.*
>
> *I will never forget Nurse Katie. She made sure my dad had the coveted reclining chair floating on the hospital floor, which was safely tucked away in my mom's room with a "do not remove from this room" sign on it. Nurse Katie made sure my eight sisters and I were allowed to see my mom at the same time during visiting hours, despite the hospital rules. Nurse Katie was 8 months pregnant, wore her sandy, blond hair in a ponytail, and made sure my mom was comfortable. The pain and sorrow I experienced losing my mom was worse than any physical pain I had ever endured. I miss my mom so much and wish she was around to give me a hug. Despite the emptiness I feel not having my mom here, I am grateful my dad had the courage to sign those DNR papers. My mom would've hated spending her remaining days in the hospital, hooked up to a machine while her loved ones suffered, keeping vigil at her bedside.*
>
> *We brought Nurse Katie a bagful of candy and other treats to show her how much we valued the care she gave to my mom and all of us during our 6 days at the hospital. She cried and hugged us all when my mom's heart stopped beating. Nurse Katie was a gem, and it's nice and reassuring to know that there are other gems just like her out there.*

NURSES: PRIMARY TRANSFORMERS IN HEALTHCARE

A question many individuals might ask at this juncture in our professional history, "What is a nurse?" is difficult to answer. Multiple entry levels into practice—the diploma and associate, baccalaureate, master's, and doctorate degrees—combined with so many different titles can leave even the most well-learned on the subject of nursing unable to easily articulate who we are and what it is we do.

In the early days of professional nursing role development, the idea of being "called to care" was readily discernible. Today, for some people, coming into nursing may not be so much a "call to care" as it is about other things, such as job security, a good salary, flexible working hours, multiple opportunities, and so forth. Yet, those of us in nursing and people in the public sector will easily recognize that this student's sustaining memory of Nurse Katie epitomizes what it means to be a nurse.

Nurses assist with healing and are the primary transformers in healthcare. We are agents of change for individual, group, community, and societal health and healing. Health and healing, in this instance, include all aspects of the life process from birth to death, neither living nor dying being more important than the other, for both are integral with our human becoming.

How do we, in nursing, transform health and assist with healing? While working in critical care, I came to wonder about what it was we were doing, and to me, it appeared related to the idea of energy. *Energy* is one of those terms that we use all the time, but rarely do we ever stop to reflect on its meaning. It has been identified as a foundational concept for all sciences, and as nursing is considered to be a science, it seemed important to be able to understand and explain what it is we mean when we use the word in our work (Todaro-Franceschi, 1998, 1999).

In the ICU, we were often doing things that, to me, did not make much sense. For example, nurses would obtain daily weights, no matter how critically ill our patients were. This meant using a Hoyer lift to do bed scale weights. What a frightening experience for those patients who were alert enough to be aware of what was going on, being lifted up on a machine over the bed! What a scary experience for the nurses, too, when the patients were already so unstable!

During my time working in this one ICU, several patients coded during bed scale weighing, and one of them actually died. Consequently, many of us refused to do daily weights on those we believed were unstable, and this resulted in ongoing unpleasant discourse with some of the physicians who wanted those weights everyday no matter what. Thankfully, today, most places have weight scale devices that are built into the beds. However, I would bet that if you reflect on your practice, you could identify similar kinds of practice issues that remain unaddressed and may be contributing to your discontent at work.

The insistence on daily weights and other ongoing events in the ICU setting had me pondering the goals of care, which at the time seemed to me should encompass conserving energy rather than depleting it. Notably, these kinds of experiences frequently set the backdrop for nurses working in our unit to suffer from what is commonly referred to as moral distress. We had frequent spurts of sick calls, but we all knew that, most of the time, the person calling out sick was really taking a much-needed "mental health day."

After taking my own share of mental health days while working on this particular unit—something I had never felt inclined to do before and for which I was feeling extremely guilty—I changed my workplace and eventually went back to graduate school, where I set out to explore ideas of energy. My journey led me through the literature from antiquity up into current-day writings in philosophy, chemistry, physics, cosmology, medicine, psychology, religion, and, of course, nursing (Todaro-Franceschi, 1998, 1999, 2001, 2008). The takeaway from that exploration is very relevant to the topics in this book, for what emerged was an ethic of care grounded in philosophy but also ubiquitous in the various scientific disciplines.

The Enigma of Energy: A Brief Synopsis

There are two ideas of energy in the literature: a traditional view of energy as part of causal processes, and a more progressive or modern view, where energy is a phenomenon—a thing (Todaro-Franceschi, 1998, 1999). Various disciplines use the term in both ways, but everyone today pretty much agrees that energy is *the* phenomenon that manifests itself into everything we can and cannot see. As Einstein (1954) pointed out in his special theory of relativity, matter and energy are interchangeable. That is to say, for example, that you and I are both manifestations of energy, as is the space between us—with all that is in it—whether we can see whatever is in it or not. It is all essentially *one* thing. He also emphasized that we, the observers of everything around us, are participants in everything around us and, therefore, to a certain degree, we create our reality.

The idea that everything is energy is quite profound when one thinks about it, for it means that there is absolutely no real separation between anything. It implies, too, that "I" or "me" is an utter illusion; one could say there is only "us" or "we." Yet, words cannot quite capture and elucidate the meaning of this enigmatic phenomenon, energy.

It—energy—never stands still. It is always changing forms. Some are natural, like when a caterpillar becomes a butterfly or a fertilized egg becomes a baby, and others are human-instigated, like taking gasoline and using it in fuel lines to transform energy into the motion of a vehicle. Accordingly, one can see that energy transformation occurs *purposefully* and not haphazardly. The changing nature of things is really organized, even when it appears chaotic, and occasionally, if we are lucky, we glean from what appears to be unpredictable and meaningless behavior, a movement toward something greater than ourselves, an underlying pattern of wholeness—oneness. When one senses this pattern in the whole, it can be a spiritual awakening of sorts for many individuals. I know that I cannot look at anything today without a sense of wonder.

After years of study, I ended up ultimately noting that while the phenomenon of energy will never be fully explained, its mysterious nature nevertheless implies that there is an underlying reason for it all. For how else can you explain something that is every single moment changing purposefully?

HEALTH AND HEALING

Given a pristine appreciation of what I perceived to be the unity and purposeful nature of the universe, I set about exploring health and healing with my new set of glasses. It was no surprise to me that ideas of oneness and purposeful action were there in various writings in medicine and nursing. Hippocrates and Nightingale both wrote about a healing force of nature that seems to cure from within; they were astutely aware of the purposive character of health and healing.

Nightingale (1859/1946) noted, "It is a curious thing to observe how almost all patients lie with their faces turned to the light, exactly as plants always make their way towards the light . . . ." (p. 49). When discussing healing, she reflected,

> It is often thought that medicine is the curative process. It is no such thing; medicine is the surgery of functions, as surgery proper is that of limbs and organs. Neither can do anything but remove obstructions; neither can cure; nature alone cures. (p. 74)

She also claimed that it is the nurse's responsibility to "put the patient in the best condition for nature to act upon him" (p. 75).

Health and healing are purposeful manifestations of the one. Health does not mean the absence of disease: One can heal as he or she is dying; one can live until he or she dies, with a good quality of life and in peace. In that sense, one can die healthy. Today, in many sectors of healthcare, we emphasize healthy aging, as if everyone will live forever; yet, as human beings are living longer and dying slower, there is no doubt that we need to be concerned with "healthy dying" as well as healthy aging. Basically, we must be concerned with healthy *living–dying*, or, if you prefer, the *quality* of living and dying.

Nurses, physicians, and other healthcare professionals, as well as loved ones, participate in the actualizing of human potential for the individual who is seeking to heal, as they are a part of the whole—the one (Todaro-Franceschi, 1998, 1999). It is in and through all of our purposeful actions that healing arises. That there is unity and purposeful action in all things little and large throughout the universe is the foundation of my ethic of care, for, if it is all essentially one, whatever I do or you do is not just reflected in the whole; *it is the whole.*

In nursing, educators and leaders, of necessity, focus on and emphasize quality and safety issues related to the provision of care. Yes, we all need to be concerned with that; however, one can teach, talk about, and continuously act to try to ensure quality and safety, but if the nursing workforce is compassion fatigued and/or burned out, quality and safety concerns will *never* be adequately addressed. It is impossible to disentangle the quality of care for the patient from the carer's professional quality of life; they are one. Health for the cared for and the carers is directly related to the care rendered and received; *how* we care transforms *our* professional quality of life (and our overall quality of life), and how patients receive care transforms their quality of living and dying.

Nurses, as transformers in healthcare, need that sense of oneness, that connectedness to other.[1] We also need working environments that support the caring aspects that allow us to maintain and enhance our humanistic connection to those we care for and also those with whom we work. This caring connection is what enables most of us to discern meaning and purpose in our work and to be content at the end of the day.

THE FLAP OF A BUTTERFLY'S WINGS

Edward Lorenz (1993), a meteorologist, reiterated an old Chinese proverb when he asked, "Does the flap of a butterfly's wings in Brazil set off a tornado in Texas?" The answer is yes and no. We all know that subtle changes happen all the time. There are changes occurring that we are not even aware of; we are also not cognizant of the relationships among what seem to be different things. Chaos theory and new physical theories of the universe tell us that everything is irrevocably connected to everything else, they are inseparable, and we can rest assured that the flap of a butterfly's wings is contributing to change elsewhere in the world, although perhaps we will never quite know how or be able to quantify it. This incredible idea is called the *butterfly effect* (Lorenz, 1993), and it is relevant to any discussion on just about anything.

Nurses frequently do not recognize our enormous power. For many reasons, each of us might go through day-to-day work without ever being fully aware of how our actions contribute to transforming the lives of other people; we facilitate health and healing. We assist with life and living, dying and death. We *are* butterflies flapping our wings, so small and yet so powerful, seemingly insignificant and yet. . . . Did you know that the monarch butterfly manages to migrate thousands of miles each year back and forth from Canada and parts of North America to Mexico? It takes four generations of monarchs to manage this migration. It is definitely not a chance happening, although if one were to find a roost of monarchs (a large number of them resting together in a tree or bush) without knowing about their migratory pattern, one might just think, well how lovely, here is a bunch of butterflies. However, once one is aware of what the monarchs are doing, it takes on a very different meaning, does it not?

Some of you may know that the monarch migrates, and then it would not surprise you to come upon a roost of them. But what if you came upon a great many common buckeye butterflies? Would you think it was a chance happening? I can tell you that it is not; they, too, have a migratory pattern, although they are only heading south, not to Mexico. There is pattern and purpose in what they do, but what makes it even more amazing is that they have the ability—the power—to do it! It is a remarkable wonder of nature.

Many of us perceive our work and what we do as inconsequential, just so with a butterfly flapping its wings, but in actuality, what we do is momentous. It is not just a matter of what we do, but *how* we go about doing it that matters. If we are task-oriented, for instance, focused on administering medications but not on the human-to-human connection part of our work, many of us will probably find that we feel less satisfied. Most patients will also tell us they are less satisfied with the care received when there is no person-to-person engagement. A thank-you note addressed to the staff on a unit is not for medication received; it is for *care* received. Meaningful are the words, thank you for *caring*.

On occasion I am asked to write something for senior yearbooks, and one time I shared the following story, trying to impart to the students the importance of cultivating and maintaining a connection with their patients. One day, while I was speaking with one of the most influential bioethicists of our time, he shared his hospitalization experience with me. He said that some nurses were "chatty," while others "just went about doing their job," and that he repeatedly tried to engage several nurses in conversation, telling them about his work. He was so surprised that none of them showed any interest whatsoever in his life, who he is, or what he does. He wanted to know if this behavior (being distant) was the "norm" for nurses.

Upon hearing his comments, the thought that immediately came to my mind was that the nurses seemed to have provided his care a bit *dispassionately*. Noticeably, he got the impression that his work was not important or impressive to the nurses who were caring for him. He was quick to say that he was not actually complaining about the care he received, but I certainly felt and relived his sense of disconnect and isolation as he spoke about it with me.

Unfortunately, I have witnessed, far too often and increasingly of late, the rendering of dispassionate care. We are facing a crisis in healthcare as we are being asked to do much more with much less, and consequently, it seems that many healthcare professionals (NOT just nurses!) are suffering varying degrees of compassion fatigue or burnout. So, having been invited by the students to write for their yearbook, reflecting my take on pressing issues in nursing today, I reiterated something I have often said in various practice, supervisory, and educator roles over the years. Safe, competent practice is *not* the be-all and end-all of what nurses must do. Nurses should provide care not only with competence but also with compassion; otherwise one risks hindering, rather than enhancing, healing.

Briggs and Peat (1999) discuss "butterfly power" in their work on how chaos theory can inform and provide spiritual wisdom to those who pay attention to the underlying patterns of wholeness. Butterfly power means that whether we wish to or not, we are *always* part of whatever changes are occurring throughout the universe. We are participating, just by our very existence, and our participation is powerful. They noted the following:

> When we're negative or dishonest, this exerts a subtle influence on others, quite aside from any direct impact our behavior might have. Our attitude and being forms the climate others live in, the atmosphere they breathe.... If we're genuinely happy, positive, thoughtful, helpful, and honest, this subtly influences those around us. (p. 41)

Put the idea of positive subtle influence into the context of healthcare. It fits beautifully with many models that are based on the concept of "care."

NOTIONS OF GOOD: WHAT IT MEANS TO CARE

What does it mean to care? Caring is all about having a relationship with someone or something; it is about forming bonds between things, especially living things. You can care about your home but you are likely to care more about your husband, children, dog, or cat.

Many of our nursing frameworks and theories capture the essence of nursing and compassionate caring practices (see Smith & Parker, 2014, where a number of theories are detailed). While space does not permit discussing all of them, I want to briefly highlight how well our theorists have articulated the caring aspects of the science and art of nursing. The most prominent work on the nature of "care" has been written by nurse scholars Jean Watson (1988, 1999, 2008), who developed a theory of human caring, also referred to as the theory of transpersonal caring, and Madeline Leininger (1984, 1994), who developed the theory of transcultural caring.

Leininger (1984) was one of the first in modern-day nursing to reflect upon, write about, and research *care* and caring practices in nursing. She noted that "care is the essence and the central, unifying, and dominant domain to characterize nursing" (p. 3) and went on to clarify the terms *care* and *caring*:

Care in a generic sense refers to those assistive, supportive, or facilitative acts toward or for another individual or group with evident or anticipated needs to ameliorate or improve a human condition or lifeway.

Caring refers to the direct (or indirect) nurturant and skillful activities, processes, and decisions related to assisting people in such a manner that reflects behavioral attitudes which are empathetic, supportive, compassionate, protective, succorant, educational, and others dependent upon the needs, problems, values, and goals of the individual or group being assisted. (p. 4)

Anyone familiar with Leininger's (1984, 1994) work knows that she emphasizes that although caring is a universal phenomenon, patterns of care can vary among cultures. A discussion on culture is not within the scope of this book; however, a notion of what it means to *care* is paramount to the discussion here; my own informal studies of how the majority of nurses respond to any discussion on human suffering and our own concurrent feelings of despair indicate that there is a subculture—a "nurseculture." We may not speak the same language and we may not all provide healthcare in the same manner, but we all feel compassion. As compassionate carers we, ourselves, are vulnerable to cosuffer with others and to become compassion fatigued.

In our line of work, caring makes all the difference. How one goes about providing care is paramount to healing; we always need to be cognizant of how we relate to others. There are two types of care in nursing: the instrumental, which refers to the technical and physical aspects of care, and the expressive, which relates to the psychosocial and emotional aspects (Woodward, 1997). In nursing, our ability to act in a compassionate manner entails using both kinds of caring. Hence, I intentionally use the word *carers*, rather than caregivers, because it seems to me that the word *carers* more effectively denotes who we are and what we do—not what we *give*; we do not just give care, we *care*.

Watson noted that

it is when we include caring and love in our work and in our life that we discover and affirm that nursing, like teaching, is more than just a job, it is also a life-giving and life-receiving career for a lifetime of growth and learning. (Watson & Woodward, 2010, p. 354)

In her theory of human caring, Watson (2008) describes the transformation that can arise within a single caring moment, a time when there is a deep connection between the person who is being cared for and the one who is the carer. Throughout her work, Watson emphasizes the important link between compassion for others and self, noting that when we bear witness to and ease the suffering of others, we are contributing to our own well-being and self-actualization.

Martha Rogers' (1970, 1992) nursing framework, the science of unitary human beings, formed the foundation for many other theoretic models; it was she who first conceptualized the idea in nursing that human beings and their environments are inseparable. In a little-known 1964 book titled *Reveille in Nursing*, Rogers wrote that as nursing evolved as both a science and profession, "knowledgeable compassion replaces emotional naiveté" (p. 77). Women, and nurses, became more knowledgeable through erudition, but they did not let go of their compassionate nature; instead, what had been perceived before as perhaps a weakness or naiveté was noted to be a strength of our profession, when combined with higher education.

In 1964, many of Rogers' ideas were revolutionary; her advocacy for our profession a pulsing, vibrant voice:

> Society's health demands that nursing stand firm in its conviction of its own social worth. Nursing alone is responsible for determining the core and boundaries of its education and services within the context of human needs and changing times. . . . The new tomorrow demands flexibility. Nurses must be able to adapt to the unknown. They must be receptive to new ideas and practices. They must reach out and grasp the unexpected with enthusiasm and with courage. Respect for human differences and for human endeavor must be a dominant value. (p. 92)

Rogers' description of nursing written in a New York University newsletter in 1966 clearly denotes nursing as both a science and art (Rogers, as cited by Malinski & Barrett, 1994, p. 338):

> Nursing's story is a magnificent epic of service to humankind. It is about people: how they are born, and live and die; in health and in sickness; in joy and in sorrow. Its mission is the translation of knowledge into human service. Nursing is compassionate concern for human beings. It is the heart that understands and the hand that soothes. It is the intellect that synthesizes many learnings into meaningful administrations.

In Rosemarie Rizzo Parse's humanbecoming theory, nursing is all about enhancing quality of life and the nurse's *true presence* in bearing witness, being with and connecting to others during their living–dying experiences (Parse, 1994, 1998, 2007, 2014). Parse's development of this school of thought is noteworthy for its clear depiction of how we go about appreciating and caring for people. Meaning, rhythmicity, and transcendence, the major themes of human becoming, all get at universal wholeness, pattern, and transformational change (Parse, 2014).

From theorist Margaret Newman's (2008) perspective, nursing is about being fully present to explore with patients their evolving patterns of health exhibited by the process of expanding consciousness, which she defined as "a process of becoming more of oneself, of finding greater meaning in life, and of reaching new heights of connectedness with other people and the world" (p. 6). It is through the nurse's relationship—our connection with others—that consciousness expands both for the patient and for the nurse. It is a unitary process.

Another nurse scholar, Marlaine Smith (1999, 2010), noted converging ideas of caring in the work of Rogers, Watson, and Newman and developed a theory of unitary caring. She describes the phenomenon of unitary caring with five concepts: (a) manifesting our intentions, (b) appreciating patterns, (c) attuning to dynamic flow, (d) experiencing the infinite, and (e) inviting creative emergence. Thus, we manifest our intention to assist with healing; we appreciate patterns of wholeness—oneness; we pay attention to our ways of being in the world; we acknowledge that this human-to-human connection is bigger than each of us separately—it is beyond us, it is sacred; and last, through our recognition of caring and our acts of caring we inspire ourselves and others "to birth oneself anew in the moment" (Smith, 2010, p. 499).

All models of care applied in practice are based on relationships and are sometimes referred to as Relationship-Based Care (RBC). Nurse expert Mary Koloroutis (2004), one of the founders of RBC, notes that it is composed of (a) the carer's relationship with patients and their loved ones, (b) the carer's relationship to self, and (c) the carer's relationship with coworkers. She emphasizes that the relationship between the patient and the nurse is the foundation of nursing, and that "it is anchored in the simple truth that care happens between people. It is in these relationships that patients and families receive support and guidance necessary for them to recover and heal" (Koloroutis, 2004). No matter which theory or model of care one looks at, the emphasis is really on the inseparable nature of the cared for and the carers.

Nursing, as a caring practice, has ethical comportment and notions of good embedded in our actions; as nurse scholar Patricia Benner (1994) wrote, it is "a way of knowing and not knowing" (p. 42). She suggested that, through our stories, the narratives of our experiences as nurses, we can gain a better understanding of the significance of our work. It is *care* that provides the foundation for a meaningful world; without it, the world is meaningless—"nothing really matters" (p. 44). Yet, Benner also pointed out that "caring practices continue to be rather invisible, devalued, and typically inadequately accounted for in our institutional designs and public policy" (p. 43).

Benner (1994) noted that any professional practice "is a socially embedded organized activity with notions of good inherent in the practice and character of the practitioner" (p. 43). Without adequate recognition of *care* as an integral part of nursing practice, and undoubtedly, that it should be paramount in all health*care* professions, one chances its ultimate disappearance. Along this line of thought I am reminded of working on units where care acuity determined staffing and where viability (when the patient prognosis is good) was taken as indicative of higher acuity—which, in turn, equates with better staffing. To me, that always seemed a bit skewed. What of the family and friends of our patients, those people who were hoping for a cure, bearing witness to their loved one's suffering? Those people walking up and down the halls, sleeping in the waiting room, standing at the bedside, watching helplessly as their loved one slipped away. Why didn't they ever factor into the patient acuity level? How could they *not* be considered?

With an increasing emphasis on outcomes, there must be additional focus on the ways in which we in nursing work to make quality and safety come about, and whether it meets our moral and personal standards. Florence Nightingale, one of the most influential people of healthcare to date, emphasized quality and safety (and positive outcomes), but they were never the sole focus of her work.

Nurse scholar Margretta Madden Styles (1992) wrote of Nightingale's enduring symbolic representation of what it means to be a nurse:

> . . . fragments pieced together form a collage of Nightingale as feminist, practitioner, politician, scientist, environmentalist, visionary reformer—a striking noble portrait. But I hold still another, a more personal, intimate picture in my mind.
>
> Displayed within a showcase at the entrance to our school is a letter written by Nightingale in 1855 to the parents of a young soldier who died of typhus in the Crimea. She describes his last moments. I fancy that she wrote it late at night fighting to overcome despair and fatigue, after she had finished her rounds with the lamp that, in turn, became her symbol. And I fancy that she wrote similar letters to the loved ones of all those for whom she cared so deeply and felt so profoundly responsible. (p. 75)

First and foremost for Nightingale, nursing was about compassionate caring for people. Her legacy lives on today in modern nursing. So why is it that many of us in nursing do not seem to know how essential our caring work is, or how vital our unique contribution is, to healthcare? How is it that we do not recognize our *own* importance? Whether intentional or not, it is in part the fault of our educational system and the systems in which we work where there continues to be demeaning and devaluing of the basic *caring* practices of nursing.

I am not laying the blame for this at anyone's feet; rather, I am asking for us to individually and collectively assume the responsibility. As a nurse and educator of nurses, I share some of my own mistakes and perceived failures quite honestly on these pages. I am certain that nurses who seem to be apathetic and dispassionate were *not* always that way. For why would individuals choose to come into a *caring* profession and then choose not to *care*? On units where care is dispassionately rendered and where healing often seems to be hindered rather than helped, it is clear that there is a collective wound. Staff and leaders who work in these areas are frequently fighting an uphill battle, perhaps sometimes even a losing battle.

FIGHTING AN UPHILL BATTLE

Taking a position as a clinical coordinator in a long-term care facility, I was assigned to cover an area that had a reputation for being the worst unit in the place. Some of the staff were not providing quality care. It seemed they were *un*caring, and in a few instances, even abusive toward the patients, their families, and coworkers. I spent more sleepless nights while employed there than I have during my entire career. I lasted in that particular job less than a year.

I went to work dreading each day, and I went reluctantly home at night worrying about what I would find on returning the next day. I realized fairly quickly that I was hired to clean house and not only was this a difficult task, it was more than a little unpleasant. What kept me centered and able to do what was needed during the time I was employed there was my ever-present focus on the well-being of those who were entrusted to our care. I recall how nurses and nursing assistants, who had themselves been seemingly battered for so long by their burnt-out coworkers and by the environment they were working in, seemed to rise to the task of assisting me to overcome some of the many obstacles that were preventing the rendering of compassionate, competent care. Still, the constant confrontations with difficult staff and union members finally wore me down; I could not sleep at all and my husband begged me to quit. Subsequently, I gave my 4-week notice and resigned.

Many of the staff were genuinely sorry to see me go and gave me a farewell party. I still have the plaque with the serenity prayer on it, given to me by a nurse who truly did care. You know, the one that begins with "God grant me the serenity to accept the things I cannot change . . . ." It was very fitting, but at that time, I felt so guilty about having failed those people—both the residents and the staff. I remember thinking, I should stay and try to make things right.

Over the years, I have heard many stories like mine where colleagues were in staff or leadership positions that they had to leave. For some, the experiences they had were so unbearable that it prompted them to leave nursing entirely. For others, perhaps those who did not recognize the choices they may have had, the experience became a catalyst for illness or apathy or both. The stark reality is that the environments in which we work are not always conducive to health and healing for everyone, and it is not just a matter of insufficient staffing, which has always been perceived to be a big part of the problem. There is an increasing database of knowledge that indicates overall quality of care, clinical outcomes, and patient satisfaction are directly related to the workplace environment (Aiken, Clarke, Sloane, & Sochalski, 2001; Aiken, Clarke, Sloane, Sochalski, & Silber, 2002; Aiken et al., 2011), and we know that in poor work environments, there is a significantly higher incidence of nurse burnout and overall job dissatisfaction.

It is ironic that many of us in healthcare work in unhealthy environments where we are often forced to ignore our own needs and our own health—but for whom do we do this? Is it for the sake of the patient or the sake of the systems in which we are working? From the many years of Magnet® studies (Drenkard, Wolf, & Morgan, 2011) in the United States, we know that a healthy workplace for us needs to be an inclusive, patient-oriented care environment in which nurses are valued for what we contribute to the healing process on a multidimensional level, and where we are provided with the resources to do it in a way that leaves us feeling like we are doing our work well—where we can feel compassion contentment. The success of the Magnet initiative has shown us that we—nurses—are unquestionably the people who can and do make it happen. It is up to us to lead the effort to transform care. So, how can we do it? By remaining cognizant of the meaning and purpose of our work. How do we do it? With compassionate and competent caring, and perhaps with our code of ethics and Nightingale's (1859/1946) *Notes on Nursing* in our pockets.

KEY POINTS

- Everything is a manifestation of energy, purposefully transforming all the time.
- It is all essentially one, so whatever I do or you do is not just reflected in the whole; It is the whole.

- Subtle influences contribute to both positive and negative transformation.

- Nurses do not only provide care, we care. We are the primary transformers in healthcare for people during both living and dying.

- Health and healing for both the cared for and the carers is directly and simultaneously transformed by how *we*, individually and collectively, go to work each day.

NOTE

1. The word "other" is used instead of "others" in various places to emphasize that all is essentially one and not separate entities (Todaro-Franceschi, 1999).

REFERENCES

Aiken, L., Clarke, S., Sloane, D., & Sochalski, J. (2001). An international perspective on hospital nurse's work environments: The case for reform. *Policy, Politics, and Nursing Practice, 2,* 255–263. doi:10.1177/152715440100200402

Aiken, L., Clarke, S., Sloane, D., Sochalski, J., & Silber, J. (2002). Hospital nurse staffing and patient mortality, nurse burnout and job dissatisfaction. *Journal of the American Medical Association, 288*(16), 1987–1993. doi:10.1001/jama.288.16.1987

Aiken, L. H., Sloane, D. M., Clarke, S., Poghosyan, L., Cho, E., You, L., . . . Aungsuroch, Y. (2011). Importance of work environments on hospital outcomes in nine countries. *International Journal for Quality in Health Care, 23*(4), 357–364. doi:10.1093/intqhc/mzr022

Benner, P. (1994). Caring as a way of knowing and not knowing. In S. S. Phillips & P. Benner (Eds.), *The crisis of care: Affirming and restoring caring practices in the helping professions* (pp. 42–62). Washington, DC: Georgetown University Press.

Briggs, J., & Peat, D. (1999). *Seven life lessons of chaos: Spiritual wisdom from the science of change.* New York, NY: HarperCollins.

Drenkard, K., Wolf, G., & Morgan, S. H. (Eds.). (2011). *Magnet®: The next generation—Nurses making the difference.* Silver Spring, MD: American Nurses Credentialing Center.

Einstein, A. (1954). *Ideas and opinions.* New York, NY: Wings Books.

Koloroutis, M. (Ed.). (2004). *Relationship-based care: A model for transforming practice.* Minneapolis, MN: Creative Health Care Management.

Leininger, M. (Ed.). (1984). *Care: The essence of nursing and health.* Detroit, MI: Wayne State University Press.

Leininger, M. (1994). *Transcultural nursing: Concepts, theories and practices.* New York, NY: McGraw-Hill.

Lorenz, E. (1993). *The essence of chaos.* Seattle, WA: University of Washington Press.

Malinski, V. M., & Barrett, E. A. M. (1994). *Martha E. Rogers: Her life and her work.* Philadelphia, PA: F. A. Davis.

Newman, M. (2008). *Transforming presence: The difference that nursing makes.* Philadelphia, PA: F. A. Davis.

Nightingale, F. (1946). *Notes on nursing: What it is, and what it is not* (Facsimile of 1st ed.). London: Harrison and Sons. (Original work published 1859)

Parse, R. R. (1994). Quality of life: Sciencing and living the art of human becoming. *Nursing Science Quarterly, 7*, 16–21. doi:10.1177/089431849400700108

Parse, R. R. (1998). *The human becoming school of thought.* Thousand Oaks, CA: Sage.

Parse, R. R. (2007). The human becoming school of thought in 2050. *Nursing Science Quarterly, 20*, 308–311. doi:10.1177/0894318407307160

Parse, R. R. (2014). *The human becoming paradigm: A transformational worldview.* Pittsburgh, PA: Discovery International Publications.

Rogers, M. E. (1970). *An introduction to the theoretical basis of nursing.* Philadelphia, PA: F. A. Davis.

Rogers, M. E. (1992). Nursing science and the space age. *Nursing Science Quarterly, 5*, 27–34. doi:10.1177/089431849200500108

Smith, M. C. (1999). Caring and the science of unitary human beings. *Advances in Nursing Science, 21*, 14–28. doi:10.1097/00012272-199906000-00006

Smith, M. C. (2010). Marlaine Smith's theory of unitary caring. In M. E. Parker & M. C. Smith (Eds.), *Nursing theories and nursing practice* (3rd ed., pp. 495–504). Philadelphia, PA: F. A. Davis.

Smith, M. C., & Parker, M. E. (2014). *Nursing theories and nursing practice* (4th ed.). Philadelphia, PA: F. A. Davis.

Styles, M. M. (1992). Nightingale: The enduring symbol. In F. *Nightingale's Notes on nursing: What it is and is not.* Commemorative Ed. (pp. 72–75). Philadelphia, PA: J. B. Lippincott.

Todaro-Franceschi, V. (1998). *The enigma of energy: A philosophical inquiry.* Doctoral dissertation, New York University (UMI No. 9819881).

Todaro-Franceschi, V. (1999). *The enigma of energy: Where science and religion converge.* New York, NY: Crossroad.

Todaro-Franceschi, V. (2001). Energy: A bridging concept for nursing science. *Nursing Science Quarterly, 14*, 132–140. doi:10.1177/08943180122108328

Todaro-Franceschi, V. (2008). Clarifying the enigma of energy, philosophically speaking. *Nursing Science Quarterly, 21*, 285–290. doi:10.1177/0894318408324332

Watson, J. (1988). *Human science and human care.* Norwalk, CT: Appleton-Century-Crofts.

Watson, J. (1999). *Post modern nursing and beyond.* Edinburgh: Churchill.

Watson, J. (2008). *Nursing: The philosophy and science of caring* (Rev. ed.). Boulder, CO: University Press of Colorado.

Watson, J., & Woodward, T. K. (2010). Jean Watson's theory of human caring. In M. E. Parker & M. C. Smith (Eds.), *Nursing theories and nursing practice* (3rd ed., pp. 351–369). Philadelphia, PA: F. A. Davis.

Woodward, V. M. (1997). Professional caring: A contradiction in terms? *Journal of Advanced Nursing, 26*, 999–1004. doi:10.1046/j.1365-2648.1997.00389.x

Unity, Purpose, and the Good: An Ethic of Caring

A human being is part of a whole, called by us the Universe . . . . He experiences himself, his thoughts and feelings, as something separated from the rest—a kind of optical delusion of his consciousness. This delusion is a kind of prison for us . . . . Our task must be to free ourselves from this prison by widening our circles of compassion to embrace all living creatures and the whole of nature in its beauty.
—Albert Einstein (1879–1955)

3

Compassion and Contentment: Being Heartful and Happy at Work

A commitment to kindness can be the thread that twines throughout our various successes, disappointments, delights, and traumas, making our lives seamless, giving us ballast in a world of change, a reservoir of heartfulness to infuse our choices, our relationships and our reactions.
—Sharon Salzberg

KEY TOPICS

- Compassion and compassionate caring
- Actualizing potentials as nurses
- Contentment
- Productivity and quality care

INTRODUCTION

In the book, *Ruby's Imagine*, written by Kim Antieau (2008), Ruby, a teenager, lives in the heart of New Orleans in a small cottage with her grandmother. A

© Springer Publishing Company DOI: 10.1891/9780826155214.0003

hurricane, which Ruby refers to as The Big Spin, comes, and in its immediate aftermath, amid terrible devastation and flooding, Ruby goes around the town in a raft with her friend Jay El and some others trying to help people:

> The day was so hot and humid and stinky that it was hard to breathe. We couldn't go fast because there was so much debris and tangled wires. We went to the first building we saw. . . . We helped one old man and woman, tiny and frail, step off their porch into our boat. They had a little dog about the size of a rat. He came too. . . . Next we got a family: a mother and her three tiny children. The mother couldn't stop crying. The babies just look at her and us. I about start crying then too. The babies didn't hardly have any clothes on them. I held the youngest one on my lap close to me and said, "I'm sorry dawlin'. I loves you, I loves you, I loves you." The baby rested her head on my shoulder. (p. 140)

Ruby is a gem and the author's choice of a name is fitting. I have read this book several times and I always get teary-eyed. Written in first person, the portrayal is one of *compassionate caring* for others. Sharing her story makes readers—us—more compassionate, for as we read, we recognize in Ruby a generosity of spirit that always gets beyond herself, away from her own pain and sorrow, to help others. We know it would be far easier for Ruby to stay in a safe place and not bear witness to anyone else's suffering.

COMPASSIONATE CARING—RUBIES AND GEMS

In nursing, we rarely acknowledge that we, too, are rubies, like the student who called Nurse Katie "a gem." Nursing is much more than physical assessment, pathophysiology, pharmacology, and medical treatments. Among my often-evoked memories of the many patients cared for over the years, a male patient named Eddie comes to mind (Todaro-Franceschi, 2012). I encountered Eddie while working as a staff nurse in critical care. He had been admitted to our cardiac ICU with an inferior wall myocardial infarction, and was placed on several intravenous (IV) medications; an arterial line and Swan–Ganz were inserted, and oxygen therapy was started. He was critically ill, but he was also alert and what everyone referred to as difficult.

Over the course of several days, Eddie became outright belligerent. He would pull on his lines while angrily telling us he did not want any of it; all he wanted was to get out of bed. The physicians said he was becoming confused; the nursing staff, for the most part, agreed. A prescription was written to use four-point restraints as needed. Placed in restraints, Eddie began to be combative, pulling at his tubes and screaming to be "let loose."

Nurses took turns going into his room and repositioning him, fixing his lines, and trying to calm him down. Antianxiety medications were prescribed and administered. Not quite to the point of involuntary sedation but looking very much like it was in his future, Eddie was still adamant that he wanted out of bed, and finally, I asked him why. He answered, "I don't want to die in a hospital bed all alone. I'd rather be sitting up in a chair." I responded by saying that everyone was trying to help him get better. He quieted down a bit while I moved around his room doing all the things a nurse does. Then, he said to me, "I know I am dying." I didn't know how to respond to that at the time; it was years later that I learned a remark like that was an invitation—an opportunity to pull up a chair and be present with someone who is suffering, but his comment certainly got me thinking about ways we could perhaps better meet his needs.

All of us—the nurses, residents, and interns—discussed this patient's wishes with the attending physician when we made our rounds, after which we changed his activity level so that Eddie could get out of the bed to a chair. We procured a geri-chair, and when we got him into it, he was so grateful and pleased to have finally gotten through to us his basic need to get out of that bed. He remained out of bed, alert, and oriented, and he was a totally different person, no longer difficult or belligerent, no longer requiring restraints or antianxiety medication. At the end of that shift, we all felt pretty good with ourselves—the carers and the cared for. Our hearts were full. The patient was heartful because we had, like in the motion picture *Avatar*, finally been able to really "see him," and we were heartful because we recognized that we had gotten beyond ourselves and had actually "seen him."

This patient eventually did die on our unit, despite our attempts to save him. This was not surprising; many individuals have some foresight of their impending death. The eye-opener for me was that he was only comfortable and content when we stopped doing what *we* thought was most important (and admittedly the textbook picture) and instead listened and acknowledged his really small request to "allow" him to get out of the bed. We briefly turned our focus outward toward the whole of the person, rather than focusing on what seems in retrospect to have been *our* need and intent to *cure* the person, in a manner that we, and not the patient, believed was the right way to go about providing care. We moved beyond the rendering of competent care to compassionate care.

When nurses make choices and act on those choices as the intelligent, compassionate carers we are, when we are authentic and true to our purpose, it is clear that nursing is not just about following "orders" and ensuring that a proper medical regimen is followed. It is evident that our purpose is not solely about administering medications and measuring outcomes.

Through our purposeful actions, we actualize our potential as nurses, assisting people to maximize their potential for health and healing in living and in dying. Herein we come to an ethic of care, which emphasizes the foundation underlying our very being. We are connected, *one* with those we care for—and it is this unity and purpose that manifest the potential to heal.

In looking back at this case, I recognize now how fortunate all of us were to be on the same page; it could have been a battle between the few and the many, had anyone thought it was not clinically feasible to get the patient out of bed. I wonder, would I then have been courageous enough to fight that battle?

HAVING A SENSE OF "WE-NESS"

Compassion, a topic of great interest in both the Eastern and Western traditions, is considered to be a human emotion; however, it is also labeled a virtue, a good feature or desirable quality of people. The word *compassion* is taken from Latin, where it means to cosuffer. As with most aspects of human nature, it is always worthwhile to begin any discussion in this area by going back to the ancients. It is Aristotle (n.d./1984) who, through his conceptualization of "pity," is credited with the modern-day idea of "compassion." Pity is said to manifest as feelings of compassion for the suffering of others, and it can also be seen as a feeling of grief, mercy, or sorrow (Angeles, 1992). On the other hand, physician Larry Dossey (2007) emphasized that "compassion doesn't mean feeling sorry or pity for people but feeling with the other, learning to dethrone yourself from the centre of your world and put another there" (p. 1). Concern for others makes us selfless in a way; we are less likely to focus on ourselves. Consequently, compassion is not just something that one feels in relation to another's suffering; it is the experience of feeling *with* another (Blum, 1980).

Physician Eric Cassell (2005) stated that compassion "appears to be an emotion that is specifically social or communal, in the same family, perhaps, with the feeling of patriotism or group-specific feeling" (pp. 434–435). I like the term *communal* and use it frequently in my own work, since it gets at the inseparable nature of all things—the inextricable connection we have to everything else. Indeed, as Cassell pointed out, the core of compassion is connecting, and identifying, with others:

> . . . the compassionate share the same universe with the sufferer—dark and light, air, gravity, noise, and quiet. Also shared are worlds of common values, ideas, beliefs and aesthetics. We know each other through proximity . . . . In other words we share community—a "we-ness" where all are joined . . . . (p. 441)

People differ in the intensity of their emotions, and thus compassion varies; how one relates to and identifies with another will differ from person to person, as Cassell (2005) wrote: "What brings tears to the eyes of one is a matter of indifference to another" (p. 438). While this is surely the case, I believe that the majority of us who go into what are sometimes referred to as the "helping" professions do so as an act of compassion. It is our compassionate nature that provides the impetus for us to enter into service to begin with—for most, it is an impelled act.

Whereas many discussions on compassion emphasize the notion of cosuffering, I believe that suffering is not necessary, nor do we need to recognize it, if it is present, in order for us to feel compassion. It is an emotion and act of love. Compassion provokes action (need I say virtuous action?), which shows appreciation for something that seems outside oneself. It is knowing that something outside ourselves contributes to who we are and what we do. It is intuiting that whatever it is really *is not outside* of us at all.

Compassion Provokes Purposeful Action

In one of the most poignant articles on the importance of compassion, organizational behavior educator and researcher Peter Frost (1999) shared an experience he had in a hospital while being treated for cancer. He described witnessing the compassionate care of a nurse for a fellow human being who was suffering tremendously and who literally felt that he had come to the end of his life. Over the course of just one day, the nurse turned this patient's perspective so completely around that, later, the patient seemed like a different person. Frost, only an outside observer, was so moved by her compassionate actions that he claimed it changed the direction of his life. He began to study compassion in earnest, as a means by which organizations can be transformed. In his talks, published papers, and research, he repeatedly acknowledged the nurse. His witnessing of the compassionate care she provided to the other patient also later led him to write a letter commending her to the hospital administration.

I would bet that nurse was, and still is, not even partly aware of how significant her actions were that day. In that one instance, not only did she transform that patient's life, she changed Frost's life, and he, in turn, has transformed the lives of countless other people with his writings and research on compassion. There is no way of telling how many people have been motivated to change their behaviors and practices because of the purposeful actions of this *one* nurse with that *one* patient. Multiply that number by millions of nurses around the world and billions of purposeful actions over the course of our careers. WOW!

As I shared this story with a loved one, who recently underwent major surgery and came as close to death as one can come without dying, he tearfully recalled how, at a time when he felt himself slipping away, he heard one of his nurses keep saying to him, "stay with me, stay with me," and how the nurse had held his hand. He believes to this day that, without that act of compassion, he would have died.

Frost (1999) pointed out that one needs to have courage to act with compassion, for "one must often go beyond the technical, the imperative, the rules of organizations and beyond past practice—to invent new practices that have within them empathy and love and a readiness to connect to others" (p. 129). In nursing, to act with compassion frequently means fighting uphill battles; calling the physician 16 times to get scripts changed; calling the pharmacy for medications that have not come up; waiting for escort to take a patient down for a test for which the patient is NPO, or heck, taking a patient down for a test because escort is not available and the patient is NPO! It might mean tweaking or blatantly ignoring the visiting hour policy for loved ones and getting into arguments with administrators over it. Or it could mean sitting in a patient's room when you really do not have the time for it, and then getting chewed out for "wasting" time, by coworkers who have lost their vision of what nursing is all about.

Nurse leaders are called upon to look at the things impacting on quality of care and to analyze all the factors to get at the source of a problem; in today's jargon, we call this "root cause analysis." We have always done this when looking at quality and safety issues. What we have not done consistently, and need to do, is spend more time exploring and appreciating the root cause of *heartfulness* in nursing, and then identify ways to foster and teach compassionate care. We need to explore more fully how we get contentment doing our work.

CONTENTMENT: A MATTER OF PURPOSEFULLY ACTUALIZING POTENTIAL

Most people spend the majority of the time, their entire lives actually, engaged in work. In essence, our professional quality of life *is* our quality of life, period. Consequently, everyone should begin each day, or at least the vast majority of our days, looking forward to going to work. Since we spend so much time at work, it should be a requirement that we be content or happy most of the time. That is a reasonable expectation, and yet so many people go to work and dislike what they do. But they keep doing it anyway.

When I began to think about writing this book, I was focused on two intertwining issues: (a) the quality of care being provided to patients who were very ill, perhaps dying, and their loved ones; and (b) the quality of the nurse's professional life. Little did I realize that I was really revisiting earlier works of mine. I mentioned my inquiry into ideas of energy in Chapter 2; in that work I was also led to explore ideas related to how people go about actualizing their potential (Todaro-Franceschi, 1998, 1999).

In trying to come to terms with what it means to actualize one's potentials in a purposeful way, I found that there was a general consensus among countless individuals who have studied human nature. The actualizing of human potential that manifests itself in happiness or contentment for people individually and collectively is directly related to an awareness and appreciation of things outside of ourselves and a perceived connection to other—other people and/or things (Todaro-Franceschi, 1998, 1999).

Whenever we use the terms *actuality* and *potentiality*, we are speaking the language of Aristotle. In fact, it was he who coined the term energy— *energeia*—and he defined it as both potential and actual things that are capable of change (Aristotle, n.d./1991; Aristotle, n.d./1996; Todaro-Franceschi, 1998, 1999). Aristotle also stressed that change comes about in a purposeful way. In his doctrine of four causes, he sought to answer the question of how and why a thing comes to exist—why there is a tendency on the part of things to actualize into whatever they eventually become.[1] Although he felt that things in nature have a tendency to become what they do, when it comes to the actualizing of human potential, Aristotle noted that there was always an element of choice; as rational beings we work by choice and not by necessity. Hence, according to Aristotle (n.d./1991, n.d./1996), everything has a purpose and *energeia*—when it becomes an actuality, is a realization of that purpose. Purpose, generally speaking, implies meaning and intention, or a reason why something is being done. People are capable of actualizing potentials, and they do so in a purposeful, intentional manner.

When linked with happiness or contentment, the actualizing of human potential is frequently referred to as *self-actualization*. Self-actualization has been postulated as the one true motive for human existence (Goldstein, 1963). Psychologist Abraham Maslow (1968, 1971), who most readers are likely familiar with, explored the idea of self-actualization in depth, proposing a whole hierarchy of human needs, going from the most basic needs for survival—"safety and protection, to belongingness, love, respect, self-esteem, and identity"—and culminating, finally, in "self-actualization" (1971, p. 22).

Maslow (1971) defined self-actualizing people as individuals who are "without one single exception, involved in a cause outside their own skin, in something outside of themselves" (p. 43). Self-actualizing people tend to be happy, autonomous individuals. There is a long list of attributes for self-actualizing individuals, the most important of which is that they have an almost intuitive kind of feeling of *oneness with the rest of the world*. That feeling appears to motivate them into purposeful action.

In addition to feeling joyful or happy, creativity is another attribute that appears to exist in self-actualizing people. Maslow (1968) noted this characteristic and in his writings he referred to it not just as creativity in the usually depicted sense of art, music, writing, invention, and so forth, but also in very down-to-earth ways, such as "one woman, uneducated, poor, full time housewife and mother . . . was a marvelous cook, mother, wife and homemaker" (p. 136). In nursing we have an overabundance of creativity. Consider the nurse who has a patient complaining of discomfort related to being bedridden and immobile, and as a result creates makeshift pillows to alleviate pressure points. Or the nurse leader who innovatively makes assignments because she is cognizant of her staff's strengths and weaknesses. And the nurse, Susie, in the story *Wit*, who hands her patient, Vivian, a popsicle and sits down beside her to eat the other half, while providing presence. All these nurses are creatively actualizing potentials in ways that help sustain their ability to do the difficult work they do, enabling them to remain connected to their work and the people in their environment, thereby ensuring quality care. The idea behind self-actualization is quite similar to Aristotle's (n.d./1984) notion of *eudaimonia*: ". . . happiness is an activity of the soul in accordance with complete excellence" (p. 1741),[2] where it is noted that "to be *eudaimon* is to flourish, to make a success of life" (Barnes, 1982, p. 78).[3]

Second Wind, Peak, and Optimal Experiences

So why is it that many people who work in healthcare do not appear to be happy? We choose to work in service to others, helping them to actualize their potential to heal and be healthy, to live a good life, and to die well; we should be happy or at least content most of the time. Perhaps it is time to cultivate more optimal experiences in our everyday life.

In an especially striking essay, "The Energies of Man," psychologist William James (1907/1987) discussed what he referred to as the phenomenon of *second wind*, the ability of human beings to go beyond their normal capabilities on various occasions. For instance, how is it that we can care for someone who is critically ill, stabilize that person after many, many hours, and leave work feeling wide awake and full of energy? Conversely, we can work an entire shift and, even though everyone has done fine, we may leave work feeling drained, disappointed somehow, bereft of that good feeling.

James (1907/1987) attributed the phenomenon of second wind to the idea that we have excess stores of energy that can be called upon as the need arises. He speculated that most of us rarely, if ever, tap our reserve store of energy. Still, by using our individual resources, we can actualize innate potentials—we can push ourselves to transcend feelings of fatigue without suffering any permanent, negative consequences. We sometimes go beyond what one could call the "normal" range of human ability.

Maslow (1971) wrote of *peak experiences*, wherein people feel extremely joyful, happy, or ecstatic. He noted that "any experience of real excellence, of real perfection, of any moving toward the perfect justice or toward perfect values tends to produce a peak experience" (p. 175). Peak experiences are similar to mystical experiences and meditative states, where one gets a sense that all is one. The person who has a peak experience displays many of the characteristics of the self-actualizing individual (Maslow, 1968, p. 97).

In a similar theory, psychologist and educator Mihaly Csikszentmihalyi (1990) detailed *optimal experiences* based on accounts of "how people felt when they most enjoyed themselves" (p. 4). Optimal experiences occur because one *makes* them happen: "The best moments usually occur when a person's body or mind is stretched to its limits in a voluntary effort to accomplish something difficult and worthwhile" (p. 3). Optimal and peak experiences are both characterized by two important things: choice and a sense of exhilaration or a feeling of accomplishment. By being in control of one's actions and using a conscious effort to meet preset goals, one can experience great happiness.

Optimal experiences are based on the concept of *flow*. Csikszentmihalyi (1990) defined flow as, "the state in which people are so involved in an activity that nothing else seems to matter; the experience itself is so enjoyable that people will do it even at great cost, for the sheer sake of doing it" (p. 4). In order to be happy, we must *consciously* pursue the attainment of goals: "Creating meaning involves bringing order into the contents of the mind by integrating one's actions into a unified flow experience" (p. 216).

People can transform negative experiences into positive events if they possess an *autotelic self*—"a self that has self-contained goals" (Csikszentmihalyi, 1990, p. 208). This means that we can take negative or potentially negative things and transform them into challenges that we enjoy, and in doing so, maintain a sense of meaning and purpose. When a person's goals are threatened, Csikszentmihalyi noted that one can develop a "condition of inner disorder, or *psychic entropy*, a disorganization of the self that impairs its effectiveness" (p. 37). Surely, from his stance, compassion fatigue and burnout would be characterized as manifestations of psychic entropy.

Csikszentmihalyi (1990) likened the human psyche to what are referred to in science as dissipative structures, since the mind has the ability to turn destructive events into positive ones.[4] He wrote of "transformational skills" and the inherent ability people have to consciously unify experiences toward the attainment of their goals: "Those who know how to transform a hopeless situation into a flow activity that can be controlled will be able to enjoy themselves, and emerge stronger from the ordeal" (p. 201). Can you think of instances where things were wild on your unit, when it may have been terribly short-staffed, and yet you still managed to make good your intent to assist your patients with their healing? In all likelihood, the cohesiveness of the healthcare team helped to make it happen. Everyone being on the same page, with the same intent and purposeful effort, resulted in feelings of contentment, despite the enormity of the workload.

We have optimal experiences because the intention is there—to do something—to work purposively toward the actualization of some potentiality. In other writings, flow has come up as a powerful means of actualizing human potential to live fully and contentedly. Synchronicity or meaningful coincidence, which I discuss in Chapter 5, is also connected to flow—each builds on the other. Flow activities in nursing come about through purposeful, and often communal, caring actions.

OPEN HEART, OPEN MIND

The Dalai Lama explains that in Buddhism, "the kind of love we advocate is love you can have even for someone who has done you harm" (Weber, 1986, p. 129). This reminds me of speaking with an Israeli nurse colleague, who shared her stories of caring for those who would (and sometimes did) kill her brethren, and yet, she was still able to feel compassion for those wounded soldiers. Being able to feel this way about those individuals who she considered enemies of her people surprised her. It is an unconditional love, born out of a sense that we are all one somehow.

Scholar Martha Nussbaum (1996, 2001) noted that the cognitive requirements of compassion hinge in part on the eudaimonistic philosophy of Aristotle. Intrinsic to the Aristotelian idea of human flourishing and happiness is a valuing of what it means to flourish and be happy (Nussbaum, 1996). For each of us, it means something different. Thus, in order to portray compassion, one must be able to empathize and identify with another; one must be able to picture himself or herself in the person's place. As she said, one must acknowledge that *this could be me.* Unfortunately, the acknowledgment that "this could be me" can sometimes lead to fear and distancing, if one is not careful. This is where dispassionate care might replace compassionate care.

A nurse who is actualizing her potential as a carer is one who can feel compassion, who can put herself in the patient's place—repeatedly going to places that scare her. In some of the literature related to compassion, one comes across the word loving-kindness, used to denote an opening of the heart. This opening of the heart leads one to show kindness for another. It is sometimes associated with the Greek term *agape,* commonly used in

Christian theology to refer to acts of kindness, motivated by love. It is love that impels us to care and to act with purpose, in essence, to show compassion.

In the Eastern philosophic tradition, there is a concept called *bodhichitta*, which is similar to the idea of compassion. Chodron (2001), explained that *bodhi* means "awake" or enlightened and *chitta* means both mind and heart or attitude (p. 4). The completely open heart and mind of bodhichitta can be equated with "the soft spot, a place as vulnerable and tender as an open wound" (p. 4). Human beings have a tendency to put up barriers to protect ourselves from feeling the pain of others, yet our bodhichitta—our soft spot—can overcome our fear of pain and suffering and instead allow us to embrace it.

Bodhichitta can be further described on two levels (Chodron, 2001). There is unconditional bodhichitta—"a just is" experience of "wow, this is good!" Then there is relative bodhichitta, which is of particular importance here, as Chodron notes this is the "ability to keep our hearts and minds open to suffering without shutting down" (p. 5). Kobat-Zinn (1994), when explaining mindfulness, noted the interchangeability of the words *mind* and *heart*: ". . . when we hear the word mindfulness, we have to inwardly also hear heartfulness" (p. 2). To be compassionate is to have an open heart and to be heartful. For nurses to be content at work we need to have both levels of bodhichitta, appreciating what is, and remaining open to our feelings of love and caring.

COMPASSION CONTENTMENT, PRODUCTIVITY, AND MAGNETISM: PEAS IN A POD

Work satisfaction comes about by meeting individual personal goals and feeling like we have accomplished something meaningful. When goals are set and met, this is referred to as productivity. In the case of nursing, work productivity basically means being able to provide quality care to our patients. But nurses are not in control of the multiplicity of things that feed into the provision of care. So can one be content or happy in the workplace but still feel dissatisfied? Conversely, might one be satisfied at work but still feel unhappy or discontent? I believe both are possible and that they are different constructs.

When I worked as a staff nurse on a medical unit, I would often be in charge and have 26 patients on a 52-bed unit. We would have no more than three nursing assistants working with us. At the end of our tour, none of us would leave on time, and I was frequently on the unit for an hour or more after the shift ended. Most nights I went home feeling content, knowing that I did everything I could to provide quality care. My patients felt cared for, often voicing their satisfaction. But was I satisfied? At the time, my salary was $18,500. I did not get paid any overtime and my husband was sure I was having an affair because I came home so late every night. I felt that none of the nursing staff were being acknowledged for the hard work we were doing and that we were expected to do far too much with far too little. I might have been content at the end of the day, but I was not satisfied with my work environment. My students who are out there in practice right now voice the same kinds of feelings; although they earn more money today, they are not satisfied. Why does this need to be a concern for everyone, especially nurse leaders? For starters, job satisfaction is one of the strongest predictors of an employee's intent to stay in a workplace (Böckerman & Ilmakunnas, 2008). What is more, the relational aspects of the workplace contribute significantly to job satisfaction (Hill, 2011).

Jessica Pryce-Jones, cofounder of a British-based company that works with organizations around the world to enhance employee happiness, distinguishes between employee satisfaction and employee happiness. Pryce-Jones notes that the major difference between the two is control: "Satisfaction is determined by factors such as pay, working environment, and benefits. Happiness is a part of job satisfaction but really concerns what you can control and influence" (Scott, 2008, p. 9). What is more, she notes that "what people are in most control of is reaching their own potential" (p. 9).

According to Buerhaus (2008), we could expect that the reduced supply of and increased demand for nurses would lead to a shortage of 500,000 RNs by 2025. However, more recent workforce predictions actually foresee a surplus of nurses in some areas and shortages in others by the year 2030 (U.S. Department of Health and Human Services, Health Resources and Services Administration, National Center for Health Workforce Analysis, 2017). Projections show a wide variability throughout the United States; if the current level of healthcare does not change, seven states are predicted to have a significant shortage of RNs, including very large deficits (greater than 10,000 full-time equivalent employees [FTEs]) in California, Texas, New Jersey, and South Carolina. In addition, 33 states are projected to have licensed practical nurse (LPN) shortages, which offers a dire picture for long-term care, where many LPNs are employed.

Shortages lead to heavier workloads, forcing higher nurse-to-patient ratios, which in turn affect nurse turnover and retention and ultimately creates an environment that hinders, rather than promotes, the provision of quality patient care. Clearly, anything that contributes to an inability to provide the quality of care we want to give our patients will lead to work dissatisfaction, and over time, perhaps burnout, which then impacts the provision of care even more. It is a vicious cycle impacting the entire healthcare system and one that healthcare organizations are only just beginning to understand. Of all people, though, it is those of us in nursing who really need to understand this, because it is not just affecting our content-ment at work and the quality of patient care that we are providing; it is much bigger than that. It is affecting us individually at work and at home, and collectively, as a profession. In addition, that butterfly effect goes out into the community of people that we serve and has increasingly become a societal issue as well.

From its inception, the Magnet® hospital program rested on criteria that stressed the importance of the nurse in the creation and maintenance of a healthy work environment. Facilities that had a low turnover of nursing staff and seemed to attract nurses (like a magnet) were studied to identify what made them so attractive (McClure, 2011). Based on the findings of that original study several decades ago, at the onset, the Magnet model focused on the attraction and retention of nurses, nurses' job satisfaction, and quality patient care productivity (Drenkard, Wolf, & Morgan, 2011; Schmalenberg & Kramer, 2008). However, when these criteria were more closely explored by nurse researchers and others over time, it was found that up to 86% of attraction, retention, and job satisfaction were in fact related to the nurses' perceptions that they were providing quality care. Consequently, productivity became the main emphasis in the Magnet model.

In 2001, when nurses from 14 Magnet hospitals were asked what makes for a satisfying and productive work environment, they named eight main attributes: coworkers who are clinically competent, collaborative interdis-ciplinary relationships, autonomy in clinical decision making, supportive nurse leaders, personal control of nursing practice, support for education, a perception of adequate staffing, and a culture where concern for patients comes first (Schmalenberg & Kramer, 2008). It was noted that "a healthy work environment is a group-level phenomenon," and in healthcare organiza-tions, this is especially so (Schmalenberg & Kramer, 2008, p. 66). Whether individuals perceive their work environment as conducive to their content-ment is largely contingent upon how people interact with each other and how patient care is provided. Structural processes alone are not enough to render a happy workforce.

The modern Magnet model focuses on "proven outcomes" and has five components: transformational leadership; structural empowerment; exem-plary professional practice; new knowledge, innovations, and improvements; and empirical outcomes (Wolf, Triolo, Reid-Ponte, Drenkard, & Moran, 2011). The first four all lead up to the last one, which is important in that it is understood that every single one of them is a necessary component to the overall goal of providing quality care. Unfortunately, many places are so focused on outcomes that they cannot see the tree for the forest, and what happens is that they fall short of the mark. And who is often blamed? The nurse!

It might be that the Magnet model, which depicts empirical outcomes at the core, seems to highlight outcomes more, at the expense of all the others. Yet, that is clearly not its intent; it is meant to put the emphasis on all of the components that feed into change, and can transform outcomes from substandard to optimal. In order to get it all to work, we know that transformational leadership is necessary, and the main ingredients for transformational leadership include one having vision, along with influence, people skills, and clinical and leadership expertise. In nursing, we have many transformational leaders, but we have a lot more "would-be" transformational leaders. They "would be" transformational if they perceived themselves as having power. I would suggest that one's role or position does not preclude his or her ability to be a transformational leader and that, in fact, staff nurses can be transformational leaders, individually and collectively. I will return to this line of thinking a bit later (and often).

QUALITY CARE OR QUALITY CARING?

If we define quality care with work productivity or with outcomes, we fall short of the mark in each case. Nurses can be considered productive because we complete all of our nursing tasks within the time allocated, but we may not have been able to provide quality caring—compassionate care. We may have a positive outcome of care such as curing an infection, but we may not meet our own expectations of quality caring if, for example, the patient and/or family does not know how to prevent future occurrences of the infection because we did not have the time to sit with the patient and/or family to discuss healthcare practices.

The quality of patient care is important to us—a necessary prerequisite for contentment. Inherent in quality care is quality *caring*. The nurse who can connect with her patients and not feel as if she is a robot is more likely to go home at the end of the day feeling heartful and more content.

A while back I had looked in cyberspace for a few pictures to portray the idea of compassion. I went to a Creative Commons site to find pictures and did a search on the word "compassion." The pictures that came up to denote compassion were mostly of "doctors," "nurses," and "kittens." Recently I revisited the site and found that it is still pretty much the same. Obviously, it is believed to be an inherent characteristic of physicians and nurses that they are compassionate and that they emanate caring in their practice. One must ask, then, why many of us frequently find ourselves wondering about "that abrupt physician" or "that apathetic nurse." We find ourselves thinking, "something is wrong." Well, something *is* wrong. The bad and the ugly are taking the place of the good.

The crux of the matter is that attainment of happiness and contentment is achieved through the recognition of the interrelatedness of everyone and everything and our ability to appreciate it all as we go about our day-to-day nursing work. This knowledge encourages many of us to take purposeful action. One could say, then, that the actualizing of our potential as nurses is contingent upon feeling compassion for others—it is a requisite characteristic for *our* happiness, human flourishing, or contentment. Our sense of connectedness feeds our contentment as human beings and carers. Purposeful actions that foster and enhance our connectedness—our sense of we-ness—are the essence of nursing, and they are powerful in that they enhance the quality of living–dying for our patients, their loved ones, and for *us*, the carers.

When we recognize that all things and people are inextricably connected, and that whatever we do transforms all else, we are more likely to act in ways that consider the whole. This, in turn, leads to acting with moral comportment. It is here that compassion becomes a virtue as well as an excellence and is valued as a requisite characteristic of the "good" nurse.

KEY POINTS

- Compassion is the ability to put oneself in another's place, and to "feel with" that person. It emerges from a sense of connection to others and other things and it provokes purposeful action.

- Actualizing our full potential as nurses entails acting purposefully and with compassion to assist in health and healing and, ultimately, to enhance the quality of living–dying for people.

- Compassionate caring is an act of love that facilitates feeling heartful. Happiness, human flourishing, or contentment for nurses arises from our caring practices.

- A healthy work environment does not emerge solely from quality care and positive outcomes; it is borne out of, and sustained by, *quality caring* for both the cared for and the carers.

NOTES

1. Any "thing" is made of some stuff—this stuff without form is called the "material cause." In this stuff a change can occur. The pattern or form into which this stuff can be or is changed is called the "formal cause." The "efficient cause" is simply the thing that brings about change or initiates the activity whereby the change takes place. The

purpose or reason for which the change takes place, "that for the sake of which," is called the "final cause" (see Aristotle, n.d./1991, n.d./1996).
2. Also see Aristotle's (n.d./1911) *Nicomachean Ethics*.
3. Aristotle's *eudaimonia* is an end, an actuality (*energeia*), toward which one strives.
4. Prigogine (1980) discovered that certain chemical reactions self-organize into complex patterns. Like chaos theory, the premise underlying this theory is that order can and does arise from disorder.

REFERENCES

Angeles, P. A. (1992). *The HarperCollins dictionary of philosophy* (2nd ed.). New York, NY: Harper Perennial.

Antieau, K. (2008). *Ruby's imagine*. Boston, MA: Houghton Mifflin.

Aristotle. (n.d./1911). *The Nicomachean ethics* (D. P. Chase, Trans.). London: J. M. Dent & Sons.

Aristotle. (n.d./1984). *The complete works of Aristotle: The revised Oxford translation* (Vols. 1–2; J. Barnes, Ed.). Princeton, NJ: Princeton University Press.

Aristotle. (n.d./1991). *The metaphysics* (J. H. McMahon, Trans.). Buffalo, NY: Prometheus Books.

Aristotle. (n.d./1996). *Physics* (R. Waterfield, Trans.). New York, NY: Oxford University Press.

Barnes, J. (1982). *Aristotle*. New York, NY: Oxford University Press.

Blum, L. (1980). Compassion. In A. M. Rorty (Ed.), *Explaining emotions* (pp. 507–517). Berkeley, CA: University of California Press.

Böckerman, P., & Ilmakunnas, P. (2008). Interaction of working conditions, job satisfaction, and sickness absences: Evidence from a representative sample of employees. *Social Science & Medicine*, *67*(4), 520–528. doi:10.1016/j.socscimed.2008.04.008

Buerhaus, P. I. (2008). Current and future state of the U.S. nursing workforce. *Journal of the American Medical Association*, *300*(20), 2422–2424. doi:10.1001/jama.2008.729

Cassell, E. J. (2005). Chapter 31: Compassion. In C. R. Snyder & S. J. Lopez (Eds.), *Handbook of positive psychology* (pp. 434–445). Cary, NC: Oxford University Press.

Chodron, P. (2001). *The places that scare you: A guide to fearlessness in difficult times*. Boston, MA: Shambala.

Csikszentmihalyi, M. (1990). *Flow: The psychology of optimal experience*. New York, NY: Harper & Row.

Dossey, L. (2007). Compassion. *Explorations*, *3*(1), 1–5. doi:10.1016/j.explore.2006.08.004

Drenkard, K., Wolf, G., & Morgan, S. H. (Eds.). (2011). *Magnet®: The next generation—Nurses making the difference*. Silver Spring, MD: American Nurses Credentialing Center.

Frost, P. J. (1999). Why compassion counts. *Journal of Management Inquiry, 8*(2), 127–133. doi:10.1177/105649269982004

Goldstein, K. (1963). *The organism: A holistic approach to biology derived from pathological data in man.* Boston, MA: Beacon Press.

Hill, K. S. (2011). Work satisfaction, intent to stay, desires of nurses, and financial knowledge among bedside and advanced practice nurses. *Journal of Nursing Administration, 41*(5), 211–217. doi:10.1097/nna.0b013e3182171b17

James, W. (1987). *William James writings 1902–1910.* New York, NY: The Library of America. (Original work published 1907)

Kobat-Zinn, J. (1994). *Wherever you go, there you are: Mindfulness meditation in everyday life.* New York, NY: Hyperion.

Maslow, A. H. (1968). *Toward a psychology of being.* New York, NY: Van Nostrand Reinhold.

Maslow, A. H. (1971). *The farther reaches of human nature.* New York, NY: The Viking Press.

McClure, M. L. (2011). The first generation. In K. Drenkard, G. Wolf, & S. H. Morgan (Eds.), *Magnet®: The next generation—Nurses making the difference* (pp. 1–8). Silver Spring, MD: American Nurses Credentialing Center.

Nussbaum, M. (1996). Compassion: The basic social emotion. *Social Philosophy and Policy, 13,* 27–58. doi:10.1017/s0265052500001515

Nussbaum, M. (2001). *Upheavals of thought: The intelligence of emotions.* Cambridge, UK: Cambridge University Press.

Prigogine, I. (1980). *From being to becoming: Time and complexity in the physical sciences.* San Francisco, CA: Freeman.

Schmalenberg, C., & Kramer, M. (2008). Clinical units with the healthiest work environments. *Critical Care Nurse, 28*(3), 65–77.

Scott, D. E. (2008). Nursing that works: Happiness at work. *New Jersey Nurse, 38*(6), 3, 9.

Todaro-Franceschi, V. (1998). *The enigma of energy: A philosophical inquiry.* Doctoral dissertation, New York University (UMI No. 9819881).

Todaro-Franceschi, V. (1999). *The enigma of energy: Where science and religion converge.* New York, NY: Crossroad.

Todaro-Franceschi, V. (2012). *A dying man and a chair. [A digital story].* Jackson, NJ: Author.

U.S. Department of Health and Human Services, Health Resources and Services Administration, National Center for Health Workforce Analysis. (2017). Supply and demand projections for the nursing workforce 2014-2030. Rockville, MD. Retrieved from https://bhw.hrsa.gov/sites/default/files/bhw/nchwa/projections/NCHWA_HRSA_Nursing_Report.pdf

Weber, R. (1986). *Dialogues with scientists and sages: The search for unity.* New York, NY: Routledge & Kegan Paul.

Wolf, G., Triolo, P., Reid-Ponte, P., Drenkard, K., & Moran, J. (2011). The next generation. In K. Drenkard, G. Wolf, & S. H. Morgan (Eds.), *Magnet®: The next generation—Nurses making the difference* (pp. 23–30). Silver Spring, MD: American Nurses Credentialing Center.

4

Values and Excellences in Nursing

Morality means living with intentions that reflect our love and compassion for ourselves as well as our caring for others.

—Sharon Salzberg

KEY TOPICS

- Code of ethics
- Compassionate care
- Commitment to self and other

INTRODUCTION

Every profession has core values and excellences that provide an ethical code, a reference point for how we go about acting professionally. In nursing education, the learning of this content may be relegated to the clinical practicum experiences, and little time is spent on seminar discussions; thus, it often seems an obscure aspect of the curriculum. Yet, it is this more esoteric "stuff" that for me and many other nurse educators has been, and continues to be, a challenge to teach to nursing students. Things like, for instance, how to question a prescription that does not seem necessary or correct (and the many other times when our advocacy

© Springer Publishing Company DOI: 10.1891/9780826155214.0004

is needed); bear witness to a dying person's anguish and comfort grieving loved ones; handle the bioethical issues you will face on an almost daily basis; remain connected to your patients while juggling the slew of tasks associated with your practice; and, of equal importance, how to care for yourselves and take the time to appreciate each day. It is the combination of a multitude of things (the whole!) that comprises the foundation for professional nursing practice, and all of it is so essential for both the cared for *and* the carer.

Introductory courses in nursing provide an overview of what professional practice is, what our code of ethics means, and how nurses are supposed to function. They usually outline the values and excellences held at the core of our being and becoming nurses. But very little time is allowed for dialogue and self-reflection. It is not enough to outline the values and excellences of nursing to those who are entering into the profession; each person must be able to reflect upon and understand how those values and excellences fit with his or her individual set of values and beliefs, as well.

When I was growing up, I was told that children do not question their elders; they do as they are told. That dictate has never worked for adults. Of course, it is also no longer the case for children. Yet, here we are in nursing teaching adults how to care for others, and in doing so, we briefly touch upon our professional code of ethics, but we never give our students time to question and truly understand those values. Instead, we emphasize the importance of quality and safety and skill sets such as assessment, wound care, medication administration, and the like, all the while taking for granted that the values and excellences emphasized in our professional code of ethics will be subsumed into our students' core through osmosis. It just does not happen that way.

OUR CODE OF ETHICS

I have had a bookmark from the American Nurses Association (ANA) since I graduated with my associate degree in 1982 that bullets 11 statements (referred to as provisions) of the Code for Nurses, dated 1976. Since then, the code has undergone three successive revisions, one in 1985, another in 2001, and most recently in 2015. While the number of provisions has changed over time, the core elements have remained. That bookmark has traveled with me to various places I have worked over the years. I continue to revisit it on a regular basis. It is a reminder of who we are and what we are individually and collectively always striving to attain. No one has captured the essence of our ethical code in a few words better than nurse ethicist Marsha Fowler (2008):

Within the Code for Nurses, whatever the version, there is a deep and truly abiding concern for the social justice at every level; for the amelioration of the conditions that are the causes of disease, illness, and trauma; for the recognition of the worth and dignity of all with whom the nurse comes into contact; for the provision of high quality nursing care in accord with the standards and ideals of the profession; and for just treatment of the nurse. (p. xviii)

These words beautifully depict what the code is about, what *we* are about. And while the word compassion is not evident here, undoubtedly without it we would have no basis for any concern whatsoever.

COMPASSION: A VIRTUE AND AN EXCELLENCE

Compassion is unquestionably at the heart of the mission of the nursing profession; in our code of ethics, it is identified as both a *virtue* and an *excellence*. In the very first provision of our code, it is noted that "the nurse practices with compassion and respect for the inherent dignity, worth, and unique attributes of every person" (American Nurses Association, 2015, p. 1). It is made clear, in the interpretive statements regarding our code, that the use of the term "health problems" encompasses all aspects of human living–dying; both those who are well and those who are ill are the recipients of care.

The ANA specifically addressed the core values of the profession of nursing, noting that "excellences such as compassion, patience, and skill are habits of character of the morally good nurse" (Fowler, 2008, p. 161). We value compassion as a virtue—a requisite characteristic of the "morally good nurse," and we also acknowledge its function as an excellence—a compassionate carer does her work well. It is not enough to be able to do the technical skills of nursing competently. *Sine qua non*, both competent *and* compassionate care have to be the basis for a nurse's work ethic; one without the other simply is not nursing.[1]

ALTRUISM: RENOUNCING NEEDS OF SELF, A MISNOMER

Nursing exists to serve society, as do all professions. Foundational to all professions is an ethic that is noted to be altruistic, and in a way, we are expected to lay aside or renounce our own needs in order to do for others. Basically, altruism equals renunciation of the self. However, this is problematic because we cannot take care of others unless we are healthy and fit; we must first care for ourselves in order to be able to care for others.

The best example that comes to mind are the instructions on an airplane: In the event of a loss of cabin pressure, oxygen masks will drop down and you are told that you need to apply the mask to yourself first, before you assist your children, loved ones, or others. There is an ANA provision in our code of ethics that shares a comparable message: "The nurse owes the same duties to self as to others, including the responsibility to promote health and safety, preserve wholeness of character and integrity, maintain competence, and continue personal and professional growth" (ANA, 2015, p. 19). We need to preserve our *own* well-being, caring for ourselves as we would care for others. In the biblical passage, we are told to do unto others as we would have them do unto us. In nursing, we need to realize this must go both ways; we must do unto ourselves as we would do unto others.

Preserving wholeness of character and integrity encompasses the physical, psychological, and spiritual parts of human well-being. If we value caring for others and it is the impetus behind our work as nurses, then by our purposeful acts of caring for others we are also caring for ourselves. Conversely, by not doing so, we are hurting ourselves. Thus, if nurses are to do for ourselves, we must be true to our authentic selves; we must always remember our purpose.

PRESENCE AND AUTHENTICITY

In their classic text, Bishop and Scudder (1996) discuss what it means to have a therapeutic caring presence, showing the relationship between compassion and authenticity. They note that a good nurse is one who is not only competent but is also obviously concerned with the well-being of those she is caring for. A caring presence

> is a way of being with others that assures them of personal concern for their well-being. This way of being fosters trust, mutual concern, and positive attitudes that promote good health. When caring presence pervades a healthcare setting, the whole atmosphere of that setting is transformed . . . . (p. 41)

A good nurse may also be referred to as an "exemplary nurse," someone who "did their work in a remarkable way and achieved outstanding outcomes for their patients and, subsequently, were positively affected themselves" (Perry, 2008, p. 88). In Perry's study of exemplary oncology nurses who seemed to avoid compassion fatigue, she found several common themes: moments of connection, making moments matter, and energizing moments, which all refer to caring practices (p. 87). Notably, the new Magnet® model emphasizes the notion of "exemplary nurses" and links it to both job satisfaction and positive clinical outcomes. What needs to be stressed more is that when we do our work well, we feel good, yes, but a main part of nursing work is the human-to-human connection that takes place: "The precursor to caring is connecting" (Clayton, Murray, Horner, & Greene, 1991, p. 155).

Why do people choose to go into nursing? In one of her early works, Watson (1985) identified that "human caring is the moral ideal and origin for nursing's professional role and 'calling,' with the goal of protection, enhancement, and preservation of human dignity" (p. 74). I believe that the vast majority of people who choose to enter into nursing do so because they feel compelled to care; they have an affinity for the work. It may not always be that nursing is/was a first choice, but that caring for others in some manner is their calling.

In his writing on the attributes of a profession, Ernest Greenwood (1982) emphasized that "professional work is never viewed solely as a means to an end; it is the end itself. Curing the ill, educating the young, advancing science are values in themselves" (p. 30). He noted that there is devotion to the work; so much so, that on occasion, the "work-life invades the after-work life, and the sharp demarcation between the work hours and the leisure hours disappears" (p. 30). I am reminded here of Maslow's (1968) notes from his studies of the self-actualizing individual: "Duty became pleasure, and pleasure merged with duty. The distinction between work and play became shadowy. How could selfish hedonism be opposed to altruism, when altruism became selfishly pleasurable?" (p. 140). The bottom line is that professionals who exist to serve society also serve themselves in that they so enjoy (*or should enjoy*) what they do that their altruistic nature is not really a renunciation of self—rather, it is an embracing of one's authentic self.

DOCTOR'S ORDERS

So here we have a nursing workforce that has an affinity for the work and wants to help people actualize their potential for health and healing. BUT the system will not let us do it, right? One must ask, is it the system that gets in our way, or is it us? I believe that it is neither alone; it is a combination of both.

Nurses are still predominantly socialized during basic education and in the workplace to be subordinate to others. This is not always intentional; rather, it seems that old habits die hard. For example, when teaching pharmacology to baccalaureate students, I always emphasized that nurses do not "take orders" from others but are responsible for our actions. One of the ways I tried to get students to realize this was by telling them on the first day of class that every time I used the phrase "doctor's orders," they were to raise their hands, and the first five or so students to do so would receive extra credit on their lowest exam grades. This worked superbly, although, one day, a student told me how angry another faculty member had gotten when all the students raised their hands every time she said "doctor's orders" during her lectures. I just laughed and said I would speak with my colleague. It was fine; when I did speak with her, we laughed together.

The following year, when I had this same cohort of students for a senior-level preceptored practicum, I noticed that many of them actually used the term "doctor's orders," themselves, in their speaking and writing. When I think of this, I cannot help echoing nurse ethicist and educator Joan Liaschenko's (2008) words, "I no longer know what nursing academia is doing—the logic escapes me. I wonder what identities are being produced and against which nurses will evaluate themselves" (p. 201). She asked, "What moral resources is academia providing?" (p. 201).

Liaschenko (2008) noted that the current day-to-day experiences of nurses in practice are alarmingly similar to those of practicing nurses from years ago (when she began nursing school in 1967). Her own experiences in practice from 1970 through 1996, along with the stories she has continued to hear from her nursing students, reflect that the moral concerns of students mirror those of practicing nurses in the way they center on the conflict between themselves and others who are involved in the care of patients. Unsurprisingly, the majority of their shared concerns involved end-of-life care issues and/or times when a patient was critically ill. During these times, conflict often arose when other members of the healthcare team were not hearing the voice of the nurse.

What leads Liaschenko (2008) to question the logic of academia is that her graduate nursing students continue to question their own abilities and blame themselves for not being heard. She reflected that:

> . . . students frequently wrote that they should have known more, the implication being that if they did, they would have been able to convince the physician to alter the course of clinical actions. The knowledge they feel they should have known was always scientific. (p. 196)

She goes on to note that "nurses fail to claim credit for their nonscientific knowledge that is absolutely necessary for patient care" (p. 198). Like Liaschenko, I believe that this is in large part due to the way we continue to educate nurses.

Going back to "doctor's orders," some readers may think, well, after all, that is what they are called in practice; yes, but, we all know that "orders" are not what they really are. Nurses are responsible first and foremost to those we serve—our patients and their loved ones—and not to those who work beside us. Accountability goes in both directions; the nurse is accountable to the physician and other members of the healthcare team concerning the provision of quality care to people who need it. The physicians and other healthcare professionals, including administrative personnel, are also accountable, to us—nurses. Yet, somehow, many nurses do not get that message in their basic nursing education, or if they do, many of them seem to be quickly socialized "out" of it.

One year, a very upset student shared with us in class a sign that she had seen posted on a nurse's locker door by an administrator. I do not recall the exact wording, but it said something along the lines of "I will not change or question doctor's orders." She was being publicly flogged! Back then, and *then* is about a decade ago, all I could think of were the words in the New York State Nurse Practice Act that said we should not vary an existing medical regimen.

I recently revisited the New York State Nurse Practice Act, which is posted online, and in 2017 it still says this: "A nursing regimen shall be consistent with and shall not vary any existing medical regimen" (NYSED. gov. Office of the Professions, 2018). But just what does that really mean? One must question the logic of that statement if we are indeed to uphold the basic premises of our code of ethics through our actions. How can we purposefully act with moral comportment and courage if we think that we are subordinate? How will we ever move away from this archaic view if our formal nursing education continues to reinforce this way of thinking?

Questioning "Orders"

I had assigned one of my senior baccalaureate students to work with a patient named Joe, who had a primary diagnosis of colorectal cancer (Todaro-Franceschi, 2010). Joe had been admitted for further diagnostic testing, and just the day before, it had been discovered that he had widespread metastasis. He was alert, oriented, and conversant. The first day of our clinical rotation, he was walking with minimal assistance and verbalized feeling very little pain; MS Contin was effectively controlling any discomfort. The second day, in the early morning, I saw the student by the nurse's station around the time that breakfast trays were being delivered to the unit. I inquired about Joe and she informed me that he was still asleep. I asked about his vital signs and all the other normal things that an instructor might ask, like whether he was easily awakened, how his skin color looked, and so forth. As we walked to the patient's room, she assured me that he was okay.

At the patient's bedside, we found that his breakfast tray had been set up in front of him. Although he was in a semi-Fowler's position, Joe was fast asleep, his food untouched. Leaning in, I gently nudged his arm, while asking him if he wanted to eat his breakfast. With obvious effort he responded to me, opening his eyes slowly and saying, "yes, I am hungry . . ." and without completing the sentence, he was again asleep. After several attempts to speak with Joe, during which time he said he "just couldn't keep his eyes open," I asked the student to get his medication record. We found that at 6 p.m. the evening before, a fentanyl (Duragesic) patch had been applied for pain management. A potent opioid-derivative narcotic, fentanyl skin patches are very effective pain relievers; however, in Joe's case, the medication was sedating him.

Further exploration revealed that although Joe had requested pain medication in the late afternoon the previous day, his requests for pain relief had been infrequent during his 5-day hospitalization. Thus, the use of pain medication, which resulted in Joe's sedation, seemed extraordinary rather than ordinary care, and prompted many questions. Was the health-care provider who had prescribed the medication aware that Joe was being sedated with its use? Was it really necessary to sedate Joe to manage his pain? Was pain management along with sedation the intended outcome of the medical treatment? More importantly, what were this patient's wishes regarding what was to be *his* "dying" experience?

The nurse assigned to Joe that day had floated to the unit and was not familiar with Joe; she felt uncomfortable calling the physician to question the prescription for the fentanyl patch. I offered to make the call and spoke with the physician who had prescribed the medication. He informed us that Joe had been adamant that he did not want to have any pain. But, I wondered aloud, did the patient want to sleep the rest of his life away? I noted that he could not even stay awake long enough to eat his breakfast. The physician did not answer that question and instead indicated his irritation with my questioning his "orders." After a brief discussion with the primary nurse, the student and I went back into Joe's room, removed the fentanyl patch from his arm, and I asked the student to pull up a chair to wait for the patient to fully awaken, at which time she was instructed to inform me.

Later in the day, when Joe was awake and after he had eaten, the student and I sat down to speak with him. I asked him what he knew about his illness and he told us, "Well now, I'm dying." He explained to us that his cancer had spread, and that they—the doctors—could not get rid of it. I proceeded to ask him if he was currently in a lot of pain. Joe informed us that he was not in much pain and a wonderful discussion ensued during which time Joe shared a lot of things with us: He had been a widower for several years and he had two daughters who lived in Florida but were currently up North to see him. He told us that both of his daughters were insisting that he move to Florida to live with them, but because he did not want to be a "burden" to his children, he had not entertained the thought of relocating.

We discussed his living–dying options at some length and then I went to the nurse manager of the unit where we planned a meeting for Joe and his family, with the physician, nurse manager, and case social worker, the following day. Ultimately, Joe chose to move to Florida with his daughters, where hospice services were put into place.

There are several practice issues here that are directly related to compassionate caring and the concomitant moral comportment with which nurses go about our purposeful actions. In this case, the purpose of the pain medication that had been prescribed was to alleviate suffering, but it was not meant to sedate the patient. Had "doctor's orders" been followed, rather than questioned, and had we not taken the initiative to remove the patch, it would have remained on Joe, and he would have been left to sleep. In all due likelihood, Joe's daughters would have thought his sleeping was due to the natural progression of his illness.

Had the nurse, who was caring for the patient that day, and the prescribing physician put themselves for a moment in the place of either Joe or his family, they probably would have taken a different approach to his pain management; in other words, their purposeful actions would likely have been more compassionate and morally sound. The significance of the issues related to the physician's practice is beyond the scope of this book; however, the issues related to the nurse's practice must be more fully explored.

It is difficult to float to a unit where one is not familiar with the patients and the staff; I know this because I worked full time in the float pool of a 600-bed hospital for 2 years. Still, had I been in that nurse's shoes, I would have picked up the phone to call the physician. This is not because I am a better nurse, but because I have always been able to put myself in the place of the patient. I cosuffer well. I also know that somehow I did get the message early on in my professional career that without *us*, the system does not work at all. In addition, and perhaps most important here, is that I have always felt *free* to be moral. I have always believed that because I am a licensed registered nurse, my practice is autonomous—I answer to myself and my patients. Sadly, many nurses do not feel free to be moral.

Nursing practice must be collaborative, yes, but ultimately, it is autonomous in nature; the morally good nurse should intuit that she is free to act always in the best interest of her patients and their loved ones. Going back to Joe and to the float nurse, had she called the physician and questioned the medication, what would have been the worst-case scenario? I am sure the physician would have said the same things to her that he said to me. Had she pulled the patch off and sat down to speak with Joe, he would have shared the same things with her that he shared with the student and me. The outcome would have been the same; however, I would be telling the story from the nurse's voice instead of my own. It would have been *her* story.

I have no idea if the nurse who floated to the unit that day ever went back to the unit and became aware of the outcome for Joe. I do know that I feel *heartful* every time I recall how we were able to act purposefully to help him. Compassion is a virtue and an excellence that makes all the difference. How many family memories would have been lost had Joe been allowed to sleep through that day and the days thereafter?

VALUING COMPASSION AS A REQUISITE CHARACTERISTIC

While we spend very little time speaking directly about it in nursing education, as previously noted, compassion is a requisite characteristic for those who enter into the health*care* professions. Nurse educator Maria Schantz (2007) claimed that the meaning of the concept *compassion* has not been adequately defined in nursing, and it is not widely promoted or emphasized in contemporary nursing practice. In a concept analysis, she detailed the differences among terms we commonly use in nursing, such as *empathy* ("a vicarious participation in other people's emotions, ideas, or opinions"), *caring* ("a state of mind, which is related to troublesome worries, anxiety, or concern"), and *sympathy* ("an overall kinship with someone's feelings, regardless of the feeling"; p. 51). Schantz noted that although these terms are related to compassion, compassion is the only one that "impels and empowers people to not only acknowledge, but also act toward alleviating or removing another's suffering or pain" (p. 51). And, in this connotation, there lies a clear demarcation between the idea of compassion as an emotion—a feeling—and the idea of it being a virtue and an excellence. It is in our *purposeful actions* to assist in healing that the characteristic of compassion as both a virtue and excellence becomes prominent.

In a recent concept analysis of *compassionate care*, repeating themes were identified in the literature, which seem to be the prevalent characteristics (of compassionate care) (Burnell, 2009):

a. A dimension of caring
b. Sympathetic consciousness of another's distress
c. Sensitivity to the pain and brokenness of another
d. Suffering alongside another
e. A spiritual connection with another person
f. Attempting to comfort or alleviate the suffering
g. A demonstration of the fruit of the Holy Spirit[2] (Burnell, 2009, p. 321)

To be a compassionate nurse essentially means that we feel for others, display kindness to others, and act on behalf of others for their benefit. We have an awareness of the interconnected nature of everyone and everything; it is all essentially one (Todaro-Franceschi, 1999). So, when someone is distressed, a compassionate carer acknowledges and bears witness to that suffering and will seek to lessen if not completely obliterate that anguish. Compassionate carers are concerned for the well-being of those entrusted to their care *and* will also willingly acknowledge that the significant others of our patients are also entrusted to our care (for they are suffering with, and sometimes more than, their loved ones). Yet, a compassionate carer also intuits that, by caring for others, we are also caring for ourselves; it is virtually indistinguishable where one ends and the other begins.

KEY POINTS

- Compassion is both a value and an excellence in nursing.
- Competent and compassionate care is the basis for our work ethic; one without the other is not nursing.
- By serving others compassionately, we serve ourselves and are authentic to our altruistic nature.
- Acting purposefully with moral comportment and courage entails being accountable to ourselves and expecting accountability from other members of the healthcare team. Thus, there is no such thing as "doctor's orders."
- Valuing compassion as a requisite characteristic for the profession means we need to embrace our compassionate caring practices and foster caring for self and other. We must do unto ourselves as we would do unto others.
- It is all one.

NOTES

1. One could make an argument that overall competency in nursing practice must include compassion.
2. This, Burnell (2009) noted, is a biblical reference to nine attributes: "love, joy, peace, longsuffering, gentleness, goodness, faith, meekness, and temperance" (p. 321). Burnell identified these visible attributes to be significant as they "embody the heart of compassionate care" (p. 321).

REFERENCES

American Nurses Association. (2015). *Code of ethics for nurses with interpretive statements*. Silver Spring, MD: Author.

Bishop, A. H., & Scudder, J. R. (1996). *Nursing ethics: Therapeutic caring presence.* Sudbury, MA: Jones & Bartlett.

Burnell, L. (2009). Compassionate care: A concept analysis. *Home Health Care Management and Practice, 21,* 319–324. doi:10.1177/1084822309331468

Clayton, G. M., Murray, J. P., Horner, S. D., & Greene, P. E. (1991). Chapter 12. Connecting: A catalyst for caring. In P. L. Chinn (Ed.), *Anthology on caring* (pp. 155–168). New York, NY: National League for Nursing.

Fowler, M. D. M. (Ed.). (2008). *Guide to the code of ethics for nurses: Interpretation and application.* Silver Spring, MD: American Nurses Association.

Greenwood, E. (1982). Attributes of a profession. In B. Baumrin & B. Freedman (Eds.), *Moral responsibility and the professions* (pp. 20–32). New York, NY: Haven Publications.

Liaschenko, J. (2008). ". . . to take one's place . . . and the right to have one's part matter." In W. J. E. Pinch & A. M. Haddad (Eds.), *Nursing and health care ethics: A legacy and a vision* (pp. 195–203). Silver Spring, MD: American Nurses Association.

Maslow, A. H. (1968). *Toward a psychology of being.* New York, NY: Van Nostrand Reinhold.

NYSED.gov. Office of the Professions. (2018). Education law. Article 139, Nursing. Retrieved from www.op.nysed.gov/prof/nurse/article139.htm

Perry, B. (2008). Why exemplary oncology nurses seem to avoid compassion fatigue. *Canadian Oncology Nursing Journal, 18*(2), 87–92. doi:10.5737/1181912x1828792

Schantz, M. L. (2007). Compassion: A concept analysis. *Nursing Forum, 42*(2), 48–55. doi:10.1111/j.1744-6198.2007.00067.x

Todaro-Franceschi, V. (1999). *The enigma of energy: Where science and religion converge.* New York, NY: Crossroad.

Todaro-Franceschi, V. (2010). *Choices [A digital story].* Washington, DC: Author.

Watson, J. (1985). *Nursing: The philosophy and science of caring.* Niwot, CO: University Press of Colorado.

The *ART* of Reaffirming Purpose: A Healing Model for Carers

So many people walk around with a meaningless life. They seem half asleep, even when they are busy doing things they think are important. This is because they're chasing the wrong things. The way you get meaning into your life is to devote yourself to creating something that gives you purpose and meaning.

—Morrie Schwartz

KEY TOPICS

- *ART*©: A Model to Enhance Professional Quality of Life

INTRODUCTION

When caring work becomes just work, and one is dreading going to work each day, it is time to *Acknowledge* that there is a problem. It is time to *Recognize* and explore one's options, reexamine intentions, and reaffirm purpose. And, it is time to *Turn* toward self and other.

What nurses need is to have a practice that emulates connection with ourselves and with others. Most of us start out that way. Like children are

© Springer Publishing Company DOI: 10.1891/9780826155214.0005   **63** more aware of their connection to things, the majority of us, as nursing students, are very aware of the human-to-human connection. Later on in school, students are taught to distance themselves, to apply a "therapeutic use of self," and they are essentially told to be empathetic while always remaining objective. This kind of classic teaching may inadvertently set the stage for the development of burnout later on; disturbingly, some nurse researchers have reported findings that suggest that the nursing educational process may lead to a reduction in caring behaviors (Murphy, Jones, Edwards, James, & Mayer, 2009).

The reduction of caring behaviors, by whatever means, brings us further away from compassion contentment because it encourages disconnection and distancing rather than connection and presencing. Still, I remain convinced that nurses know more than most that "everyone needs to feel a sense of belonging, in living, and in dying" (Todaro-Franceschi, 1999, p. 130). Watson (2008) emphasizes that we need to consider an ethic of "belonging before being" (p. 304). This ethic, I believe, has been the light that propels most of us to choose a nursing vocation; however, somewhere along the way, many nurses seem to forget our reason for *being* what we are. We deny that sense of connection to other. The nature of the healthcare system contributes to this sense of disconnect, and it often prevents us from remembering the reason for our *being* during our day-to-day living–working.

Years ago, when I recognized that many RNs who were coming back to school were not content with their work, I began to incorporate this knowledge into many of my classes. In an elective offering I wrote and regularly taught for over 15 years, I did a lot of work trying to bring compassion contentment back into the nursing practice of my RN to BSN pathway students. The course was about changing death experiences in healthcare. However, teaching this content for so many years taught me the profound applicability of Virginia Woolf's words when she wrote, "I meant to write about death, only life came breaking in as usual" (Woolf, 1922). No discourse on dying and death is very meaningful without equal attention to life and living.

I always began the course by telling the students that they were there for a reason and that no matter what brought them to enroll in the course, their lives would be forever changed by the end of the term. At the end of the course I asked them to identify one AHA!, a moment where things seemed to come together to make more sense for them. The majority of the students shared more than one, and sometimes many, AHA! moments like the following one written by an RN to BSN pathway student:

My second AHA! moment happened when one more time I got inside myself and I was able to reflect on the real me. That was when we spoke in class about finding some time in our busy work schedule to pull up a chair and talk with our patients. After this class, I realized how much I have changed since I became a nurse—to tell the truth, for the worse . . . . I still remember how passionate I was about my work, how very eager I was to stay one or two hours after work to finish documentation for which I never had time during my normal work hours because I had chosen to spend all this time with my patients. Many times I was ridiculed by other nurses and was told that I had a problem with time management . . . . I also recall my conversation with one of my coworkers who asked me why I like to work on Medical–Surgical units and not in the Emergency Department. I told him that I really enjoy talking with my patients and I don't have time when working in such a busy place as the ER, where you work like a robot that only follows orders.

After taking this class, I realized that working for 2½ years as a floater on many different units has changed me a lot. Now I am no longer willing to stay after my regular work hours, no longer am I getting into long conversations with my patients, and the place that I like the most is . . . . Emergency Department, the place where I became one of those robots . . . . Am I happy with who I have become? I am not sure about it. But I am certain about one thing—I am glad that I have taken this class because it has opened my eyes to myself; I am more aware of myself, my unresolved conflicts, my hidden angriness, my current preferences and who I am right now . . . .

Nurses need to reawaken what most of us intuited when we first entered into nursing—that it is all essentially one. We need to reaffirm a sense of both unity and purpose. What is deemed negative or bad—compassion fatigue—is a pattern of the whole, a pattern which indicates that transformation is needed. When we get to the ugly—burnout—we have become automated, apathetic, and are working mindlessly rather than mindfully.

WHAT PURPOSE?

Some of you may be asking yourselves: Is there a purpose in the things I do as a nurse these days? You may be wondering exactly what it is that I am referring to when I write of reaffirming purpose. You might think, "I am running around for 12 hours, with barely a moment to myself; it seems all I do is administer medications and check prescriptions for accuracy. In between, I document, and document, and document. Occasionally I empty a bed pan, or turn a patient, but most of the time the only interaction I have with my patients is when I am giving meds. I might speak collegially with a physician or therapist, but more often than not I feel like I am being spoken *to* and not *with*. Increasingly, of late, I find myself avoiding having to speak with patients and their family members; who has time for them and what can I say to them that will make any difference, anyway?"

Does any of this sound familiar to you? If so, then you are right to question what I mean by *our purpose* in nursing, and most assuredly, you need help to recognize and reaffirm your sense of purpose. It is not easy, and I will not claim that anything *will* be fixed; I only claim that it *can* be fixed and that each of us always has a choice in how we go about being in the world, both personally and professionally.

What I mean by reaffirming purpose is that nurses who have forgotten or lost enthusiasm for nursing *can* recover zeal for who we are and what we do. Individually and collectively, we can heal from and/or possibly avert compassion fatigue or burnout, and at the same time, reaffirm purpose in nursing, by following certain steps depicted by the acronym *ART*.

ART: A MODEL FOR ENHANCING PROFESSIONAL QUALITY OF LIFE

ART is an acronym for *A*cknowledging, *R*ecognizing, and *T*urning. Over the years, as I have taught and presented on this topic, I have come to think of the *ART* of reaffirming purpose as a healing model for our wounded workforce (Todaro-Franceschi, 2008, 2013, 2015). Following these steps can help you enhance your professional quality of life.

You first need to *acknowledge* your feelings and that you may have wounds, wounds that you have not been aware of and that are festering. With this newfound knowledge, *recognize* the choices that you have and reexamine your intentions. Then, through your purposeful actions based on the choices you make, you can *re-enchant* yourself with the nature of your work. Last, you must *turn outward toward* yourself and other. It is through reconnection rather than *dis*connection that we can prevent and/or overcome feelings of compassion fatigue and burnout. In Auden's classic 1940 poem, he notes we must "love each other or die." We must love ourselves as we love others, too. In healthcare, it is through our connection to self as well as other that we can maintain and enhance our individual and collective professional quality of life; I call this my *reconnect contention*. Understanding and practicing mindful awareness (also referred to as mindfulness practice or meditation) can broaden your ability and make it easier to use *ART*.

Mindful Awareness

Mindful awareness is an ancient Buddhist practice that can be acquired through study. It denotes a way of being connected with the rest of the world by making a conscious effort to do so. Mindful awareness really entails *being aware of being* and doing it while you are in the moment. Some people might get turned off when they hear it is a form of meditation, but it is not the kind of meditation that requires one to drop everything. It is actually more like embracing everything, by being attentive and aware of it; accepting it, just as it is.

I became enamored with mindful awareness in 2003 when I was diagnosed with uterine cancer and one of my daughters bought me an audiotape of the book, *Wherever You Go, There You Are: Mindfulness Meditation in Everyday Life* (Kabat-Zinn, 1994). Although I had a vague idea of what it was, I had never practiced mindful awareness. It was fitting at the time that I learn the lesson that mindfulness meditation expert Jon Kabat-Zinn was teaching. When I was diagnosed with cancer, I became worried about the future, about having surgery, surviving surgery, developing complications from surgery, learning I might have advanced cancer, and ultimately, I was worried about dying and what would happen to my family. I was so fixated on what *might* happen that I could not appreciate what *was* happening, right there in each moment. Consequently, I was losing all of my moments.

Mindful awareness helps one appreciate the present, and as Kabat-Zinn (1994) noted, the present is really all we have; what is past already happened, but what is happening right now will transform our future. In light of that he asks, should we not pay more attention to our *now*?

> In every moment, we find ourselves at the crossroad of here and now. But when the cloud of forgetfulness over where we are now sets in, in that very moment we get lost . . . . By lost, I mean that we momentarily lose touch with ourselves and with the full extent of our possibilities. Instead, we fall into a robotlike way of seeing and thinking and doing . . . . If we are not careful, those clouded moments can stretch out and become most of our lives. (Kabat-Zinn, 1994, p. xiii)

Who has not, at one time or another, gotten caught up in a robotic way of being? It is, as Kabat-Zinn (1994) noted, our nature to be habitually unaware as we go about our lives.

In just the past few years, there has been an increasing emphasis on the use of mindfulness in nursing and other health-related professions. Since 2015, the American Nurses Association (ANA) has been working to promote awareness of the ways that nurses can incorporate mindfulness into daily life. Not only is it a way to improve the well-being of the nursing workforce, but there is also a butterfly effect; improving our lives in turn transforms the lives of our patients, coworkers, and loved ones outside the workplace.

Mindful awareness stops the mechanical activity of the mind, because once you are aware of what you are doing, you are "thinking" about the moment you are in, rather than unthinkingly acting. When applying *ART*, being mindfully aware will help you to complete each step of the process. In the following chapters, I often encourage you to be mindfully aware of your feelings and thoughts; you will be prompted to "capture your moments" (Kabat-Zinn, 1994, p. 17).

Step 1: Acknowledgment

Acknowledgment of our feelings is accomplished by self-reflection and mindful awareness. How do you feel, right now, in this moment? If you are reading this book, chances are that you are already unhappy with your work and are searching for ways to improve your professional quality of life. Or perhaps you are a nurse leader and are searching for ways to increase staff retention or help them improve productivity. Acknowledging that there is a problem and identifying what is contributing to it involves looking back and trying to discover turning points, accompanied by in-the-moment reflection on one's current experiences and behavior.

Narrative storytelling is a useful way to identify turning points. In some instances, it may also entail exploring the behavior and experiences of others who are sharing or have shared your moments. As you go about your work, try to look toward yourself, your actions and reactions to others, coworkers, patients, and the environment. Jot down your thoughts and feelings. Identify patterns of behavior and any negativity. Has the way you go about your practice changed for the better or worse since you began nursing? If so, can you identify when it started to change?

The Dalai Lama emphasizes that "If you directly confront your suffering, you will be in a better position to appreciate the depth and nature of the problem" (Dalai Lama & Cutler, 1998, p. 136). The problem with us in nursing is we often do not realize we are suffering. We have to learn how to be mindfully aware, as Madeline Ko-I Bastis (2000) shared with us how she learned to "sit in the midst of my suffering, feeling my feelings" (p. xiv).

There is this great little book written by Kent Keith (2003), *Do It Anyway: The Handbook for Finding Personal Meaning and Deep Happiness in a Crazy World*. He writes about overcoming adversity and making our lives have meaning through personal efforts to do good and to be kind, no matter what happens. He notes that in order to move forward, we need to acknowledge the past, and if we are stuck, we need to get unstuck (p. 18). No matter what is in our way, his message is that we can get beyond it. What's more, we *need* to do it, for our own sake.

On the flip side, it is also helpful to acknowledge things that are *good* for you: things that contribute to a sense of well-being and wholeness. When we acknowledge the gifts inherent in our lives, it fills us with joy. There are many aspects of our work as nurses that can make us feel heartful.

The environment in academia, as many will attest, is fraught with issues that can make the workplace unhealthy at times. Sometimes I really miss being with patients, but the students sustain me and my sense of purpose. Teaching end-of-life care, there are times when I am notably feeling compassion fatigued. You simply cannot help cosuffering when teaching about dying, death, and bereavement. But I love what I do. I love teaching this topic and could not imagine doing anything else. It is the emails, notes, cards, and occasional visits from students who tell me what a difference my teachings have made for them that remind me when I seem to get overwhelmed and forget: The work I am doing *is* meaningful.

Think about the lives you have touched. You have no idea how far your reach has gone with your purposeful actions. One of my daughters told me she bought an extra cup of coffee while in Dunkin' Donuts and "put it on the ledge." Just picturing that cup of coffee makes me smile. This act of kindness is thanks to students in a leadership class who, when I assigned an unguided teaching–learning creating change project, took it upon themselves to go around town to coffee shops to get store managers to institute the practice of "hanging coffee." Essentially, a customer goes into a coffee shop, and buys an extra cup of coffee. The store management then makes it known to the community (usually by posting signs) that extra cups of coffee are "hanging around" for those who cannot afford to buy one. This great idea came from a coffee shop in Prague called The Hanging Coffee Café and Pub. A student had gone to this café while visiting Prague and she shared the idea with her group members. They in turn shared the idea with their families, friends, and classmates, who shared the idea with others . . . it is about 15 years later and in local cafes, thanks to student efforts, they are still "hanging" cups of coffee. Random acts of kindness, paying it forward; these things are purposeful acts of caring that can make a huge difference.

If you think about it, nursing is a continual process of sometimes random, sometimes intentional, but always purposeful, acts of kindness. Our compassionate caring actions in nursing practice come at some of the most significant times of our patients' lives. What we do is so meaningful. Being mindfully aware and acknowledging the contributions we make in our day-to-day work nourishes and enhances our compassion contentment, leading us to feel ever more heartful.

Step 2: Recognition

The second step of *ART* is the *R*ecognition that we always have choices, and then, with intention, we are able to choose those actions that will reaffirm our purpose. In this way, one may achieve a re-enchantment with one's life (and our life's purpose). Our lives are full of choices; they not only shape the path of each person's present and future, but also inform and transform the lives of others. And it is important to note that "from a conventional viewpoint, we make 'bad choices.' But from a transcendental perspective, there are no wrong decisions, only different lessons" (Millman, 2000, p. 138).

Things are happening in our day-to-day living that are very meaningful and could help us along our life journey, but many times we miss them entirely because we are not paying attention to our moments. I am referring to magical moments such as when a child smiles at you or when you walk out into a gloriously beautiful day and are met with melodious birdsong or a butterfly nectaring on a flower nearby (or perhaps flapping its wings!). However, I am also referring to what we may deem to be insignificant moments, events that we tend to shrug off as chance happenings, but which in actuality may be very important, if only we would recognize them as such. As Henry David Thoreau (1854/1995) noted, "We should be blessed if we lived in the present always, and took advantage of every accident that befell us" (p. 203).

Meaningful Coincidences

"Chance" happenings can be very meaningful, especially when we stop to reflect upon them. When something that is unlikely to happen does happen, and it is appreciably connected to some other thing, this is referred to as synchronicity or meaningful coincidence (Jung, 1973; Peat, 1987). I am a firm believer in synchronicity and have studied the phenomenon as it relates to grief healing (Todaro-Franceschi, 2006). Meaningful coincidences are purposeful changes—energy transformation—that emerge out of our wholeness; our oneness (Todaro-Franceschi, 1998, 1999). People who pay attention (to the changes occurring) can be directed in momentous ways to actualize their potential; in other words, the synchronicity is transformative!

For years I had a *Celestine Prophecy* poster in my office to remind me to pay attention to my moments (Redfield, 1993). I no longer need the reminder to pay attention to the synchronicity occurring in my life, although I do not always follow up as I should. A case in point was when my husband and I traveled to Maui for our 25th wedding anniversary. While there, we hiked to one of only a few red beaches in the world, Kaihalulu (Roaring Sea) or Red Sand Beach. It was a difficult hike, very hilly and slippery, and parts of the trail had drastically eroded

The trail wound through a very old cemetery, and many headstones had fallen below into the surf. It was very scenic and sad. As we rounded the last bend of this rugged trail, there was the most magnificent place—a bright red volcanic sand beach—contrasted against the turquoise blue ocean, with frothy white waves rolling into the shore. I immediately noted that there were only six other people there; one was a man who had carried his child there on his back in an infant carrier. He had passed us along the trail, obviously much more comfortable with the rough terrain than we were. As we waded in the ocean, awestruck by this glorious place, a newlywed couple approached us and asked us to take a picture of them. We spoke with them briefly. Imagine our surprise to find that we lived less than a mile from each other, in Brooklyn, New York! I would have pursued the meaning of this synchronicity; however, it was their honeymoon, after all, and it seemed intrusive to prolong our goodbyes. Still, I often wonder why we met when we did, for how unlikely was it that we had? It really is a small world; when synchronicity occurs like this, we realize that it is all one.

Have you ever had a day where everything went smoothly and things you did not expect happened to make it all come together in a profoundly good way? Belitz and Lundstrom (1997) referred to these synchronicity events as "being in the flow":

> In those times, we know we're in the right place at the right time doing the right thing. We feel both exhilarated and at peace, somehow connected to something larger and greater than ourselves. Life is rich with meaning, magic, and purpose. (p. xi)

When things *seem* to go wrong, I think perhaps it is synchronicity, too. There are messages in everything, if only we take the time to recognize and reflect upon them. Realizing that things are connected can lead us to make choices we would never have thought of making.

We Always Have a Choice in the Matter!

Even when we think we do not have any choice in the matter, we always do. Doing nothing is a choice, too! It is all one, and as such we are always participating, whether knowingly or unknowingly (Todaro-Franceschi, 1998, 1999). As nurse scholar and friend John Phillips always says, you cannot *not* participate! Recognition of choices can be enhanced by paying particular attention to what is going on in your moments and trying to keep track of them through such things as journaling or recording events and memories. Once you recognize the possible choices you have, then you can choose to take purposeful action to actualize some potentials rather than others. Always know that making a decision does not necessarily mean you cannot change your mind later. In fact, in most cases, you can easily change your mind and then make another choice. Of course, if you have carefully thought through your options and make a radical decision, it is unlikely you will want to go back and renege after the fact. What do I mean by radical decision? I mean a decision that results in a big change in your way of being in the world, and make no mistake, one that will transform other people's ways of being in the world, too.

A Radical Decision

I worked for a time in a small community hospital first as per diem nursing staff and then as a full-time clinical supervisor of the ICU and a medical–surgical unit with some dedicated telemetry beds. Dedicated telemetry beds in this hospital meant that we had portable units, which were hooked up to patients, and strips were obtained on a regular basis. It did not mean that they were actually being monitored; in fact, most of the nursing staff who worked there had not been taught how to read rhythm strips and were only required to print out strips and place them in the patient's chart.

It was a rough place to work because the nurses were not well respected by many of the physicians. It was one of those places that had what we call an "old boys' club," a group of physicians who considered nurses to be hand-maidens and little else. Even the top hospital administrator was one of those old boys. Naturally, staffing was a *big* problem. The hospital administration not only had a problem with bedside nurse retention, they also had difficulty keeping their nurse leaders. While I was working there, the director of nursing (DON) retired and the administration hired a new director. It immediately became apparent who buttered her bread. When she was not kissing up to her boss, she was "enforcing" rules and regulations.

One day, we had a code in the ICU, and there was only one regular staff member along with two per diem nurses on duty. It was already a terrible day in that unit. There were seven patients and every one of them should have been one-to-one assignments. Having a code made it all the more horrific, putting both the patients and the staff at risk. Of course, I went up to the unit to assist the other nurses; there was no way I was staying out of there. Shortly after I arrived and was up to my neck multitasking, I was called to the phone because the DON wanted to speak with me. As I listened agape, she proceeded to tell me that I was to—right now!—go around the hospital and count the number of wheelchairs that did not have safety belts. I simply informed her that "now" was not a good time for me to leave the unit, that there was a code going on and they were short-staffed, and then I quickly hung up the phone. That woman actually called back to yell at me! I was pretty disturbed by her behavior; I waited until things calmed down in the unit and then did what she asked.

Not too long after, I had another experience, which left me reeling yet again. I was the weekend administrator on duty, meaning that all emergencies over the course of the weekend had to come to me. I received a call from one of our ED nurses who was concerned about a new admission; he told me he wanted to give me "a heads up" that there might be a problem. The nurse proceeded to tell me that the patient came in with chest pain. He believed that the patient was experiencing a myocardial infarction (MI) and, although he had told the physician this, the physician on duty had insisted the patient be admitted to the telemetry unit. To this I responded, "We cannot do that"—but in fact, it had already been done. I immediately went to the telemetry unit and found this patient alone in a private room, with a portable telemetry monitor at his side. What good was that, I thought? One look at the patient told me that the ED nurse was correct and that we needed to quickly get this patient up to the ICU where he could be properly monitored and cared for.

I was upset with the physician who knew it was our hospital policy that all patients being ruled out for MI were to be directly admitted to the ICU. I notified him via phone that the patient would have to be moved. His response was to scream into the phone that I was "just a nurse" and that I had no right whatsoever to question him or to make any decisions regarding patient admissions. I had no choice but to call the chief of cardiology, who lived nearby. Before I could blink my eyes, it seemed, the chief had arrived to assess the patient. Of course, the patient had to be sent to the ICU and that meant the physician on call, who was already so irate, had to transfer one of the patients out of the ICU to make room for this new patient.

Later on in the day, when I was making rounds, I was confronted by the physician who asked me to step into the lounge area to speak privately. He proceeded to literally scream at me and swung his hands in my face. I was perceptibly shaken but determined to hold my ground. So I told him he had no right to speak to me like that and I walked away. I wrote up the incident and submitted it to our DON the following Monday.

Never hearing anything further about it from the DON, I assumed that it was being taken care of and that the physician would at least be reprimanded for his inappropriate behavior. Imagine my dismay and anger when I heard from one of the other clinical supervisors that the director was investigating the way I related to physicians, by asking the MDs whether my responses to them "were appropriate!" I went to a few of the nurses and physicians to confirm that this was indeed occurring and left work at the end of the day fuming. I sat down that evening, acknowledged that there was a problem, and made a list of my possible choices:

- I could go to work and act like nothing had happened (yeah, right).
- I could go to work and ask the director why she would choose to investigate one of her staff rather than support and advocate for her (and nothing would happen).
- I could take it over her head to the hospital administrator, who was an MD and had been in the position for years (and nothing would happen).
- I could quit the position.

So, what did I do? You guessed it; I quit. I am proud to say that I did it with real flare. I wrote my resignation, to be effective at 3 p.m. the next day. In it, I shared my concerns for a hospital administration that did not put the best interests of the patients first and foremost. Of course, I also shared my concerns for a workplace that did not sufficiently support its nursing staff and leaders.

The next morning I went in at 8 a.m., left the resignation letter for the director, who was not yet in her office, cleaned and packed up my office, and then made my rounds. While I did so, I informed everyone I would be out of there for good at the end of the day. I then spent the remainder of the day saying "hell no!" to physicians and staff alike who stopped by my office begging me to reconsider.

To leave that place the way I did was a radical decision and one I have never regretted, although I did lose my sick time and a few weeks of vacation pay because I did not give the mandatory 2-week notice. Some folks thought I cut my nose off to spite my face; I thought it was well worth it. I am a firm believer in the "take this job and shove it" mentality, when the job is putting you at risk. That job was putting me at risk for a lot of ugliness. Had I stayed, the ugly head of burnout would surely have surfaced eventually—and when I think about it, of all the possible ugly issues that could have surfaced, that might have been the prettiest of the bunch. Composing another list of the possible changes, depending upon making different choices, is helpful too. In this case, here are a few possibilities, had I chosen to stay there:

- Having units with inadequate staff could result in serious errors or omissions, causing more harm than good to the patients and as the covering supervisor I could be jeopardizing my RN license (e.g., if something were to happen to a patient as a result of being admitted to the wrong unit, I could be charged with negligence).
- Emotional, physical, and spiritual exhaustion (compassion fatigue and/or burnout) can lead to altered health status and serious, perhaps even life-threatening, illness.

At the end of the day, the job was not worth it!

If you are having difficulty recognizing the choices you have and you have no one to be a sounding board, you can try pulling up a chair and having a chat with yourself. In fact, even if you have others to talk with, occasionally it is helpful to just talk to yourself. Indeed, I do it often and consider it a sign of normalcy. Eric Maisel (2005), famed creativity coach, suggests pulling up two chairs and alternating your position, first being yourself and then being your coach. When you sit in the first chair you can be you, and when you sit in the second chair you become your own coach. In this way, you can coach yourself to make choices that will lead you toward a plan of action to reaffirm your purpose in nursing.

Step 3: Turning Outward Toward Self and Other

The third step, like the others, is meant to be ongoing and entails a *Turning outward toward self and other*. It is when one becomes aware that through reconnection, not only with self but also with other(s) (our loved ones, coworkers, and patients), we can remain content in our work and feel heartful. If we are compassion fatigued, reconnecting with ourselves and other(s) can help us to heal (the reconnect contention!).

Nurses are human beings taking care of human beings. We need to frequently remind ourselves of this as we go about our day-to-day work. Reiterating my earlier words, we are *not* robots. When discussing how to keep compassion fatigue at bay through the reconnect contention, I accentuate making time to see things you normally would not notice. We can use this practice in both our personal and professional lives. At the end of a work day, how often do we go home at night and barely notice our loved ones? The dog's tail is wagging as you walk through the door and you tell him to get out of your way. Your husband, wife, or children are trying to tell you things and you are completely zoning them out. Does this sound familiar?

In our work environment, oftentimes we lose sight of the person in the bed, so intent are we to do all the multitasking that needs to be done. Nurse Doris Hines (1992) noted that we should "enfold the skills and technologies within the relationship rather than performing the task according to safety requirements and as the main function of the time spent together" (p. 303). I regularly ask my fellow nurses, "What if, when we are with a patient, taking care of IVs, Foleys, and wounds, we make the focus the *patient*, rather than the things associated with the person? What if we encourage our patients to talk to us as we take care of the mundane day-to-day activities of nursing, the things we barely think about as we are doing them because they have become second nature to us?"

It is important to take time to *see* our patients, really see them. How often do we notice the color of a patient's hair or eyes? These are small things, perhaps, but nevertheless a beginning step in reconnecting with others. Our purpose as professional carers is to provide care, to heal, and we cannot do that effectively without forming some *connection* with those we care for every day. To remain disconnected only feeds the illusion that all things are separate. It is unrewarding to feel this way and over time can only generate a growing discontent with work and life in general.

It may be a human defense mechanism to distance oneself from painful experiences; however, to keep loving what we do in nursing, we need to remind ourselves time and again that we are *allowed to feel*; essentially, we need to get closer to others rather than put more distance between us. We need to *Turn outward*, toward ourselves and other(s), even when doing so means that we feel *more*, not less.

Nussbaum (1996) pointed out that:

Equipped with her general conception of human flourishing, the spectator looks at a world in which people suffer hunger, disability, disease, slavery, through no fault of their own or beyond their fault. In her pity she acknowledges that goods such as food, health, citizenship, freedom, do all matter. Yet she acknowledges, as well, that it is uncertain whether she herself will remain among the safe and privileged ones to whom such goods are stably guaranteed. She acknowledges that the lot of the poor might be (or become) hers. This leads her to *turn her thoughts outward* [italics mine], from her own current comfortable situation to the structure of society's allocation of goods and resources. For, given the uncertainty of life, she will be inclined to want a society in which the lot of the worst off—of the poor, of people defeated in war, of women, of servants—is as good as it can be. (p. 36)

Through our empathetic concern, we recognize that "I" is "we"—it is all one. Mindfully remaining aware of our "we-ness" can keep us loving what we do.

Healing our workforce must entail a reawakening of what Capra, Steindl-Rast, and Matus (1991) referred to as a sense of belonging to the universe. Studies on how spiritual experiences and practices can lead to a transformation of consciousness suggest that "altruism and compassion may arise as natural consequences of experiences of interconnectedness and one-ness" and that these transformational experiences "appear to lead to shifts in perspective and changes in one's sense of self and self in relationship to others" (Vieten, Amorok, & Schlitz, 2006, p. 915).

By encouraging experiences of connectedness and oneness, we may enhance our altruistic compassionate nature, which is integral to the nurse's authentic self. We do not have to accept compassion fatigue and/or burnout as the costs of caring; with intention, we can make choices that help us to reaffirm our purpose and actively sidestep feeling dissatisfied and disenchanted with our work.

Eckhart Tolle (2005) wrote that all of us have both an inner purpose and an outer purpose. Our inner purpose is for each of us to awaken; it is a collective purpose for all human beings: "Your inner purpose is an essential part of the purpose of the whole, the universe and its emerging intelligence" (p. 258). To awaken means to become aware of the connectedness–oneness. It means to be able to rid oneself of the ego or what he refers to as the "illusory self" (p. 27), along with the corresponding idea that we are separate from everything else. With true awakening, we can perceive the patterns of the whole and the words "I," "me," "my," and so forth, disappear, and in their stead it is "we" and "us." On the other hand, each of us has an outer purpose that is unique—it varies from one person to another and it is fluid—it changes over time.

When both our inner purpose and outer purpose are in alignment, we are in a state of "awakened doing," which essentially means our acts are more closely in tune with the purposeful actions of the universe (Tolle, p. 294). Tolle (2005) suggests that we can purposefully do "awakened doing" through the use of three modalities: (a) acceptance, (b) joy, and (c) enthusiasm (p. 295). Each of these modalities is appropriate at different times and all of them can help us tap into what he calls "the creative power of the universe" (p. 295).

APPLYING *ART* FOR COMPASSION CONTENTMENT

Having considered the positive aspect of professional quality of life—compassion contentment—in previous chapters, we can take the *ART* model (Todaro-Franceschi, 2008, 2013, 2015) and apply it to hold and augment a sense of heartfulness. When you use *ART* to enhance compassion contentment, you are, in essence, doing an appreciative inquiry or self-interview. Appreciative inquiry is a means to mindfully identify the positive aspects of our lives so that as we move through life we can repeatedly experience and appreciate what brings us joy and happiness (also see Chapter 13).

Try the following:

- *Acknowledge* a good feeling from an experience you had at work, something that made you feel glad to be a nurse. What did you choose to do that day that made it all seem worthwhile and that had you leaving at the end of the day feeling content about your day's work? Did you look forward to going to work the following day? Acknowledge how good you felt while you were in a specific moment. What were you doing and how did you feel while doing it? Jot down the things that contributed to your good feeling.

- *Recognize* that one always has choices and then choose appropriate actions to reaffirm purpose. Going back to that good day at work, can you identify the choices you made that contributed to the day turning out the way it did? Is having a good moment or day an anomaly in your work life? If so, why? What are the obstacles? What can you *do* to make it a regular happening? What did you choose to do that day that made it all seem worthwhile? Can you make the same or similar choices today? If not, why not? If so, what is preventing you right now, this moment, from doing it?
- *Turn* outward toward yourself and other. Can you take the positive experience you had and reproduce it? Were you able to connect with your patients, loved ones, and coworkers? Grasp your sense of well-being from that time. Reconnect with those feelings.

Hopefully, as you read and work on each of these steps, they will encourage you to be present with *yourself* and to be aware of your connection to others. *Combined ART can be thought of as awakening.*

TURNING POINTS EXERCISE: LOOKING BACKWARD TO LOOK FORWARD

When applying *ART*, you focus on awareness of turning points, connection to others (and the environment), and one's place (individually and collectively) in the unfolding present.

Find a quiet place, a pen and paper, and about 15 minutes of "me" time. Sit and reflect upon your career. Did my story of applying for a job at Macy's resonate with you? Has there been a time when you seriously considered leaving nursing? What about right now? When you first entered the profession of nursing, what goals did you have? What did you think you would be doing? Are you doing it? Have you met your goals? Have your goals changed? Make a list as shown in Table 5.1.

The goal is to get clarity about what your priorities are and then act on them. While many of us feel we have no choice, remember, we always do. It is a matter of being able to recognize what choices we have and which ones are more important for each of us at particular points in time. What are your priorities? Through mindful awareness of what is going on right now, in this moment, you can discover your options and act accordingly.

Table 5.1 Career Goals

Goals	Met	Not Met
1. _____	___	___
2. _____	___	___
3. _____	___	___
4. _____	___	___

If you have not met the goals that you previously set for yourself, you will need to explore the reason(s) why. The following chapters help you to get further clarity (see Chapters 12 and 13 for more on mindfulness).

KEY POINTS

- *ART* is a healing model composed of three steps designed to help address professional quality of life issues: (a) *Acknowledgment* of a feeling or problem; (b) *Recognition* of the possible choices one has and then choosing which actions to take to reaffirm purpose in one's work life; and (c) *Turning* outward toward self and other. This Is done by making a conscious effort to reconnect with oneself and others (aka, the "reconnect contention").

- *ART* is ongoing and steps may overlap. The key is to be mindfully aware of our moments and actions.

- With intention we can find meaning in our work and be heartful (at least most of the time!).

REFERENCES

Belitz, C., & Lundstrom, M. (1997). *The power of flow: Practical ways to transform your life with meaningful coincidence.* New York, NY: Harmony Books.

Capra, F., Steindl-Rast, D., & Matus, T. (1991). *Belonging to the universe: Explorations on the frontiers of science and spirituality.* San Francisco, CA: Harper & Row.

Dalai Lama & Cutler, H. C. (1998). *The art of happiness: A handbook for living.* New York, NY: Riverhead Books.

Hines, D. R. (1992). Presence: Discovering the artistry in relating. *Journal of Holistic Nursing, 10*(4), 294–305. doi:10.1177/089801019201000403

Jung, C. (1973). *Synchronicity: An acausal connecting principle* (R. F. C. Hull, Trans.). Princeton, NJ: Princeton University Press.

Kabat-Zinn, J. (1994). *Wherever you go, there you are: Mindfulness meditation in everyday life.* New York, NY: Hyperion.

Keith, K. M. (2003). *Do it anyway: The handbook for finding personal meaning and deep happiness in a crazy world*. Maui, HI: Inner Ocean.

Ko-i Bastis, M. (2000). *Peaceful dwelling: Meditations for healing and living*. Boston, MA: Tuttle Publishing.

Maisel, E. (2005). *Coaching the artist within*. Novato, CA: New World Library.

Millman, D. (2000). *Living on purpose: Straight answers to life's tough questions*. Novato, CA: New World Library.

Murphy, F., Jones, S., Edwards, M., James, J., & Mayer, A. (2009). The impact of nurse education on the caring behaviours of nursing students. *Nurse Education Today, 29*, 254–264. doi:10.1016/j.nedt.2008.08.016

Nussbaum, M. (1996). Compassion: The basic social emotion. *Social Philosophy and Policy, 13*, 27–58. doi:10.1017/s0265052500001515

Peat, F. D. (1987). *Synchronicity: The bridge between matter and mind*. New York, NY: Bantam.

Redfield, J. (1993). *The Celestine prophecy: An adventure*. New York, NY: Warner Books.

Thoreau, H. D. (1854/1995). *Walden, or, life in the woods*. Mineola, NY: Dover.

Todaro-Franceschi, V. (1998). *The enigma of energy: A philosophical inquiry*. Doctoral dissertation, New York University (UMI No. 9819881).

Todaro-Franceschi, V. (1999). *The enigma of energy: Where science and religion converge*. New York, NY: Crossroad.

Todaro-Franceschi, V. (2006). Synchronicity related to dead loved ones: A natural healing modality. *Spirituality and Health International, 7*, 151–161. doi:10.1002/shi.257

Todaro-Franceschi, V. (2008). Preventing compassion fatigue and reaffirming purpose in nursing. *Proceedings on the 3rd European Federation of Critical Care Nursing Congress and 27th Aniarti Conference, Influencing Critical Care Nursing in Europe*, Florence, Italy (October).

Todaro-Franceschi, V. (2013). *Compassion fatigue and burnout in nursing: Enhancing professional quality of life*. New York, NY: Springer Publishing.

Todaro-Franceschi, V. (2015). The ART of maintaining the "care" in healthcare. *Nursing Management, 46*(6), 53–55. doi:10.1097/01.numa.0000465407.76450.ab

Tolle, E. (2005). *A new earth: Awakening to your life's purpose*. New York, NY: A Plume Book.

Vieten, C., Amorok, T., & Schlitz, M. M. (2006). I to we: The role of consciousness transformation in compassion and altruism. *Zygon, 41*(4), 915–931. doi:10.1111/j.1467-9744.2006.00788.x

Watson, J. (2008). Caring science: Belonging before being as ethical cosmology. *Nursing Science Quarterly, 18*, 304–305. doi:10.1177/0894318405280395

Woolf, V. (1922, February 17). *Diary*. Retrieved from http://www.readprint.com/author-91/Virginia-Woolf-books

III

The Bad: Compassion Fatigue and Moral Distress

There can be no transforming of darkness into light and of apathy into movement without emotion.

—Carl G. Jung

6

Compassion Fatigue: A Heavy Heart Hurts

Heavy hearts, like heavy clouds in the sky, are best relieved by the letting of a little water.

—Antoine Rivarol

KEY TOPICS

- Compassion fatigue
- Primary and secondary trauma
- Substance abuse

INTRODUCTION

The very same qualities that make us excel as carers also put us at risk for compassion fatigue. Fundamentally, being compassionate and feeling compelled to care sets us up to be hurt.

While I was writing the first edition of this book, I attended a conference sponsored by the National Institute of Nursing Research, where a number of brilliant people gathered together to explore where we have been and where we are going with palliative and end-of-life care. The title of the conference, coincidentally, was "The Science of Compassion." The kickoff for this summit was a town hall discussion on ethical issues in end-of-life care. The topic turned to the vulnerability of people who are

© Springer Publishing Company DOI: 10.1891/9780826155214.0006

dying; however, it became glaringly apparent during the discussion that in designating some people as more or less vulnerable, we might be doing a disservice to some or all. Who is it that decides who is vulnerable and who is not? The bottom line is that all people are vulnerable at different points in their lives, and that, of course, includes us nurses. Our recognition of human vulnerability is in large part the basis of compassionate caring and is also the source of compassion fatigue.

DEFINING COMPASSION FATIGUE

Compassion fatigue is a syndrome that carers may develop when they internalize pain or anguish related to other people in their work environment. As noted earlier, the term *compassion fatigue* is ambiguous and is often used interchangeably with secondary traumatic stress (STS) and, on occasion, vicarious trauma.[1] It is sometimes referred to as a lesser (or unique) form of burnout.

Some of the most inclusive work on the subject has been written by trauma study pioneer Charles Figley (1995, 2002a, 2002b), who thinks that compassion fatigue is a more user-friendly term than STS, which is closely aligned with posttraumatic stress disorder (PTSD).[2] He believes that the modern-day description of this syndrome is equivalent to his early depiction of secondary victimization as well as the similar concept of "emotional contagion."[3] Basically, when carers become preoccupied with another's experience (of being traumatized), we, too, are traumatized (Figley, 1995, 2002b).

Figley (2002a) also describes compassion fatigue as a chronic lack of self-care, and this definition is in keeping with Joinson's (1992) portrayal of compassion fatigue. It has been said that the most basic thing nurses provide in the delivery of care to others is ourselves, and unless we can find ways to continuously renew ourselves from the drain associated with our nursing practice, we will not only lose energy but also enthusiasm for our work (Joinson, 1992). What is always implicit in any description of the syndrome is that those who develop compassion fatigue are, on some level, internalizing pain and suffering from their relationship with others in the workplace, usually cosuffering with another human being, and it is manifesting itself in harmful ways on a multidimensional level. If it is not recognized and tended to, it can spiral out of control and may eventually result in burnout (Benson & Magraith, 2005; Figley, 2002b).

Who Is at Risk?

Nurses who work in areas where patients usually do not return to a previous level of wellness are especially at risk of compassion fatigue; however, it is important to realize that we bear witness to suffering in all areas of healthcare. Palliative care nurse pioneers Betty Ferrell and Nessa Coyle (2008) emphasized this in a book on the nature of suffering and the goals of nursing. Suffering is part of the human condition, and while we each may be able to describe some universal idea of what it means to suffer, the lived experience of suffering is unique for every person. Consequently, none of us can ever assume that suffering is or is not taking place; we need to look deeper than the surface.

People with chronic, and what are referred to as life-limiting illnesses, as well as acute, life-threatening illnesses, are often treated aggressively, and treatments can result in additional suffering for them and their loved ones. Their suffering is a part of the nurse's daily work, and whether or not the nurse acknowledges it, he or she internalizes at least some of the anguish. Even a seemingly benign task such as obtaining bed scale weights might be quite traumatic for both the cared for and the carer. And, while I may still shudder to recall those bed scale weight days in the ICU (and really I do!), other coworkers may not; such is the uniqueness of human beings.

Since what is traumatic to one person may not be to another, it is imperative to recognize the possibility that someone might be traumatized, even when we think not. It is also important to explore what the term *trauma* implies to you. You may realize that some of the experiences you have had were very traumatic, although at the time you did not realize it (see also Chapter 11).

BUTTERFLY POWER: SUBTLE INFLUENCES AND BEING TRAUMATIZED

Traumatic stressors are described as those things that might contribute to the development of the syndromes of compassion fatigue and burnout, and they can be primary or secondary in nature (Stamm, 2002, 2010). Primary trauma can be anything that directly affects us. In the workplace, experiences such as getting hit on the job or being browbeaten (mentally abused) or bullied by colleagues and/or management count as primary trauma, whereas witnessing the suffering of others is considered secondary trauma.

Repeated or prolonged exposure to trauma that is relational in nature can lead to the sudden occurrence of compassion fatigue. This is similar to that night I broke down in tears and could not take one more night of caring for John, or that WHAM! I experienced years ago, when I woke up one day and abruptly realized I no longer looked forward to going to work.

Not too long ago, while speaking with some nurse colleagues, I was surprised to find out that a few of them did not consider working with people who are in the ICU to be a source of trauma. This goes back to the point about our unique perceptions of who may or may not be vulnerable and what may or may not be traumatic. It is also indicative of the continuing lack of knowledge related to the syndromes of compassion fatigue and burnout. Not being able to recognize and understand what might contribute to these syndromes puts everyone at a disadvantage.

It has been noted that, "All of us who attempt to heal the wounds of others will ourselves be wounded; it is, after all, inherent in the relationship" (Hilfiker, 1985, p. 207). How is it that some nurses might not think that working with ill people is at all traumatizing? Perhaps it is for the very same reason that many of us in healthcare continue to use terms like "passed away" or "expired" instead of "dead" or "died." Technologizing or dehumanizing suffering makes it commonplace and distant rather than up front and center. After all, it is our job to provide care *no matter what*, to get all the medications in, to chart everything, to change the dressings, and so forth; never mind that we are walking in and out of rooms full of people who are scared and deathly ill.

There are a lot of things in the profession of nursing that can contribute to the development of compassion fatigue; basically, anything that results in one's *heart feeling heavy*. Some of the contributors may be overt, while others are more covert or subtle. Briggs and Peat (1999), in their discussion on "butterfly power," describe how small subtle changes can transform things on a large scale. In relation to compassion fatigue and burnout, it is the *negative* subtle influences that occur in many systems that are a cause for concern.[4] They note that people may consciously conform to the traditional or expected workings within a system and automatically go along with the norm in order to survive. This kind of process is composed of a negative feedback loop—the same behavior pattern is exhibited over and over again. Unfortunately, the healthcare system has many such negative subtle influences and some not-so-subtle influences, too. Take, for instance, the story of a nurse who was at the top of her class upon graduation. She was hired to work on an oncology unit in a major teaching hospital renowned for excellent care. Having taken a course on death, dying, and bereavement, she felt she had something to offer this particular population of patients and was extremely happy with her first position working as a nurse. The following was shared with me shortly after she began to work on the unit:

> *Reality has officially set in and it bothers me so much. I want to sit with my patients, hold their hands, cry with them, and provide them with true presence, but my preceptor is always rushing me out of the room, saying I have too many things to do. I know she is right, but I feel so awful at times. I am fortunate in that every single patient thus far has opened up to me in so many ways, and many have cried to me, telling me things that*

they have not told other nurses on the unit. I feel so honored to have their trust and feel that I am violating my relationship with them because of my workload. My unit is one step below an ICU and I have six patients minimum every shift. I try hard but find myself going home sad many nights. It got to the point where I was waking up the last couple of weeks and telling myself how much I dislike that unit, and your words came into my mind: "When you wake up feeling like you hate your job, it's time to go."

The nurses on this unit are extremely competent, but I have seen compassion displayed by only two other nurses, who are both coincidentally leaving next week. I have stayed there because I know that I am making a difference, no matter how small, and I see the look in many of my patients' eyes when I go in to say good-bye to them at the end of my shift and when they ask me if I will come back the following day to be their nurse.

I'm trying the techniques that you taught me, such as talking to them as I give them their medications, holding their hands as I take their pulse; I cover them when they seem cold; I lower myself at eye-to-eye level to let them know I am truly listening, and I thank you so much for teaching me those skills in our class on death and dying . . . . I have spoken of you many times on my unit. I have even considered suggesting that you be brought in to show these nurses the things that you showed us, because most of the nurses are burnt out and provide no compassion whatsoever.

I love nursing, so please do not misunderstand my comments. I just need to find my own style of providing the care that my patients require without losing the three essential components that are important in nursing: compassion, caring, and commitment to my patients.

Each time a nurse shares a story such as this, I want to cry for all of us. How is it possible that some nurses have allowed themselves to harden so much?

Obviously, the harried environment of this unit did not support the new nurse's conception of what it meant to provide quality care to her patients. Despite this, she managed to withstand the negative subtle influences of her work environment and eventually made a choice to move to another place of employment rather than join in on the negative feedback loop to become one of the automated, seemingly uncaring nurses on that particular unit.

Both primary and secondary traumas are exemplified in this new nurse's situation. Secondary trauma is evidenced by her identifying with the suffering of her patients; however, she felt gifted to bear witness to that suffering. She knew that by doing so, she was doing something good for her patients and also herself. This is a buffer, really, for her acknowledgment of the contribution she was making helped to sustain her sense of purpose. At the same time, the unit pace and the other nurses working with her were not supportive and did not value her conception of what it meant to be a "good nurse."

Primary trauma arose from her frequently being the butt of negative commentary, such as being told she was too slow and not cut out for this work. She regularly overheard the staff talking about her, saying unpleasant and, on occasion, even racist things. This distressed her even more; unfortunately, her story is *not* an oddity in nursing (see Chapter 9 for further discussion).

Joinson (1992) noted that compassion fatigue can emerge in relation to how we are providing care for others, but she also emphasized that our coworkers can contribute to its development. She wrote, "When the people around you are tense, impatient, and hurried, you may be swept into the same reactions. Nurses who are tired, indifferent or cynical, can sap your own energy and enthusiasm" (p. 118). Notably, Joinson was alluding to the precursor for what we refer to in current day as bullying or incivility in the workplace; it is the indifferent and/or cynical nurse who treats coworkers, and on occasion, patients and their loved ones, with a lack of respect. Some, if not the majority, of these bullying nurses are probably themselves suffering from burnout. I return to this topic in Chapter 9.

Death Overload

Where nurses work can contribute to the development of compassion fatigue. In areas where there is a higher incidence of dying and death, suffering is more visible, and, thus, larger numbers of nurses are at risk. *Death overload*, a term used to denote having experienced the death of too many patients in a short period or having worked with a patient for too long a time prior to the person dying, is also a form of traumatic stress (Vachon, 1993). Critical care, trauma, and ED nurses and those working in oncology and palliative care are more apt to experience death overload. My firsthand experiences working in many of these areas and my years of teaching nurses prompt me to say, with some conviction, that the most troubling thing for a great number of nurses who work in these areas is to *face death* (and the suffering that often accompanies it). By this I mean not only us having to face the patient but also the family members of those patients who are dying.

There is some evidence to show that many individuals who provide care that they believe to be medically futile (care that will not lead to eventual cure or a better quality of life) develop compassion fatigue and burnout. For instance, Meltzer and Huckabay (2004) studied 60 critical care nurses' perceptions of futile care and their effect on the development of burnout. They found a positive correlation between the critical care nurses' emotional exhaustion scores and morally distressful situations where the care provided was considered to be medically futile. I return to this topic in further depth in Chapter 10.

MANIFESTATIONS OF COMPASSION FATIGUE

Signs and symptoms of compassion fatigue are abundant and highly individualized, but for the most part, they usually go unnoticed by those who are experiencing the phenomenon (see Exhibit 6.1). Because compassion fatigue is also considered to arise from cosuffering, we would do well to recall the manifestations of suffering, noting that it is existential and encompasses the entire being. A common response *to* suffering *is* suffering.

EXHIBIT 6.1 Some Typical Signs of Compassion Fatigue (and Burnout)

Behavior Changes
Inability to maintain balance of empathy and objectivity
Depression
Anger
Blaming
Irritability
Chronic lateness
Overworking
Exaggerated startle response (see Ch. 11 on PTSD)
Difficulty focusing or concentrating
Substance abuse
Eating disturbances
Disrupted sleep patterns
Avoiding or dreading work
Calling out sick more often
Feelings
Heart heavy (compassion fatigue)
Diminished sense of personal accomplishment
Decreased sense of purpose
Less able to feel joy or happiness
Low self-esteem
High self-expectations
Helplessness and hopelessness

(continued)

EXHIBIT 6.1 Some Typical Signs of Compassion Fatigue
(and Burnout) (*continued*)

Numbness
Empty-hearted (burnout)
Disinterested and detached (burnout)
Disillusioned
Apathy (burnout)
Physical Changes
Chronic fatigue
Exhaustion (physical, emotional, or both)
Frequent headaches
Gastrointestinal complaints
Hypertension
Cardiac symptoms such as chest pain or tachycardia
Sleep disturbances
Muscle tension, aches, and pains
Frequent or lingering illness
Difficulty focusing
Anxiety

We have no real way of knowing how our own health is transformed by the occurrence of compassion fatigue, for as nurse Brenda Sabo (2006) noted, there has been little focus on how our nursing work may be changing our health status. In fact, all the seminal research that has been done on health status using nurses as participants could not possibly have taken this piece of the *whole* into consideration, making those research findings a bit skewed. Going back to that new nurse: She has type 1 diabetes. During her time on that unit, she suffered frequent episodes of severe hypoglycemia along with loss of appetite and difficulty sleeping, in addition to the terrible emotional upheaval she experienced. Her life was literally being threatened by her work. So in answer to the question, "Can we accurately capture the consequences of caring work?" (Sabo, 2006, p. 136), it becomes clear that we cannot. The whole is far too complex and each case is highly individualized.

The list in Exhibit 6.1 is not meant to be all-inclusive. Realize too that not all of the signs and symptoms have to be evident for one to be suffering from compassion fatigue, and there is also significant overlap with the symptoms of burnout. I touch upon a few of the signs of compassion fatigue in greater depth here; others have been or are discussed in other places. Again, I am really trying to emphasize the *whole*.

Turning Away

We are dealing with a national public health epidemic—an opioid crisis of great magnitude. Large numbers of people are dying from drug overdose every single day. It is generally estimated that the incidence of substance use disorder (SUD) in nursing mirrors national levels of 10% to 15% of the population (Clark & Farnsworth, 2006; Kunyk, 2015; NCSBN, 2011), although some research suggests that it might be a bit lower or higher (Monroe, Kenaga, Dietrich, Carter, & Cowan, 2013; Ramer, 2008). Thus, the American Nurses Association (ANA) has noted that, on average, one out of every 10 nurses is dealing with substance use and a fair number of those nurses are probably not aware that they have a problem. Compound this issue with the fact that substance abuse is likely to impair work performance, which for us means that nurses may be placing people in danger. No dedicated nurse would knowingly choose to do that!

In one study, oncology nurses were found to have a higher incidence of substance abuse than other specialty groups (Trinkoff & Storr, 1998), which, when looked at from the perspective of compassion fatigue, does seem to make sense. Patients with cancer often suffer from both the disease and the treatments. Nurses who work in oncology are frequently providing care while wondering why the treatments are being continued; or they may be stopping care while wondering why it is not being continued. There is a lot to "cosuffer with" in oncology.

Substance abuse and eating disturbances, when they occur in relation to some experience or event, are considered a form of self-medicating. I consider them an indication of how people often turn *away from*, rather than turn *toward*, something. The something we need to turn toward is ourselves; we need to reconnect with or confront whatever is bothering us before the destructive behaviors harm us. We need to go to the places that scare us. This is easier said than done. Indeed, it can be very difficult to recognize that there is a problem and to face it head on.

A general rule of thumb is, if you are drinking or taking medication as a way to relax or de-stress on a regular basis, or if you turn to food, you are self-medicating and abusing the drug or overindulging in food. If you find that you cannot go without a drink or a drug, then there is a possibility that you are psychologically, if not physically, already dependent on it. If your loved ones have voiced concern over your drinking or drug habits, that is also a clue that you need to evaluate your behavior.

I once worked on a unit where quite a few of the staff were abusing alcohol; back then I did not realize it, but looking back I can see where, if things had not changed, I might have developed a problem myself. Many of the folks who were on the night shift would stop on the way home for wine coolers and/or beer. I recall that, on occasion, when I got home from a particularly difficult night I would go and sit in the garden drinking a wine cooler at 9 in the morning to unwind because I could not sleep. Did I know it was a step *away* from what I needed to be doing for myself? No. I was probably very fortunate that we had to relocate while I was still working at that particular place. I am not sure I would have been able to recognize that there was a problem endemic to the unit I was working on at the time. Eventually I left the night tour and went to work part time on the evening shift, where things were a bit less chaotic for me. Here again, looking back can help you look forward and see things more clearly. These days I easily recognize signs of trouble and I am hoping that some of you, while reading this, have an AHA! moment, too.

One of the biggest problems with individuals who are abusing drugs or alcohol is that they do not recognize they have a problem before it gets out of control. If you are leaning on a bottle (of alcohol or pills or some other form of drug), or maybe you are leaning on too many Twinkies, you have choices that you can make to work on healing. You can choose to speak with your healthcare provider about it and/or also seek help from your employee assistance program (EAP). You need not worry about confidentiality; you are protected and there is no stigma associated with seeking help for addictive behaviors. Nurses are people, too (although it might not seem like this is so, it is a mandate that all employers have an EAP). Today, employers realize that it is far more cost-effective to help impaired nurses rehabilitate rather than lose them entirely. You can also check with your state board of nursing; many of them now offer alternative-to-discipline (ATD) programs for nurses with SUD (Strobbe & Crowley, 2017).[5]

A related issue in healthcare workplaces that has not been given much attention is the associated trauma to nurses who are working with those who they know to be substance abusers. They may become morally distressed because, on the one hand, these nurses are compelled to report their concerns, knowing that it is a matter of legal and ethical obligation to do so. At the same time, they cosuffer with their coworker, and can easily become compassion fatigued.

In bearing witness to or discovering drug diversion by a coworker, nurses often feel anger, betrayal, and grief (Ramer, 2008). It is important for them to seek assistance themselves—to turn toward, and acknowledge, the problem rather than turn away from it. Needless to say, the way nurse leaders support, or conversely, do not support, the nurses on units where drug diversion has been discovered can make or break the sense of communality among staff, which in turn affects overall retention and productivity. If not adequately supported, collective wounds will fester and the environment can become toxic, but with compassionate leadership, healing will occur (see also Chapter 11).

If you are abusing substances and become addicted, or know of a nurse who is, supportive programs such as Alcoholics Anonymous, Narcotics Anonymous, and Overeaters Anonymous are tried-and-true programs with much success. In most states, there are now programs for impaired nurses, which may be called peer assistance or diversion programs. In all cases, nurses are assisted in regaining their former lives. (Please see Appendix C, Resources, for further information.)

CAN COMPASSION FATIGUE BE EVADED?

In earlier chapters, I stressed the importance of compassion—as both a virtue and excellence in nursing. Here and there I have emphasized that we do not have to accept compassion fatigue as a consequence of caring work. We can take steps to alleviate it and also sometimes prevent it. For each of us it is a matter of finding the appropriate balance.

Perry (2008) highlighted reasons why exemplary oncology nurses seem to avoid compassion fatigue (p. 87). In one study she identified seven nurses whose practice was considered exemplary by their coworkers. Four of the nurses worked on a palliative care unit; the others worked in hospice or oncology. She engaged in conversations with each of the participants on the subject of compassion fatigue, after which she analyzed the transcripts for shared themes.

The seven nurses shared three main characteristics in their practice, which I noted in an earlier chapter: moments of connection, making moments matter, and energizing moments (Perry, 2008). All of these themes resonate with ideas of peak experiences, flow, second wind, and, in general, self-actualization. All are contingent on our ability to connect with self and other and on our ability to compassionately care. When we remain true to our authentic caring nature as we go about our practice—when we keep first and foremost in our hearts and minds the meaning and purpose of our work—it can help us to recognize and heal from, as well as avert, compassion fatigue.

APPLYING *ART* FOR COMPASSION FATIGUE

If you are suffering from compassion fatigue, being mindfully aware of your actions as you go about doing things in your day-to-day activities can help to heal your wounds. Does any of the preceding resonate with you?

Having picked up this book, it is likely that you do recognize there is a problem somewhere, so the hardest step has been taken already; now it is a matter of making choices that turn you back on the path to happiness and well-being. You are already applying the *ART* model (Todaro-Franceschi, 2008, 2013, 2015) here!

Step 1: Acknowledge Feelings (or a Wound That Needs Healing)

Bearing witness to one's own feelings, especially suffering, is difficult but necessary in order to enhance professional quality of life and heal from compassion fatigue. How do you feel when you are going into work? Are you looking forward to work or are you dreading it? Do you feel tired? Review the signs and symptoms in Exhibit 6.1. Complete the secondary traumatic stress/compassion fatigue part of Stamm's (2010) ProQOL tool in Appendix A. Remember, all of this is meant as a guide to help you become more aware of your situation and whether there is a problem. It is not meant to be diagnostic but rather is a contemplative exercise.

Look *toward yourself* as you go about your day. Note how you act with others and how you react to others. Pay attention to what might be irritating or upsetting you over the course of your work day. Reflect on your moments while you are living them. Jot things down as you become aware of them.

If you have identified that you are compassion fatigued, you need to explore possible turning points and try to establish what factors in your work may have contributed to it. Looking back, can you recognize when you began to feel the way you are feeling? Depending on your circumstances, there may be more than one thing that you need to address. Once you are aware of the contributing factors, you can begin the second step.

Step 2: *Recognize Choices and Take Purposeful Action*

Depending upon your unique situation, there are any number of choices and actions that can be taken. It might take some time to identify all of them. I personally like list-making when I have problems that need to be solved. I will frequently share my list of choices with a friend or loved one, and sometimes that fresh pair of eyes will come up with a novel approach to the problem. Give yourself some time with this because, at the end of it all, you are really aiming to reaffirm purpose in your life (since work is such a big part of it!) and that is no small task. You never need to settle for anything that is making you feel compassion fatigued. Remember, it is *your* choice! To give an example, maybe you have witnessed too many patient deaths in the past few months. Think about your own situation. Writing down or sharing with others any sustaining memories you might have of experiences with dying and death can be helpful for healing.

Here are some suggestions of choices you can make (not meant to be all-inclusive):

- You can request critical incident stress debriefing.
- You can schedule some vacation time.
- You can see a grief counselor.
- You can seek employee assistance.
- You can request a transfer to a different area where dying and death occur less frequently.

Since there are so many things that might contribute to compassion fatigue, there will be lots of choices and purposeful actions that only you can identify, given your unique situation. Once you have figured out what choices you have depending upon your circumstances, you are ready to take action to begin to heal and to reaffirm purpose.

Step 3: *Turn Outward Toward Self and Other*

Stepping outside of yourself, turn toward yourself; look objectively at how you are caring for yourself. Do you make time for the important things? What *are* the important things for you? Consider your general health status, along with eating, sleeping, and maybe substance abuse patterns.

How are you interacting with others? Are you able to connect with your patients, loved ones, and coworkers? Seek support from friends and family—connect with them, talk about your feelings.

Some of the things you can do to reconnect with your own needs and with others include participating in meditation and yoga, attending specialized retreats and in-service education programs, and using employee assistance support services. (See Appendix C, Resources, for additional information.) Turn toward the things that make you smile—both little and big. It could be family, friends, pets, nature—a butterfly! Or if you prefer, music, art, a good book, a good movie; make time for the fun things.

Once you are on the path to healing you, can try to prevent the reoccurrence (or minimize the occurrence) of compassion fatigue through mindful awareness. Pay attention to how you are living. One of the greatest gifts in my life was getting (and obviously surviving!) cancer—it continues to remind me how important it is to live each moment well. Journaling can be a very effective way to stay mindfully aware of our moments. Make some "me" time at the end of each day to jot down your thoughts, emotions, and any meaningful events that occurred. Make sure to note your feelings—the most potent indicator of when things might be off . . . or on!

KEY POINTS

- Compassion fatigue is a syndrome that occurs suddenly in response to a distressing or traumatic experience. It is relational in nature in that the compassion fatigued individual is usually cosuffering with or internalizing the pain and anguish related to another.

- Trauma can be primary or secondary in nature; primary trauma is direct; for example, being mentally or physically hurt. Secondary trauma is when a person bears witness to another's suffering. What is and is not considered traumatic is highly individualized.

- Nurses are especially vulnerable to developing compassion fatigue because we are continually bearing witness to the suffering of others.

- The classic indication that one is experiencing compassion fatigue is feeling heart heavy and overburdened while continuing to do the work.

- Remaining connected to ourselves and our patients—being true to our authentic caring nature as nurses and remaining cognizant of the meaning and purpose of our work—can help to avert compassion fatigue.

- *ART* offers a framework to facilitate healing from compassion fatigue and may be helpful in thwarting its occurrence.

NOTES

1. Vicarious trauma refers to a cumulative effect of witnessing the suffering of those who are traumatized, resulting in transformative changes in the carer; it is frequently noted to involve a loss of spiritual connection—feelings of hopelessness or helplessness.
2. PTSD results from being the recipient of and/or witnessing someone else experiencing primary trauma.
3. Emotional contagion refers to the idea that someone may "catch" and feel the emotions of another, similar to how one might "catch" a cold. In this manner, the emotions of individuals and groups of people can spread to others.
4. Negative subtle influences are referred to as active collusion functioning within automatisms (Briggs & Peat, 1999).
5. The Emergency Nurses Association (ENA) and the International Nurses Society on Addictions (IntNSA) (Strobbe & Crowley, 2017) have issued a joint position statement, which has also been endorsed by the ANA. In it they address issues related to substance use not only

among nurses but also nursing students. Emphasizing that SUD is a chronic illness that can be successfully treated, the ENA/IntNSA position statement outlines the responsibilities of nurses, nursing students, nursing schools, and workplaces. The position statement calls for more education, establishment of policies and procedures, as well as adoption of ATD approaches for the treatment of nurses and nursing students with SUD.

REFERENCES

Benson, J., & Magraith, K. (2005). Compassion fatigue and burnout: The role of Balint groups. *Australian Family Physician, 34*(6), 497–498.

Briggs, J., & Peat, D. (1999). *Seven life lessons of chaos: Spiritual wisdom from the science of change.* New York, NY: HarperCollins.

Clark, C., & Farnsworth, J. (2006). Program for recovering nurses: An evaluation. *Medsurg Nursing, 15*(4), 223–224.

Ferrell, B., & Coyle, N. (2008). *The nature of suffering and the goals of nursing.* New York, NY: Oxford University Press.

Figley, C. R. (1995). *Compassion fatigue: Coping with secondary traumatic stress disorder in those who treat the traumatized.* New York, NY: Brunner Mazel.

Figley, C. R. (2002a). Compassion fatigue: Psychotherapists' chronic lack of self care. *Journal of Clinical Psychology, 58*(11), 1433–1441. doi:10.1002/jclp.10090

Figley, C. R. (Ed.). (2002b). *Treating compassion fatigue.* New York, NY: Brunner-Routledge.

Hilfiker, D. (1985). *Healing the wounds: A physician looks at his work.* New York, NY: Pantheon Books.

Joinson, C. (1992). Coping with compassion fatigue. *Nursing, 22,* 116–121. doi:10.1097/00152193-199204000-00035

Kunyk, D. (2015). Substance use disorders among registered nurses: Prevalence, risks, and perceptions in a disciplinary jurisdiction. *Journal of Nursing Management, 23*(1), 54–64. doi:10.1111/jonm.12081

Meltzer, L. S., & Huckabay, L. M. (2004). Critical care nurses' perceptions of futile care and its effect on burnout. *American Journal of Critical Care, 13*(3), 202–207.

Monroe, T. B., Kenaga, H., Dietrich, M.S., Carter, M. A., & Cowan, R. I. (2013). The prevalence of employed nurses identified or enrolled in substance use monitoring programs. *Nursing Research, 62*(1), 10–15. doi:10.1097/NNR.0b013e31826ba3ca

NCSBN. (2011). *Substance use disorder in nursing: A resource manual and guidelines for alternative and disciplinary monitoring programs.* Chicago, IL: Author.

Perry, B. (2008). Why exemplary oncology nurses seem to avoid compassion fatigue. *Canadian Oncology Nursing Journal, 18*(2), 87–92. doi:10.5737/1181912x1828792

Ramer, L. M. (2008). Using servant leadership to facilitate healing after a drug diversion experience. *AORN, 88*(2), 253–258. doi:10.1016/j.aorn.2008.05.002

Sabo, B. M. (2006). Compassion fatigue and nursing work: Can we accurately capture the consequences of caring work? *International Journal of Nursing Practice, 12,* 136–142. doi:10.1111/j.1440-172X.2006.00562.x

Stamm, B. H. (2002). Measuring compassion satisfaction as well as fatigue: Developmental history of the compassion fatigue and satisfaction test. In C. R. Figley (Ed.), *Treating compassion fatigue* (pp. 107–119). New York, NY: Brunner Mazel.

Stamm, B. H. (2010). *The ProQOL (Professional Quality of Life Scale: Compassion Satisfaction and Compassion Fatigue)*. Pocatello, ID: ProQOL.org. Retrieved from www.proqol.org

Strobbe, S., & Crowley, M. (2017). Substance use among nurses and nursing students: A joint position statement of the Emergency Nurses Association and the International Nurses Society on Addictions. *Journal of Addiction Nursing, 28*(20), 104–106. doi:10.1097/JAN.0000000000000150

Todaro-Franceschi, V. (2008). Preventing compassion fatigue and reaffirming purpose in nursing. *Proceedings on the 3rd European Federation of Critical Care Nursing Congress and 27th Aniarti Conference, Influencing Critical Care Nursing in Europe*, Florence, Italy (October).

Todaro-Franceschi, V. (2013). *Compassion fatigue and burnout in nursing: Enhancing professional quality of life*. New York, NY: Springer Publishing.

Todaro-Franceschi, V. (2015). The ART of maintaining the "care" in healthcare. *Nursing Management, 46*(6), 53–55. doi:10.1097/01.numa.0000465407.76450.ab

Trinkoff, A. M., & Storr, C. L. (1998). Substance use among nurses: Differences between specialties. *American Journal of Public Health, 88*(4), 581–585. doi:10.2105/AJPH.88.4.581

Vachon, M. L. (1993). Emotional problems in palliative medicine: Patient, family, and professional. In D. Doyle, G. Hanks, & N. McDonald (Eds.), *Oxford textbook of palliative medicine* (pp. 577–605). New York, NY: Oxford University Press.

Moral Distress: I Know What I Ought to Do!

Action may not always bring happiness, but there is no happiness without action.

—William James

Our lives begin to end the day we become silent about things that matter.

—Martin Luther King, Jr.

KEY TOPICS

- Moral distress
- Unique professional knowledge
- The importance of nursing
- Moral courage

INTRODUCTION

Are there things in your practice that you think ought to be done but feel unable to do? Is the environment you are working in hindering rather than enhancing your practice? In the original text, I asked the reader to consider the following scenario; however, this time I want to disclose that Mrs. Frank in the following was actually my husband, Michael, and this story was part of an awful hospitalization experience we had just a few years prior to the writing of the first edition of this book:

> *Mrs. Frank is in the surgical intensive care unit after having had open heart surgery. In addition to the sternal surgical wound she has three chest tubes, a Swan–Ganz, an arterial line, a femoral central line, and a Foley. It is 86 degrees in the room and the nurse is perspiring as he works. He notices that the patient's dressings are coming off due to diaphoresis, and he attempts to reinforce them.*
>
> *The nurse knows that the patient is at risk for infection and that the environment is not conducive to healing. He feels helpless, for many times in the past he and other staff have reported the excessive heat on the unit to no avail, and in fact they had been told that there was nothing that could be done about it.*
>
> *Mrs. Frank develops a high fever on her second postoperative day; the nurse wonders if it is because she is now septic and if the heat in the room may have contributed to the infection. He prays that the vancomycin they are starting will effectively treat the infection. At the end of the day he goes home worrying about his patient.*

Does this sound familiar? Are there things in your practice that you know *ought* to be different, but you feel at a loss to change? Now for more honesty; the room was hotter than hell and despite my repeated requests to the nurses to call engineering, I was met with apathy. I would like to think that the nurses did go home worrying about Michael when he started to spike a temperature. However, their behavior did not indicate moral distress, rather, it indicated something far worse: burnout. I return to this in later chapters.

DEFINING MORAL DISTRESS

Moral distress occurs "when one knows the right thing to do but institutional constraints make it nearly impossible to pursue the right course of action" (Jameton, 1984, p. 6). In essence, moral distress is a form of secondary trauma that over time can result in compassion fatigue and/or burnout. Moral distress can arise, like in the preceding clinical vignette, from any number of things in our practice environment. Corley (2002) identified that there are opposing internal and external factors involved: The nurse's values and sense of obligation (internal) can conflict with the values and views of an organization, other providers, patients, families, or even society (external).

Moral distress is also prevalent in nursing education, where faculty may find themselves in anguish for various reasons on behalf of students (Ganske, 2010). Nurse educators can contribute to moral distress in their students if they are not careful. A case in point is when a nurse faculty member tells her students that although they witnessed unsafe or substandard care in a clinical setting, because the students are students and they are all guests, they must not speak up about it.

The manifestations of moral distress are similar to those experienced by someone suffering from compassion fatigue. In fact, social worker Donna Forster (2009) has offered the idea that compassion fatigue may be more correctly understood as a *form* of moral stress. Unresolved or ongoing experiences of moral distress over time can result in burnout. The classic indication of moral distress is a sense of powerlessness due to feeling unable to carry out what one thinks is the right thing to do (Jameton, 1993). Anger, guilt, feeling unimportant or inadequate, difficulty sleeping, gastrointestinal upset, and any number of the multitude of signs and symptoms related to suffering can ensue.

THE BIGGEST CONTRIBUTING FACTOR

Nursing is predicated on a value for human life and on health and healing. It is through our service to, and connection with, others that we actualize our potential as nurses. Yet, many times nurses do *not* act the way they want to act or do what it is they know in their heart and mind needs to be done. In the literature, one reads how "nursing staff definitely appear to be experiencing moral frustration and guilt as a result of being prevented from providing the care they wish" (Schluter, Winch, Holzhauser, & Henderson, 2008, p. 318). I would point out that this has been the case for a pretty long time—it is nothing new. What I would like to know is why *we* have not been able to address the biggest contributor to moral distress in nursing, which, as far as I can tell, has always been either the nurse not being able to find (or use) his or her voice or, alternatively, working in a place where his or her voice does not seem to matter.

Many nurses cannot seem to make their voices heard. The reasons why this happens are many, but include our personal values and beliefs, our education (or lack thereof), our workplace, and the people who work with us. An overarching issue that crosses over all of it is the valuing and, conversely, devaluing of our unique nursing knowledge and skills.

When Our Voices Do Not Seem to Matter

In their classic article, Roland Yarling and Beverly McElmurry (1986) expounded upon the importance of the moral foundation of our discipline as a determinant of our professional well-being. One of the most significant deterrents to doing what we know we *ought* to do continues to be what Yarling and McElmurry (1986) referred to as *hospitalonian captivity*. The healthcare systems in which we work put restrictions upon the profession, limiting what we can and cannot do, and our voices do not seem to matter. Accordingly, we often feel powerless. Their words were applicable a quarter of a century ago and remain so today:

> . . . there is grave institutional culpability in a situation where the institutional disincentives to morally responsible action are so per-suasive that the probability of moral action by the average person is rendered minimal . . . nurses are not free to be moral because they are deprived of moral agency by the repressive character of the hospitals in which they practice. (p. 71)

There are definitely institutional disincentives that are worse than others. Take, for example, the case of the nurse who questioned a "doctor's orders" and was publicly reprimanded with a note on her locker door; that was pretty bad. But the nurse who is fired because he or she advocates for patients is much worse. There are other ways in which disincentives are covertly imposed. Having a heavy workload on a unit where patients often die does not encourage "presencing" for the nurse who feels compelled to be present with the patient and his or her loved ones. Instead, heavy workloads on these units deter nurses from doing what they feel they should be doing.

The Right to Have One's Part Matter

Nurses are not taught to be assertive, and without this skill it can be dif-ficult to find one's voice or to make one be heard. Feminist and educator Carolyn Heilburn (1988) said that power is the "ability to take one's place in whatever discourse is necessary to action and the right to have one's part matter" (p. 18). Nurses in practice may frequently find themselves in a posi-tion where they feel as if their part does not matter at all. For instance, on the unit where the heat was excessive, not only were the patients suffering, the nurses who were providing care in that less than optimal environment were, too. But none of the nurses felt that their voices were being heard—so they stopped using their voices completely about the issue.

In our code of ethics, Provision 6 emphasizes the part that we must play in cultivating an environment conducive to acting with ethical comport-ment (American Nurses Association [ANA], 2015). Specifically, Provision 6.3 notes that "nurses are responsible for contributing to a moral environ-ment that demands respectful interactions among colleagues, mutual peer support, and open identification of difficult issues, which includes ongoing professional development of staff in ethical problem solving" (ANA, 2015, p. 24). I would point out that the language used in this most recent update of the code is somewhat stronger in tone, especially in Provision 6. It is emphasized that the environment we work in can and does influence how we go about doing our work and that we have a moral obligation to ensure that the environments we practice in are safe. Taking this further, the newly revised code also notes that working in an environment where conditions are repeatedly compromising the standards of practice or personal integrity cannot be an option.

Recall the observations I shared earlier made by Liaschenko (2008), that her students—nurses engaged in practice—often felt their voices were not heard because *they* did not know enough of the science. As a result, they believed that they were at fault for not being heard. Disturbingly, the relational aspects of nursing—the caring attributes—were not factored into their concerns at all (Liaschenko, 2008). At the end of the day, being dismissed by others as "noncredible knowers" was sufficient grounds for these nurses to *believe* themselves to *be* noncredible knowers.

Liaschenko (2008) emphasized that it is because nurses continue not to have the necessary freedom that enables them to speak up and act assertively to advocate on behalf of their patients, whereas others who work in healthcare have this freedom. While other healthcare professionals claim their legitimacy to speak up, assert that they are credible knowers, and insist on accountability from other members of the healthcare team, she noted that we in nursing do not. Liaschenko claimed that this is because we occupy a social space of "gendered labor" (p. 197), because care of the sick continues to be a predominantly female occupation, and because, well, even nurse educators often do not seem to value the caring aspects of the profession, which make us unique.

Not all nursing knowledge is considered "scientific," but it nevertheless has enormous value to facilitate health and healing. With our continued silence, inability to articulate what it is we do—choosing not to use our voices either because we are oppressed in our workplaces or because we believe we cannot or should not do so—we allow others to think that our contributions to health and healing are minimal, at best. *We* allow hospitalonian captivity to prevail.

PATTERNS OF KNOWING

We are not victims; we participate in creating reality through our actions. In essence, we give up the power we have as equal participants in ensuring the quality of care received by our patients. We do this in large part by devaluing our unique ways of knowing. Nurse Barbara Carper (1978) identified patterns of knowing that are all important sources for knowledge acquisition: empirical, personal, ethical, and aesthetic. She noted that "each pattern may be conceived as necessary for achieving mastery in the discipline but none of them could be considered sufficient" (pp. 21–22). Empirical knowledge is the scientific component of nursing, based on empirics and evidence; personal knowledge arises from our self-understanding of who we are and how we feel; ethical knowledge is a matter of principles and codes, establishing what is right, and acting with moral comportment to do what one believes he or she ought to do; and aesthetic knowledge is the going beyond to seek meaning—it is fundamentally the artistic expression and comprehension of all that is and has yet to be (Carper, 1978).

Focusing solely on empirical ways of knowing—scientific knowledge—does not take into account the human characteristic of uniqueness. It is surely a cause for concern when we follow "standing orders" or "clinical pathways" without taking into account the distinct variability from one person to another. We always have outliers and everyone wonders what *we* are doing wrong. What is wrong is that the healthcare system is emphasizing one way of knowing—empirics—and not using any of the others (personal, ethical, aesthetic). Needless to say, none of the patterns of knowing can stand alone without becoming less effective. As nurse Christopher Johns (1995) noted:

> Whereas empirics encourages the practitioner to stereotype the situation according to some rule or law that predicts an outcome, aesthetic knowing involves a process of perceiving or grasping the nature of a clinical situation; interpreting this information in order to understand its meaning for those involved, whilst envisioning desired outcomes in order to respond with appropriate and skilled action, and subsequently reflecting on whether the outcomes were effectively achieved. (p. 228)

All of our ways of knowing combine to *complete us* as nurses.

The tragedy is that most nurses are not educated to believe in our inherent value and the contributions that all of our unique ways of knowing make to human health and healing. On more than one occasion, I have heard fellow colleagues as well as other healthcare professionals say that nurses were and always will be handmaidens to physicians. I have never believed myself to be that, and I do not educate "would-be nurses" to believe it either. Nevertheless, the image of the handmaiden is, without a doubt, reinforced through our language and social practices, such as is evident in the story of "doctor's orders" I shared earlier.

CHOICE AND POWER: DEVELOPING A SENSE OF OUR OWN SALIENCE

That it is a choice nurses make (to value some ways of knowing and skills more than others) is obvious, but our choices are often influenced, and then reinforced, by others. Take, for example, a female nurse practitioner (NP) who is purportedly in collaborative practice or is functioning as an independent practitioner. She is told that she must limit her time with patients to 15 minutes each visit; however, she knows that some patients require more time, others less. Still, she may choose to conform rather than say this to her administrators or the physicians she is in practice with, or perhaps she does share her concern, but it is not valued.

The NP's practice is changed based on the influence of others or the policies of the institution rather than her getting the system to accommodate her practice the way she knows it should be. More than likely, she probably feels she has no choice in the matter. One might say that the NP does not have a choice, and perhaps the individual NP does not, for if she refuses she may well find herself out of a job. But collectively, NPs *do* have a choice—it is, after all, their patients, their practice, their licenses, and it is also their right to have "their part matter."

Some may think this is a simplistic view of a complex problem and I might agree, if it were not for the fact that people who do not understand what nursing entails are making the rules for things like this in our practice and I know that many of our physician colleagues agree. An NP is not supposed to function like an MD; they are different roles. Certainly there is overlap because both are primary care providers; however, nurses look at wholes, and physicians (usually) specific parts. The two roles should complement one another.

Although I used the NP as an example, I want to stress that bedside nurses, nurse leaders, clinical nurse specialists (CNSs), and even nurse educators are all influenced by others and by the policies and procedures in our workplaces. If we are allowing others to make decisions concerning our profession and practice, it is ultimately still a choice that *we* are making.

In one of my stints as a CNS, I wanted to be on the hospital Pharmacy and Therapeutics Committee. I was the only CNS in the entire hospital, a large teaching hospital, and I thought I belonged there, but the deputy director of nursing, who I answered directly to, said that the "big boys club" would not want a nurse there; for the same reason I was told that I couldn't be the team leader of a continuous quality improvement (CQI) project that I initiated. I had to ask a physician to be the leader, even though he rarely came to meetings and I did all of the work. I realized it was still my choice and that perhaps the effort I was making—coming in the back door, so to speak—was effective, to a point. But I also recognized that it was to some degree a new take on an old game, a game that nurses have played in some fashion for decades: treading lightly, saying to the MD, "Do you think perhaps that this might be a better way?" Instead of saying bluntly, "This is a better way."

With little things, it might be okay to play that game, but with the bigger things, it is never okay because it leads us to moral distress. Over time, and especially with repeated occurrences, moral residue builds—long-lasting effects that are very hard to shake (Webster & Bayliss, 2000). We are wounded in such a way that our sense of self is compromised. Our moral concerns have not been acknowledged—we have not been acknowledged—and we begin to believe that our voices really do not matter.

Nurse scholar and practitioner Elizabeth Ann Manhart Barrett (1989, 2010) stresses that everyone has power; it is just a matter of how we go about actualizing it. She noted that there are two ways to view *power*, similar to my claim about two views of energy: Power can be defined and actualized as control, or as knowing participation (Barrett, 2010). *Power as control* is the normal way many people go about influencing change. It is predicated on domination over others and other things, whereas *power as knowing participation* entails a person's awareness, choices, freedom to choose, and involvement in creating change (Barrett, 1989, 2010). We have to be aware that we have choices we can make, and then we must feel free to choose and be involved in creating change.

In nursing, many of us have been conditioned to allow *power as control* to suppress us and devalue our very real power as the largest constituent of professionals in healthcare. It is through our knowing participation as compassionate, competent carers that people are able to actualize their potentials to live well and die well. That is *real power*—we have it, but we do not exercise it as well as we should, perhaps because many of us are kept unblissfully ignorant (unaware!) by the way we have been taught. It is time to change all that. As Shirley MacLaine (2011) notes in her writing, it is time for each of us to reiterate, "I am all over that." Try saying, I am over: being oppressed, being made to feel subordinate, being told to do what I know I shouldn't do, and being prevented from doing what I know I ought to do. It is time to *know* our power and to live it together.

Pat Benner and colleagues (Benner, Sutphen, Leonard, Day, & Shulman, 2009) wrote about the transformation needed in nursing education if we are to keep up with the fast pace of healthcare, stressing the widening gap between education and practice. They emphasized that nurses have to develop a sense of salience; that practitioners must be able to identify what is and is not important in terms of clinical priorities. But in cases where nurses experience moral distress, it is not due to them not having a sense of what the priorities are; it often appears to be just the opposite. We *know* what we are supposed to do, we know what appears to be the right thing to do, yet we feel unable to do it. Thus, it is equally important for nurses to develop a sense of our *own* salience.

At the onset of our careers, we should be taught that what we do is enormously important and that the actions we take, both little and large, make a difference in the quality of people's living–dying. To have a sense of what is and is not important will not do much for the nurse who cannot make her voice heard. Note that it is not too late to develop a sense of your own salience. The following is an AHA! shared by an RN in one of my classes:

> *To narrow my experience during this course of when I came to the realization of some meaning or understanding that I did not have before is difficult because of the many things that we covered and learned; however, it was during one session that the professor had the class complete a survey which is used to assess burnout, when I came to an epiphany that, although I was close to burnout, I did not want to be like those nurses who exhibit all the signs of burnout. During this class discussion, the professor, possibly without knowing, helped me come to the realization that, although I enjoy working with the mentally ill, the program I am working at may not be where I want to continue working.*
>
> *For some time I had been sharing my concerns about patients' medication responses with the program psychiatrist, and I felt like I hit a brick wall when I went to administration to further address the issue. I continued to witness patients demonstrating severe side effects from the psychotropic medications being administered to them. Their medications were not being monitored properly, and some patients were on unnecessarily high dosages that more than likely contributed to the worsening of their conditions. While this is not an end-of-life situation, it does contribute to the quality of life of patients and reflects the ethical decisions that nurses have to deal with in the workplace . . . . This class made me realize that, although I am not in complete control of what is happening in the place where I work, my enthusiasm and concern for the patients, as a nurse, and my efforts to expand my education in the field have an impact that is important and makes a difference.*

This nurse was in a workplace where he was experiencing moral distress on a daily basis; coming back to school was the best thing for him and for his patients—what he learned empowered him and over time he was able to develop a sense of his own importance.

Assert Yourself! You Have a Right to Be Heard

My favorite nurse author on the subject of assertiveness is Melodie Chenevert, who noted that nurses have a collective goal: "We want to make safe, sane, humane health care available" (1988, p. x). She stressed that assertiveness might be the most significant skill for nurses to learn in order to achieve that goal. I agree. Over the years I have often wondered, where does one learn this important skill? It is obvious that most nurses do not get assertiveness training while in school. In fact, Chenevert's wonderful books on assertiveness training are out of print; I emailed her trying to get her to have them republished. It amazes and disgruntles me that, over 30 years later, her words are still so applicable to us in nursing. Find a copy of one or two of her books; you will be equally amazed and disgruntled and you will learn an awful lot in a short space of time, I promise you.

Not meaning to be sexist, I must nevertheless point out the obvious (which Chenevert also pointed out): Nursing is a predominantly female profession and with it comes some very real issues. That is why, throughout this book, I most often refer to the nurse as a "she," not to be stereotypical or to leave out the men in our profession, rather, just to be realistic . . . *We* are MOSTLY women. Not every cultural tradition holds the belief that women are equal to men, and even when it is believed that this is so, not every woman is treated equally and not every woman *expects* to be treated equally.

In Carol Gilligan's (1982) groundbreaking work on the voices of women in moral decision making, she noted the following:

> As we have listened for centuries to the voices of men and the theories of development that their experience informs, so we have come more recently to notice not only the silence of women but the difficulty in hearing what they say when they speak up. Yet in the different voice of women lies the truth of an ethic of care, the tie between relationship and responsibility, and the origins of aggression in the failure of connection. (p. 173)

When nurses—predominantly women—are prevented from valuing the connection to self and other, and the caring practices inherent in our work, it is not good for us individually or collectively.

The basic premise underlying assertiveness training is that we have a right to be heard and respected as human beings. But, in order to *learn* assertiveness, we first have to believe in ourselves; we each have to turn toward the mirror and recognize our own inherent value as a person and as a professional. Because to assert oneself means, for all intents and purposes, to communicate one's opinions, values, and beliefs in such a way that others take notice, but not in such a way that it is viewed as an act of aggression. Without a sense of our own salience, we may not believe our own opinion should count and, thus, we will not assert ourselves. We will not bother to try to make our voices heard.

I was fortunate in that, early on in my career, I had an incredible nurse educator named Judy Carlson-Catalano for a nursing leadership course in my Bachelor of Science in Nursing (BSN) program (I am a firm believer in giving credit where it is due!). I took the course while I was working as a fairly new RN, having graduated not too long before from an Associate Degree (AD) program, and I was already unhappy with some of the things I saw and experienced at work. She introduced us to Chenevert and she taught us how important we were. Judy stressed that we had power—power in numbers, intelligence, and caring. It was she who talked me out of going to law school when I completed my BSN, a decision that I have never regretted. Have you ever had an educator like this one? If so, then you must already have a sense of your own salience; if not, now is a good time to learn some of the things we were taught in that class.

With wit and clarity, Chenevert (1988) asked us in her book *STAT: Special Techniques in Assertiveness Training for Women in the Health Professions*, who we would choose to be—chickens or eagles. She claimed that many of us are eagles with a chicken complex. We do not realize that we can fly; we can soar above the trees. Instead, we believe what we have been conditioned to believe, and for nurses, especially those who are women, we have been conditioned in various ways to believe that we answer to others and that our jobs consist of following "orders." As Chenevert (1988) noted, we may think we belong in a barnyard eating chicken feed, rather than using our eagle gifts—powers of flight and keen vision.

I always point out to my students that getting into nursing school is no easy task. Staying in nursing school is even less so. It takes intelligence, courage, perseverance, compassion, and incredible skill to be a nurse. We really are *wonderful* people; we should love and respect ourselves, each other, and our important contributions to the healthcare world.

What happens when we do have a sense of our own salience but others do not? When we use our voice and it is not heard? If we are working in a system where this repeatedly occurs, we may well find ourselves losing our voice—or at least no longer choosing to use it. We may begin to doubt ourselves and our importance as the moral residue builds. Or we can stand up and fight, like the two nurse administrators did in Texas, who then found themselves fired for reporting a physician who was practicing "bad medicine" (Sack, 2010).

It Is Not Whistle-Blowing, It Is Advocacy!

Ann Mitchell and Vickilyn Galle, both nurse administrators in quality improvement who had worked a combined 47 years at their hospital, began trying to get the attention of hospital administration in 2008 related to the patient care practices of a particular physician, which were clearly a cause for apprehension (Sack, 2010). Their worries fell on deaf ears and they then turned to other measures to protect the patients—sending off an unsigned letter to the Texas Medical Board detailing their concerns.

When it was ultimately discovered that Mitchell and Galle had sent the letter, both nurses were fired. Adding insult to injury, they were then indicted and threatened with 10 years in prison for misuse of official information, a third-degree felony in the state of Texas (Sack, 2010). Galle was acquitted shortly afterward, and when Mitchell went to trial, she, too, was acquitted. Both vindicated, they filed a civil suit and were ultimately awarded $750,000 to be shared between them. But no amount of money could rectify this wrong.

What did the hospital administrators hope to accomplish by firing these nurses? How might the fear of negative consequences such as this deter other nurses (and would-be nurses) from acting with moral comportment? No matter how you look at it, the entire thing was bad news for everyone.

Whistle-blowers are supposed to be protected for reporting to the authorities any bad practices and conditions that put people, and on occasion, other living things, in harm's way; however, I take offense when nurses who act with moral comportment are called "whistle-blowers." A well-meaning person might make a phone call to the authorities concerning the practices of a group of people who are cutting down trees in a forest, damaging an ecologic environment that is supposed to be protected; that is considered whistle-blowing. An office worker who calls the state environmental protection agency because he finds there is uncontained asbestos in the office ceiling and finds out that his employer has been hiding the risk from all of the office workers; that is whistle-blowing. On the other hand, nurses are patient carers and advocates; we are not whistle-blowers. We are the *first* and *last* line of defense for people who are vulnerable and who put their complete trust in us to compassionately and competently care for *and* protect them. In fact, the public routinely votes the nursing profession as one of the most trusted; we are *expected* to speak up!

Annually, the Gallup public opinion poll indicates that nurses are believed to be the most trustworthy and ethical of all groups. If we do *not* act to protect, then that line of defense is broken and we might as well throw up a white flag, surrendering our moral code along with the values and excellences deemed to be the foundational core of our profession. And that is what eventually happens when we know what we ought to do but are repeatedly unable to do it. The result: moral distress → moral residue → burnout.

When We Are the Cause of Anguish

Suffering is an ineluctable part of living and dying; however, many times we in healthcare unintentionally cause further anguish through our acts. We not only bear witness to suffering but sometimes also directly cause what is clearly unnecessary suffering. When this occurs repeatedly, we find ourselves wondering what the goals of care are, and over time, we may well find ourselves flicking the shutoff switch to the anguish in our patients' eyes. It could be what seems on the surface to be a simple matter, like bed scale weights or even little things like taking rectal temperatures in cardiac critical care, because it is considered the most accurate thing to do. How many men do you know whose heart rate would not increase when told to lie on their side so you could take a rectal temperature? Well, I remember a coworker's story of taking a rectal temperature on a male patient who went into v-tachycardia during the procedure; she did a precordial thump, which luckily converted his rhythm. Imagine the possibility of losing a patient because you asked him to turn over to get a rectal temperature? Of course, we can laugh about it now, only because we no longer do rectal temperatures . . . but I bet many nurses can think of a thing or two that is being done in their practice, which they are not laughing about, knowing that it may be causing more harm than good.

One of the common practices that really irks me in teaching hospitals is when patients are used by interns and residents for learning how to do things—such as line insertions—the day before, and the morning of, surgery. Some of these patients are going for very risky procedures, and some of them are going to die. Yet they spend their last day or so as pin cushions and guinea pigs for those who are there to learn, separated from their loved ones in the process. Where is the beneficence in that?

Unfortunately, it seems that many interns and residents who are learning how to do things (on patients) have already distanced themselves so much that they do not recognize the human beings they are oftentimes literally torturing with their unskilled hands. When I was in practice, I frequently advocated for patients to be left alone after the first stick or two and insisted an experienced nurse or physician come in to do the sticking. In the past decade I have had many occasions where I have witnessed these kinds of occurrences with loved ones (and on occasion even myself) and have wondered, "Where is the nurse?" (I return to this question again later.)

On medical–surgical and oncology units, nurses are frequently faced with knowing that a patient is scheduled for diagnostic tests or procedures that will not improve his or her quality of life and which may in fact create unnecessary suffering. For instance, I remember assigning a student to work with an older adult who was diagnosed with stage 3b lung cancer when he was admitted to the hospital for uncontrollable diarrhea due to *Clostridium difficile* colitis (*C. diff*).

Speaking with him about his choices, he shared some personal information. He was estranged from most of his family; he had eight grown children and was not sure how many grandchildren he had. He lived alone and rarely saw anyone. He said he had made some bad choices as a youngster—he "loved to drink and he loved the women." Now, he was ready to die, he said, and he opted not to receive any treatment for his late-stage cancer. He made that very clear. His plan was to return home as soon as his diarrhea was resolved. The following week when we returned to the unit, this man was being sent for radiation therapy. When asked why, he told me and the student that the MD said he had to have the treatment.

Another time, when I was working as a nursing supervisor, we had an increased incidence of postoperative infections in the cardiothoracic surgical intensive care unit. In retrospect, it was found that the staff and many of the advanced practice nurses knew what the likely cause was; several of the surgical interns and residents were not washing their hands when they were taking down and changing dressings. Yet no one had documented or acted on it. It was not until the State came in that the problem became general knowledge and was rectified. At a staff meeting a few weeks later, many of the nurses voiced having felt morally distressed about it but none of them had had the moral courage to come forward.

As an educator, I look around and I say it is no wonder. I do not see us in nursing education spending anywhere near enough time teaching our students how important *they* are and how to use their voices; rather, I see extraordinary emphasis being placed on clinical skill development.

What Do You Mean I Am Not Allowed to Be Sick?

Nussbaum (1996) pointed out that a concern for the good of others often leads one to risk his or her own contentment: "For people very often sacrifice their own interests and well-being, and in many cases even their own lives, for the well-being of those they love, or for good social consequences that they prize" (p. 49). Nurses are self-sacrificing; we go in to work when physically or emotionally exhausted (like I did when returning a fourth night to care for John Doe), we skip breaks and meals, we stay long after our shift ends to complete various tasks, and so forth. We will go to great lengths to get what our patients need, wearing ourselves out completely in the process.

We have been conditioned to sacrifice our own interests and well-being. We are informed that we must not call in sick and that our patients and unit duties come before our own needs. Even while in nursing school, the expectation is that we will not miss classes, and, consequently, students frequently drag themselves into classes sick and expose everyone else to illness. Heck, I had an emergency C-section during my senior year in nursing school and signed out against medical orders, running a temperature no less, to go to my clinical because I was certain the instructor would not allow me to pass the course if I missed it. Why did I feel that way? Because it was emphasized repeatedly that we could not miss any clinical days (and my professor showed no compassion whatsoever).

When we are conditioned for unfair expectations it leads to moral distress, because we are then torn between doing what we have always been told is the right thing versus what we intuit is needed for our own well-being. If we act in our own best interests, for example, calling in sick, we chance feeling guilty because we left our unit short of staff. We perceive ourselves as the cause or contributor of another's anguish.

ACTING WITH MORAL COURAGE VERSUS FEELING POWERLESS

There is another side to the self-sacrificing nurse. There is the nurse, who literally lays himself or herself on the line in order to advocate for others. This is the nurse who is said to have moral courage, the one who acts with moral comportment, regardless of risk to his or her own well-being. There are plenty of nurses who have a great deal of moral courage, and there would undoubtedly be more if all nurses had a sense of their own salience. Make no mistake; I am not slapping anyone's wrist here on this issue, either. It is difficult to have moral courage if you have no awareness of your own power and no confidence in your own ability. It is difficult to have moral courage in an organization that does not support it. Without a just culture, most people will not be particularly courageous about anything.

Nurse educators and leaders can encourage the development of moral courage in their students and staff, if they emulate it themselves. The nurse educator is the gatekeeper for the profession and the developer of future nursing practice. The nurse leader who supports and fosters quality caring ultimately sets the tone for a healthy work environment (Edmonson, 2010). That is why nurse educators and leaders need to be cultivated in an atmosphere where, as Barrett's (2010) power theory demarcates, *power as knowing participation* is stressed and where *power as control* is minimized. We need transformational leaders and transformational educators (see Chapters 12 and 13).

APPLYING *ART* FOR MORAL DISTRESS

Once again the *ART*© model (Todaro-Franceschi, 2008, 2013, 2015) can be readily applied. To address moral distress on an individual basis one needs to first acknowledge if there is a problem getting one's voice to be heard. However, acknowledging and making known to others our worth as nurses who contribute so much to health and healing and whose voices do matter is a task for *all* nurses, including leaders and educators. We must first recognize the importance of the profession as a whole. We need to turn toward ourselves by teaching and learning how to insist that our voices do matter and also toward others in how we approach the care of our patients, to act with assertion—with moral comportment and courage—to do what we believe is right and what is needed.

Step 1: Acknowledge a Feeling or Wound That Needs Healing

Can you think of any regular practices that you think you should or should not be doing? Or perhaps there are things that used to bother you and you are no longer paying attention to them or have given up trying to change your practice? A case in point is the nurse who knows that it is too warm on the unit but no longer asks for the temperature control to be fixed; or the nurse who continues to do bed scale weights, simply because it was "ordered," all the while knowing it may cause additional suffering; or the nurse who knows that another course of chemotherapy is not going to make things better, yet when the patient asks about it, she feels that she cannot speak up. As you go about your work, identify any uncomfortable feelings—capture your moments by writing them down so that you can reflect upon them later.

Step 2: Recognize Choices and Take Purposeful Action

If you are experiencing moral distress, depending upon the circumstances, you will have any number of choices. In addition to the specifics of each case, you need to reflect upon your

- Values and beliefs
- Relationships with the people with whom you work
- Support systems

Ask yourself, in light of these, what choices you have that might make things better for you and for your patients. List them.

1. _____

2. _____

3. _____

4. _____

5. _____

Who might listen to your concerns and support you in making the necessary changes in practice? Can you approach your administrative staff alone or do you need the support of coworkers? If there is an ethics committee in your institution, you can certainly approach them. If not, maybe you can seek support outside of your institution; such has regularly been the case with students who contact me after graduation to help them brainstorm ways to address concerns in their practice. Or perhaps you need to take a more radical action like the nurses who contacted the medical board about a physician's unsafe practices or the nurse who called in the State for an unsafe environment.

When working as a clinical specialist in a fairly large teaching hospital, there was a period of time when there was a string of medication errors on several medical–surgical units. Consequently, as is often the case, the staff nurses were being disciplined and in-serviced to no end. The morale on the units was low and nurses were scared. Some of the staff spoke with me; one told me she was looking for a new job and another said she was going back to school. I went home each night troubled and spent hours talking about the problem with my husband. It was one of the times I lost sleep over work.

On further exploration of the issue, during which time I did a retrospective study of the patient charts, physician prescriptions, and incident reports, I found that it was actually the physicians who needed in-service education regarding how they were writing the prescriptions. The majority of the nurses knew there was a problem and, in fact, a few had taken it upon themselves to just change the scripts, which of course is beyond a staff nurse's scope of practice. What the staff nurses really needed was not in-servicing on medication errors, but rather assertiveness training in order to be able to go back to the physician and say, "No, this is not right."

If you do not feel an issue can be addressed by yourself or you are unable to direct the issue to the appropriate person and there does not seem to be anywhere to turn for support, you still have choices to make. You can choose to advocate, climbing the ladder up, and mayhap not just up but also out (such as the nurse administrators who reported the physician to the medical board in Texas) until your voice has been heard. Or, if you do not see that happening, maybe it is time to move on. Weigh your choices. If you are being repeatedly put in a position where your license or health might be in jeopardy and there is nothing else you can do to make things better, start to look around for a new position. The one thing we must not do is settle; we must never choose to compromise our beliefs and values. We must never flick the shutoff switch. When the switch is flicked off, the bad is becoming ugly!

If you are unable to find your voice, another choice you have is to seek assertiveness training. There are training programs available (see Appendix C, Resources, for further information or just Google it). I mentioned earlier Melodie Chenevert's writings on the subject; she has written a number of helpful exercises that can be used individually or in group sessions. When I worked as a clinical nurse manager, I adopted one for use with staff and it was a big hit (I come back to this in later chapters).

Step 3: *Turn* Outward Toward Self and Other

In patient cases leading to moral distress, it can be helpful to ask yourself what your beliefs and values are, and then where possible, try to explore all sides of the situation. This is important because, in any given situation, others may or may not feel the same way that you do. If you can, speak with others about the issue. In the classes where I teach ethics, I frequently ask that the students dialogue in a special way put forward by physicist David Bohm (1996), where all participants must make an effort to hear one another's viewpoint. As per Bohm's basic principles on dialogue, I emphasize that we are not trying to drive the conversation in any way or to any specific conclusions; instead, we agree to suspend individual judgment during our discussions, remaining open and honest. In this way we can try to build upon one another's ideas. The end result is always that individual perspectives shift and one's beliefs and values sometimes change completely.

I have used Bohm's dialogue method in a number of classes, most notably in graduate-level bioethics courses. The majority of students in these classes are seasoned nurses, some of whom have been working for decades. The stories they share of ethical dilemmas they have faced in practice indicate that moral distress can linger and fester over time. Some of these nurses noted that they never felt there was an opportunity to talk about their concerns; consequently, they had internalized their anguish. Sharing their stories in class, and having time to reflect upon and dialogue with others about them, was a healing experience.

When discussing ethical issues, in particular, the nature of the topics is such that no discussion can yield an understanding of the human race at large; there are far too many different beliefs on life, living, death, dying, health, and healing. By understanding that the view from the looking glass can vary considerably from person to person, we can come to see the world anew, perhaps unlearning long-held beliefs, values, and ideas (or on occasion relearning things forgotten!).

Once you have explored your feelings in relation to other points of view, if your perspective does not shift, and it is making you feel helpless and/or ineffective, and you believe it is affecting patients, their loved ones, coworkers, or perchance even your loved ones, it is time to act. Think: The choices I make can change how I feel, how my patients heal, how my colleagues work together, and how I interact with loved ones. Reconnect, now. As Henry David Thoreau noted, "Only that day dawns to which we are awake."

When moral distress occurs in healthcare, it is usually a group-level happening so that turning outward toward self and other may be especially effective in group sessions. Clinical leaders and educators can try taking a specific situation and explore it from a group perspective. On occasion, it might be fitting to encourage discourse by taking it out of the unit or current moment of moral distress. I like to use short clips of events (such as those from the motion picture *Wit* or *Patch Adams*) to encourage dialogue about critical issues.

The American Association of Critical-Care Nurses (2006) put forward a model called "The 4 A's to Rise Above Moral Distress" created by their ethics work group. The four A's stand for "Ask, Affirm, Assess, and Act," and as a whole, they offer a framework to address moral distress in the workplace. Check out Appendix C, Resources, to learn more.

KEY POINTS

- Moral distress arises when you know what the right thing to do is in a given situation, but feel for whatever reason unable to do it.

- Moral distress can occur from conflicts related to our own personal values and beliefs, surfacing in the many ethical dilemmas we face, as well as from interpersonal discord between coworkers or members of the healthcare team, patients, and their families, or it can be related to environmental factors that we know are not conducive to health and healing.

- The biggest contributing factor to moral distress in nursing is nurses feeling, or being, unable to make their voice heard.

- Repeated instances of moral distress lead to the buildup of moral residue and over time can result in burnout.

- Developing a sense of our own salience as nurses individually and collectively so that we feel we have not only the responsibility but the right to speak up can help to prevent repeated instances of moral distress.

- Assertiveness skills can be developed in order to learn how to effectively use one's voice. We have a right to be heard!

- Self-reflection as well as group-level discussion of uncontrollable events that lead to moral distress can facilitate a converging of viewpoints and, in cases where that may not be possible, it can still help everyone to be more aware and participate more knowingly in changes that will benefit everyone.

REFERENCES

American Association of Critical-Care Nurses Ethics Work Group. (2006). *The 4 A's to rise above moral distress.* Retrieved from http://www.aacn.org/WD/Practice/ Docs/4As_to_Rise_Above_Moral_Distress.pdf

American Nurses Association. (2015). *Code of ethics for nurses with interpretive statements.* Silver Spring, MD: Author.

Barrett, E. A. M. (1989). A nursing theory of power for nursing practice. In J. P. Riehl-Sisca (Ed.), *Conceptual models for nursing practice* (3rd ed., pp. 207–217). Norwalk, CT: Appleton & Lange.

Barrett, E. A. M. (2010). Power as knowing participation in change: What's new and what's next. *Nursing Science Quarterly, 23*(1), 47–54. doi:10.1177/0894318409353797

Benner, P., Sutphen, M., Leonard, V., Day, L., & Shulman, L. (2009). Foreword. *Educating nurses: A call for radical transformation* (Jossey-Bass/Carnegie Foundation for the Advancement of Teaching). Kindle Edition. Retrieved from www .amazon.com

Bohm, D. (1996). *On dialogue.* London, UK: Routledge.

Carper, B. A. (1978). Fundamental patterns of knowing in nursing. *Advances in Nursing Science, 1*(1), 13–24. doi:10.1097/00012272-197810000-00004

Chenevert, M. (1988). *STAT: Special techniques in assertiveness training for women in the health professions.* St. Louis, MO: C.V. Mosby.

Corley, M. C. (2002). Nurse moral distress: A proposed theory and research agenda. *Nursing Ethics, 9*(6), 636–650. doi:10.1191/0969733002ne557oa

Edmonson, C. (2010). Moral courage and the nurse leader. *The Online Journal of Issues in Nursing, 15*(3), Manuscript 5. Retrieved from http://www.nursingworld. org/MainMenuCategories/ANAMarketplace/ANAPeriodicals/OJIN/Tableof Contents/Vol152010/No3-Sept-2010/Moral-Courage-for-Nurse-Leaders.html

Forster, D. (2009). Rethinking compassion fatigue as moral distress. *Journal of Ethics in Mental Health, 4,* 1–4.

Ganske, K. M. (2010). Moral distress in academia. *The Online Journal of Issues in Nursing, 15*(3), Manuscript. Retrieved from http://www.nursingworld.org/ MainMenuCategories/ANAMarketplace/ANAPeriodicals/OJIN/Tableof Contents/Vol152010/No3-Sept-2010/Moral-Distress-in-Academia.html

Gilligan, C. (1982). *In a different voice: Psychological theory and women's development.* Cambridge, MA: Harvard University Press.

Heilburn, C. (1988). *Writing a woman's life.* New York, NY: Ballantine Books.

Jameton, A. (1984). *Nursing practice: The ethical issues.* Englewood Cliffs, NJ: Prentice-Hall.

Jameton, A. (1993). Dilemmas of moral distress: Moral responsibility and nursing practice. *AWHONNS Clinical Issues in Perinatal & Women's Health Nursing, 4*(4), 542–551.

Johns, C. (1995). Framing learning through reflection within Carper's fundamental ways of knowing. *Journal of Advanced Nursing, 22*, 226–234. doi:10.1046/j.1365-2648.1995.22020226.x

Liaschenko, J. (2008). ". . . to take one's place . . . and the right to have one's part matter." In W. J. E. Pinch & A. M. Haddad (Eds.), *Nursing and health care ethics: A legacy and a vision* (pp. 195–203). Silver Spring, MD: American Nurses Association.

MacLaine, S. (2011). *I'm all over that and other confessions.* New York, NY: Atria Books.

Nussbaum, M. (1996). Compassion: The basic social emotion. *Social Philosophy and Policy, 13*, 27–58. doi:10.1017/S0265052500001515

Sack, K. (2010, February 10). Nurse to stand trial for reporting doctor. *The New York Times.* Retrieved from http://www.nytimes.com/2010/02/07/us/07nurses.html?pagewanted

Schluter, J., Winch, S., Holzhauser, K., & Henderson, A. (2008). Nurses' moral sensitivity and hospital ethical climate: A literature review. *Nursing Ethics, 15*, 304–321. doi:10.1177/0969733007088357

Todaro-Franceschi, V. (2008). Preventing compassion fatigue and reaffirming purpose in nursing. *Proceedings on the 3rd European Federation of Critical Care Nursing Congress and 27th Aniarti Conference, Influencing Critical Care Nursing in Europe*, Florence, Italy (October).

Todaro-Franceschi, V. (2013). *Compassion fatigue and burnout in nursing: Enhancing professional quality of life.* New York, NY: Springer Publishing.

Todaro-Franceschi, V. (2015). The ART of maintaining the "care" in healthcare. *Nursing Management, 46*(6), 53–55. doi:10.1097/01.numa.0000465407.76450.ab

Webster, G., & Bayliss, F. (2000). Moral residue. In S. Rubin & L. Zoloth (Eds.), *Margin of error: The ethics of mistakes in the practice of medicine.* Hagerstown, MD: University Publishing Group.

Yarling, R. R., & McElmurry, B. J. (1986). The moral foundation of nursing. *Advances in Nursing Science, 8*(2), 63–73. doi:10.1097/00012272-198601000-00010

The Ugly, Uglier, and Ugliest: Burnout and Workplace Violence

The very first requirement in a hospital is that it should do the sick no harm.

—Florence Nightingale

8

Burnout: Feeling Empty-Hearted and Disheartened

I suffer from nothing. I no longer know what suffering is.
I have come to an end of all that . . . .

—Graham Greene

KEY TOPICS

- Burnout
- Consequences for nurses and patients

INTRODUCTION

In his 1960 book, *A Burnt-Out Case*, novelist Graham Greene described his protagonist, a famous male architect named Querry, who, having become disillusioned with his work and life, chooses to disappear into the African jungle. There he takes on work in a colony with lepers and, in doing so, transforms his life in positive ways. The term *burnt-out case* refers to a leper whose disease has eaten away until it no longer exists and is consequently considered at the point of cure. But by that time, many lepers are missing limbs. In this story it is clear that the protagonist himself is a burnt-out case,

© Springer Publishing Company DOI: 10.1891/9780826155214.0008

although he suffers not from leprosy but from apathy. Instead of missing limbs, Querry seems numb and heartless.

A more complete idea of burnout as job stress arose in the 1970s, and today it is recognized as a global phenomenon that is of significance due to the negative changes that result from it in both people and their workplace environments (Maslach & Leiter, 2017; Schaufeli, Leiter, & Maslach, 2009). Despite the noteworthy implications of burnout, there continues to be wide variation in terms of how it is defined, what contributes to the manifestation of it, how to treat it, and how to prevent it. In some countries, for instance, *burnout* is an actual medical diagnosis, while in others it is a nonmedical label (Schaufeli et al., 2009). Imagine being able to legitimately call in sick with a diagnosis of burnout!

The term burnout really caught on as an acute form of job stress when a psychiatrist equated the emotional exhaustion and loss of commitment he and others experienced in their work with the lasting effects of chronic drug abuse exhibited in drug abusers (Freudenberger, 1975). Around the same period, a social psychologist, Christina Maslach (1976, 1982), was studying the emotions of individuals who worked in human services. In her interviews with people, many voiced feeling emotionally exhausted, had negative feelings about their patients and coworkers, and questioned their own abilities as professionals. They referred to what they were feeling as "burnout," and many of them identified it with feelings of energy depletion, hence, the idea that one is "running on empty."

While the bulk of early studies focused on burnout in the caring professions, research later extended into all kinds of workplaces and we now know that one does not have to be in a caring profession to experience burnout. As of 2009, it was estimated that there were over 6,000 publications on the topic (Schaufeli et al., 2009); by now there must be well over 10,000. A countless number of studies have been performed and various healing strategies developed to address the syndrome.

DEFINING BURNOUT

Burnout is a broad-based syndrome that develops gradually as a person interacts with his or her workplace: "When the workplace does not recognize the human side of work or demands superhuman efforts, people feel overloaded, frustrated, and well, burned out" (Maslach & Leiter, 1999, p. 50). It can also be associated with an imbalance of demand and resources along with the fact that the ideal and the real often differ to the extent that one is frequently chasing rainbows that dissipate when approached. Burned-out people feel hopeless to create change, and so over time they flick a shutoff switch.

Disenchanted and Disillusioned

In a way, burnout is a widespread disenchantment with one's work. Karl Emil Maximilian Weber (known as Max Weber, 1958), a German sociologist and political economist, discussed the concept of *disenchantment* as the manifestation of a generalized devaluing of beliefs accompanied by an increased valuing of scientific rationalization in modernity. Sadly, it often seems that this is what we are doing in both nursing education and practice. We are devaluing our core values and beliefs while elevating the scientific knowledge base of nursing. On another level, I suppose one could equate disenchantment with dehumanization, for when you remove the subjective and replace it with only the objective, you remove most of what makes us uniquely human. Disenchantment is sometimes equated with disillusionment, a rude awakening of sorts where one is faced with a reality that is less than ideal.

When we are enchanted, we are enamored with something—we value it as something worthwhile. We are more apt to be engaged, interested, and motivated because we like whatever it is we are doing or are "enchanted with." Conversely, when we are disenchanted, we are more likely to be disengaged, disinterested, and unmotivated. We are emotionally empty—heart empty—and suffer with a generalized apathy. It is a form of suffering that transforms our very being into an almost *nonbeing* kind of existence. It is when we become routinely robotic!

Of all the professions, nursing is the one that has been most studied in relation to the phenomenon of burnout. Why is that the case? Because there are so many things inherent in the profession that set us up for burnout—we are the people most at risk to develop it!

WHAT STACKS THE DECK FOR NURSES TO BURN OUT?

To list the things that put the odds in our favor, I will reiterate the obvious. We have been, and continue to be, a predominantly female profession and, as I already noted, women are *not* equal to men in all cultures and environments.

Women remain the predominant carers in the home for loved ones, where there often is unequal work distribution related to household responsibilities. As Chenevert (1988) noted, "While today's women are expected to bring home the bacon, today's men are still not expected to fry it" (p. 124). A case in point is the too-frequent occasion when I arrive home at 9 p.m., after putting in a 16-hour day, and my husband will tell me he has not eaten dinner. I might respond that I have not had a moment to go to the bathroom, let alone eat a meal, and that I ate Twinkies for breakfast, lunch, and dinner. His typical response will be something along the lines of, "You could call for a pizza." Geez, he is doing me a favor . . . I do not have to cook! To be fair, I did choose to work at a university several hours away from home—that is not his fault. But surely there is something lopsided here—just once, couldn't he cook or at least call for the pizza?!

Pecking Orders Prevail . . .

Physicians continue to be predominantly male, and this is at least partly responsible for why there seems to be a natural pecking order that goes from them to us. The "physician's order" mentality prevails in academia, practice, and also policy. A case in point is the advent of the *Physician Orders for Life-Sustaining Treatment* (POLST). In some states, advanced practice nurses (APNs) and other healthcare professionals may also use the POLST forms. Yet, they are labeled a "physician's order." To give credit where due, it should be noted that some areas are a bit more diplomatic (less paternalistic) about it and refer to the form as the *Medical Orders for Life-Sustaining Treatment* (MOLST). The point is, with the continued use of paternalistic expressions comes a message that the physician is the superior.

Who gets paid better, the physician or the nurse? Who works better hours and is able to, for the most part, choose which days can be taken off for play? And, who seems to be more respected by others both in and out of healthcare settings? For example, it is puzzling that we have so many incredible nurses with much to impart to others and who speak so eloquently, and yet there continue to be major nursing conferences where physicians are the keynote speakers . . . conversely, I have yet to hear of a nurse being the keynote speaker at a major medical conference. Why is that? I definitely do not have an answer. When nurses become regular keynote speakers at physician events, it will be a sure sign that something has fundamentally changed for the better in terms of nurses being valued as "full partners."

Please do not think that I am making this all about the male–female disparities that continue to be prominent in all business sectors, including academia, where it is well known that women do not get paid as much or advance as quickly as men. Do male nurses suffer from compassion fatigue and burnout? Absolutely! But many of the issues that prevail in nursing do so because of the male–female thing, the gender inequity that persists both overtly and covertly. Virginia Valian, professor of psychology and linguistics at Hunter College and the Graduate Center of City University of New York, has studied and written quite a lot about the subject. She had pointed out that women continue to make less money and advance more slowly in *every* field, *including nursing* (Valian, 2006). A more recently published article reports no narrowing of the pay gap between male and female nurses over time—across settings, specialties, and positions (Muench, Sindelar, Busch, & Buerhaus, 2015).

I am not necessarily advocating that nurses need to earn more money; clearly the economics of the healthcare system is such that in order to pay higher salaries one would have to decrease the number of nurses who work in the healthcare system, and that would only make things worse. What I am emphasizing is that wherever there is inequitable distribution of rewards *and* respect, there is bound to be an unhappy workforce. Society in general places higher accord to those who earn better salaries. Why this is the case has never made much sense to me. Perhaps it is because those who earn more seem to have more (from a materialistic point of view, anyway). Nevertheless, most nurses did not go into nursing because of the amount of money that we could earn, or the material things we could buy, for surely, if one can become a nurse, *one could become most anything else*.

Burnout is said to be the result of cumulative frustration with one's workplace environment, and for nurses, many of the things that contribute to our frustration are more relational in nature than anything else. They have to do with whom we work (both patients and coworkers), how we interact with each other, and whether we are respected and valued for what it is we do. Far too often, our interpersonal relationships at work are less than satisfactory. A number of factors feed into this as well, including status and role incongruities, different personalities, organizational structure, and obviously, leadership styles (see also Chapters 9 and 13).

Since a lot of the things nurses do are not valued, many who began their careers as very compassionate, competent carers, over time seem to value less the caring aspects of their own work. It is then that the technical skills and the lab values might become more important than the human-to-human connection. I think of this as *disenchantment in action*. The purported science of nursing becomes more important than the art of nursing, and, as a result, the science of nursing becomes more visible, while the art of nursing is discernibly less visible and in some cases seems to disappear altogether. When that occurs, with it comes burnout.

Nursing Education

Our nursing education helps us stack the deck against ourselves, not only by often accentuating what is deemed the science of nursing while minimizing the art of nursing (for lack of a better term to denote the caring relational aspects of our practice) in our basic education, but also because we continue to have multiple entry levels into practice. With diploma, AD, BS, MS, and doctoral-level entry programs, and then all the certificate programs, it really is difficult for people to understand the role of the nurse. We have, in recent years, shifted things yet one more time, adding in the clinical nurse leader (CNL)[1] and doctor of nursing practice (DNP) programs to confuse the public and other members of the healthcare team even more. I am not saying that there is no value in these roles; quite the contrary. Having developed the first CNL program in the New York City area, I am without a doubt committed to anything that will help enhance the quality of healthcare rendered to all.

Advanced practice nursing roles are of enormous importance in our healthcare system and I certainly support pushing their education level up to a clinical doctorate (the DNP). The intricacy of multiple diagnoses and treatments, along with the chaos and complexity of the systems themselves, is such that more education is necessary to prepare APNs. Still, there remains the fact that we have had the clinical nurse specialist (CNS) role, which has never been clearly delineated. Having worked as a CNS, I can say that far too often CNSs find themselves in positions where they are not valued and where they have to repeatedly explain what they do and how it impacts care outcomes as well as patient and staff satisfaction. Then we have had the nurse practitioner (NP), who frequently works in a medical model and feels, for whatever reason, constrained by the organizational policies, which many times conflict with nursing's core values. All of these factor into the manifestation of burnout syndrome (I return to nursing education in Chapter 12).

Devaluing of the Caring Aspects of Nursing

Minimizing what we refer to as the "art" of nursing—devaluing the importance of the compassionate caring practices of our work—along with the nondevelopment of advocacy and assertiveness skills has contributed to us having a workforce that has been relatively easy to oppress. Increasing our scientific knowledge while minimizing the study and application of the things that enable us to engage in caring practices has *not* empowered us. Instead, a vicious cycle has ensued—where the oppressed have become the oppressors, and this, in turn, has made many of our workplaces toxic, with bullying behavior rampant (see Chapter 9). All of these things contribute to stacking the deck.

The devaluing of the caring aspects of nursing includes the widespread teaching of depersonalization. Since burnout, at least in part, seems to stem from our inability to fulfill our inherent need to connect with others and to know that we are making a difference in the world, it does not make any sense to teach depersonalization. I have heard thousands of nurses and nursing students over the years say that they were taught *not* to use first names, *not* to cry in a patient's room, *not* to hug or show patients or their loved ones affection, *not* to become "emotionally" connected. Never were they taught how to just be present. Indeed, I, too, was taught in this manner. It is typically called "therapeutic use of self," and some semblance of this idea is taught in every healthcare profession. But it really is not therapeutic; it actually encourages the use of distancing when performing patient care. Pettigrew (1990) pointed out that therapeutic use of self is not the same as providing presence. He noted that a "nurse may be physically present, even attentive, and still refuse to give self in an interaction," whereas "presence . . . means making room internally for the other person, being willing to be involved, to be there wholeheartedly" (p. 503).

In the burnout literature, depersonalization is equated with cynicism and detachment from the job. And here we are, from the beginning, teaching our nurses that they need to maintain distance in order to do the job well. Some start off their careers already burned out! Or, at the very least, they become compassion fatigued early on, perhaps even while still in school. I have heard it said that we go into the profession of nursing with a naïve idealism that is quickly knocked out of us in the harshness of the workplace and that it is the real conflicting with the ideal that makes us more vulnerable to the syndrome of burnout. The fact is that naiveté alone cannot account for our vulnerability to burnout; *we* have to take responsibility for at least some of what ensues to ultimately "set us up" for these syndromes.

PHASES OF BURNOUT

Psychologists Herbert Freudenberger and Gail North (Kraft, 2006) identified a number of phases of burnout. They may not occur in any particular order, and they all do not have to manifest in order for someone to be experiencing burnout:

1. The Compulsion to Prove Oneself
2. Working Harder
3. Neglecting Their Needs
4. Displacement of Conflicts
5. Revision of Values
6. Denial of Emerging Problems
7. Withdrawal
8. Obvious Behavioral Changes
9. Depersonalization
10. Inner Emptiness
11. Depression
12. Burnout Syndrome (Kraft, 2006, p. 31)

Individuals who are developing burnout will frequently appear to be ambitious. Wanting to prove themselves, they work harder and harder, and as they try to demonstrate worthiness, they let go of other important things (Freudenberger & North, 1985), such as not taking care of themselves (eating and sleeping poorly) and spending less time with loved ones. It seems as if their values have changed—things that were important to them before no longer seem so.

At some point burned-out individuals become aware that there is something wrong, but they are unable to define it—it is at this stage that physical manifestations commonly begin to appear (Freudenberger & North, 1985; Kraft, 2006). Despite the recognition that something is wrong, many individuals will not confront the issues and instead become intolerant, cynical, and even aggressive (bullying behaviors may arise). Withdrawal, apathy, and depersonalization are characteristic and can lead to depression, with increasing feelings of hopelessness. At its most extreme, burnout syndrome can lead a person who is afflicted to thoughts of suicide and, for some, to eventual suicidal acts (Freudenberger & North, 1985).

So How Do You Know if You Are Burned Out?

Exhaustion is said to be the classic sign of burnout; however, as a stand-alone, it does not capture the essence of this complex phenomenon, especially since compassion fatigued individuals are also often exhausted physically, psychologically, and/or spiritually. Maslach (1993) identified three core dimensions of burnout: (a) an overwhelming feeling of exhaustion, (b) feelings of cynicism and detachment from the job, and (c) a sense of ineffectiveness and lack of accomplishment. Research in the area of burnout has led to the creation of various assessment tools, the predominant one being the Maslach Burnout Inventory (MBI), which measures all three dimensions (Maslach, Jackson, & Leiter, 1997).

Accumulating data suggest that there is a progression from exhaustion to cynicism over time; however, it remains unclear as to when feelings of ineffectiveness may come into play (Maslach, Schaufeli, & Leiter, 2001). Although the first and last dimensions are self-explanatory, the second—cynicism—requires an explanation. Many people take cynicism to mean sarcasm, scorn, and/or skepticism; however, as a dimension of burnout, cynicism really refers to feelings of pessimism, which then manifest as detachment and disengagement. As Leiter and Maslach (2009) noted:

> Burnout is one end of a continuum in the relationship people
> establish with their jobs, and stands in contrast to the opposite pole

Table 8.1 Burnout–Contentment Spectrum

Burnout	Contentment
Exhaustion	Increased energy
Disengagement	Engagement
Feelings of ineffectiveness	Feelings of effectiveness

of engagement, in which people experience energy, involvement with their work, and feelings of effectiveness. (p. 332)

Thus, what we have is as shown in Table 8.1.

Unlike compassion fatigue, which is sudden in onset, burnout sneaks up on you, developing gradually over time. Pfifferling and Gilley (2000) differentiate between burnout and compassion fatigue by noting that individuals suffering from burnout tend to emotionally withdraw and display diminished empathy, whereas individuals with compassion fatigue will continue to give of themselves despite it wearing them down. It is said that if compassion fatigue is recognized and addressed early enough, burnout, which is more pervasive and difficult to recover from, may be prevented (Benson & Magraith, 2005).

Chenevert (1985) noted the importance of anger, how it helps us cleanse our minds and can also help renew our interest and enthusiasm for work. She also made the astute observation that anger may well be a precursor of burnout, noting that "usually before you burn out, you have to burn up" (p. 47). Herein one can see a clear relation to the topic of moral distress discussed earlier. The morally distressed nurse will feel frustration and anger; channeled appropriately, it can lead to butterfly power of a good sort. Anger is a meaningful transformation of energy; whether it is turned inward or outward, it is very meaningful. It means that change is needed. Just as a little bit of anxiety can be a good thing, a little bit of righteous anger can impel us to seek change, and that is always a good thing when you are unhappy with a set of circumstances. What we do not want is for moral residue to build up.

It has been noted that both compassion fatigue and burnout seem to arise as a result of failed survival strategies related to the inability to achieve one's goals (Valent, 2002). It would seem that burnout is a kind of defense mechanism similar to pulling your hand away from something hot. Shut the switch, pull the plug, become numb, and protect yourself. The difference and the irony is that in flicking the shutoff switch, we actually hurt ourselves as well as others.

There are a great many signs and symptoms that may manifest when one is suffering from burnout. I especially like Chenevert's (1985) list, which includes whining and bitching, among other appropriately labeled common behavior patterns (p. 47). Typical signs and symptoms of burnout include physical and emotional exhaustion, feelings of hopelessness and/or helplessness, depersonalization–dehumanization, disenchantment, forgetfulness, apathy, irritability, melancholy, reduced efficiency, and discontent with achievement (Langle, 2003; Pross, 2006). Tack on all of the previously listed signs and symptoms of compassion fatigue noted in Chapter 6 that are not listed here and add in just about any other human indication of suffering (physical, psychological, and spiritual), and you have a pretty good picture of the enormity of the situation. Burnout is serious stuff.

The one thing that is absolutely a sure sign of burnout is when you *really* hate getting up and going to work. At that point you are in genuine trouble, and, unfortunately, so are your coworkers, your patients, and your loved ones!

To recap, compare, and contrast, the nurse who is *heartful* is manifesting love and caring; she will be a compassionate carer and in return will feel good. She still works terribly hard and rarely takes a break but does not feel fatigued at the end of the day; instead she feels energized and goes home thinking that her job has been done well. The meaning and purpose of her work are evident, from which comes a sense of contentment. Some would say she is in flow; others might call it second wind. It is all about energy transformation. This goes back to the earlier discussion on how we actualize our potentials. Conversely, the nurse who is *heart empty*, or seemingly *heartless*, is just the opposite; she is manifesting apathy and perhaps lethargy; she will be a dispassionate carer and will not feel good about herself. She feels exhausted, energy depleted, and never goes home feeling like her job has been done well. She feels disheartened, hopeless, joyless, and numb.

WHERE WAS THE NURSE?

Recently, an article came across my desk that focused on the care of "cancer survivors," prompting me to relive yet again my experience as a patient who had just had major surgery for uterine cancer. At the memory, I hemmed and hawed whether I should include this particular story here and finally my emotion won out. What follows highlights an especially horrid experience for me (Todaro-Franceschi, 2007).

I requested to have a private room postoperatively, but there were none. My roommate was very confused; she kept running over to my bed. At one point she wanted to smoke one of my mouth swabs. It was a neurological oncology unit and while it was not surprising to find confused patients there, I was a fresh post-op *total abdominal hysterectomy, bilateral salpingo-oophorectomy* (TAH BSO) with *lymphadenectomy* patient (with a suture line even longer than the name of the procedure), and I was fully cognizant although not very mobile. Needless to say, I was scared to death! I could not guard myself; it was difficult enough just to take deep breaths.

My family, having stayed until I was admitted to a unit, formed a body shield around my bed and was insistent that I be moved to a safer place. Where was the nurse who admitted me into this bed on this unit, I wondered? I recalled that as a staff nurse I had always tried to have final say as to which room on the unit my patients would be admitted. I know I would not have willingly put a fresh post-op patient in with a confused ambulatory patient.

After what seemed like an eternity, but I am sure was no more than an hour or so, I was moved into another room via bed with all the typical amount of banging into doorways and things along the way. The jarring added salt to the wound; my body already felt so badly beaten. My new room was empty, but there was room for two patients, and shortly afterward, someone was admitted into the other bed. The standard process of admitting histories, assessments, and treatments transpired. The physicians (there were two) were fairly loud and I lay there wondering, where was the nurse? The compassionate person who advocates for patients, the person who would diplomatically tell the physicians to take their discussion of their private lives outside?

After some time contemplating the idiosyncrasies of just trying to close my eyes in this unrelentingly noisy environment, I decided to try to advocate for myself. I spent some time wondering just how I should approach this. Should I tell the physicians to stop discussing their vacations while working with a patient? Should I tell them I am having difficulty getting comfortable and really need to try to sleep? Or should I quietly call the nurse and ask her to advocate for me? Finally, I just decided to use the call bell and asked the nurse if there might be an alternative place for me.

Another period of time went by. I was told that there (miraculously) was a private room and once again I was hauled via bed out of the room; of course, did you doubt? The bed banging into the doorway and down the hall, and I was unceremoniously dumped, or at least it felt so, into a private room, but I was so very relieved. For the rest of the evening and night until 8:00 the following morning, no one came to check my vital signs or to see how I was doing. It was ok, my husband and daughter were nearby, but still I could not help wondering, where was the nurse?

There was this doctor of osteopathic medicine (DO) specializing in gynecologic oncology who was covering for my surgeon and who came around every once in a while, beginning on post-op day 1. She always started her assessment by saying, "my hands are cold," immediately before she put them on me to assess my wounded, distended, hurting abdomen. Her hands were like ice, though they did not really bother me since I was in nonstop hot flash mode, but still I wondered, why could she not rub them together and warm them up prior to touching her patients? In this instance I was a patient, not a nurse, and I thought that it was not my place to tell her how to handle her patients. But I know that as a nurse, had I noticed this DO's problem with cold hands, and had she tried to touch my patients after announcing repeatedly that her hands were cold, I would certainly have mentioned to her how quickly and easily she could warm her hands prior to laying them on *my* patients. I reflected that perhaps no one else had yet noticed this little problem.

The second night postoperatively I developed acute abdominal distention. In the middle of the night I started to have dry heaves; I hadn't eaten anything. My abdomen was huge and board-like. I called the nurse and she answered via intercom; I explained to her, in between these awful dry heaves, how I felt. She did not come to the room and instead proceeded to tell me via intercom that she would inform the doctor on call. I thought, if only I had a stethoscope. Then again, I knew there would be no bowel sounds. Not one nurse had touched my abdomen or listened for bowel sounds since I had been admitted to the unit. I rationalized this by reminding myself that it was a neurological oncology unit, though assessing bowel sounds is very basic nursing.

A little time went by, actually 45 minutes, but it felt like forever to me. I called the nurse again and this time she informed me via intercom that the physician was up on another unit taking care of a patient. I told her I really needed someone to come see me. A little while later she came in with an oral dose of the antiemetic Zofran and proceeded to tell me the doctor "ordered" this for my abdominal discomfort, but that the doctor could not come to the unit to see me because she was making rounds on patients upstairs.

In between dry heaves, I tried to explain that I did not have any nausea. I pointed to my huge abdomen. Yet, she did not seem to understand or recognize the potentially serious nature of what was going on with me. She instead informed me that "there are some really sick patients on this unit" and that "it's already almost 5 a.m.; the doctor will be making rounds in an hour or so." Essentially, she implied that I could wait and finished with, "here is the medication, this is what the doctor 'ordered' for you." She put the medication on the bedside table and left the room.

At that point I was desperate, knowing well that the Zofran would not help me one bit. How could it? But I took it anyway and proceeded to vomit the pill back out with my next dry heave. As I stared at the whole pill there in my emesis basin, my tears flowed, and I put the call bell on again. This time when the nurse answered through the intercom, I insisted that someone either get a physician immediately or provide me with my surgeon's home telephone number. Another period of time went by, and finally someone came to see me. It was the DO with the very cold hands.

For three days and nights postoperatively, I cared for myself with the help of my loved ones. After I received several laxatives, I could finally pass gas and no longer had dry heaves, but then I could not eat anything without having to go to the bathroom. And with the abdominal suture line the bedpan was even less friendly than it would usually be, and my sense of urgency was such that I was sure I would not be able to move quickly enough to get to the bathroom. So, I asked for a commode and one was brought into the room.

Since I had been admitted to this unit, no one had asked if I needed anything or offered to assist me with bathing or to get out of bed and walk. I did my own I & Os and assessment. Not one person ever looked into the commode or offered to clean it out. Thank heaven for my family; they rotated shifts to be with me throughout this ordeal. My spirit was truly broken; I just could not imagine caring for anyone like this. I wondered if it was because I was not a neurological cancer patient, or because I was 47 and not elderly or younger, or because perhaps I had upset the nurses with my repeated requests for a private room.

An APN who covered this area stopped in to visit. She was lovely, compassionate, and efficient. She asked me about everything and I told her a bit of my plight; my intestinal problems were consuming me still and she empathized with me. She told me that the unit is run mostly by travel nurses because there was a very high, frequent turnover of staff and that it was a hard unit for everyone to work on. I told her I understood how difficult the work of the nurse is, and that I was a nurse myself, but in my head I was thinking that having a *hard* job could not account for the dispassionate and sometimes substandard care I received during my stay there.

Four days postoperatively, still suffering with too frequent bouts of diarrhea, my daughter noted that there was no running water in the bathroom. I called the nurse and was told that they were doing renovations on another floor and she guessed that they had to shut off the water. I was told to be patient, but in the meantime, my loved ones could carry the dirty pot from the commode across the entire unit to the soiled utility room where they could rinse it. They could also get water from there and carry it back to my room. I was horrified.

Hours into the day with no water, and several bowel movements later, my surgeon walked in on rounds with his entourage of staff. I broke down completely and in a fit of absolute despair and anger, I told him about my experience on this unit. I told him about his DO's cold hands, and about not being sick enough to warrant a nurse walking into the room or to have a physician come down to the unit to see me in the middle of the night when I was having such difficulty. I tried to explain what it felt like to have dry heaves 24 hours postoperatively with my abdominal suture line, and what it felt like to watch my loved ones, with no sleep, provide the care that I would willingly give to anyone as a nurse if he or she were my patient. What it felt like to be the recipient of such awful care, having been a dedicated nurse for so many years, advocating and caring for people, both patients and nurses alike.

I told him that I could have been anything, could have done anything, but that I chose nursing because I love what I do; I love making a difference in people's lives. I told him how I have looked forward to getting up each morning and going to work, and that the few times during my career where I did not, I knew that it was time to change jobs and I did so. I pointed out that there were way too many folks at his hospital who obviously did not like getting up and coming to work each day.

I finished my heartfelt tirade with the fact that I had no running water in the bathroom for much of the day, that I had had too many bowel movements to count, and that my family was running back and forth across the unit to go to the soiled utility room to clean out the commode and to get water. He and his group of interns, residents, and an APN were very close to tears by the time I finished. It was clear that they were all appalled. Truth be told, so was I. I had never intended "to wash my dirty laundry in public," so to speak. I was ashamed, for me and also for my profession.

Shortly thereafter, the very same day, my surgeon had me transferred up to the gynecologic oncology unit. The minute I was wheeled onto the unit I felt the change in environment. It was far less stressed, the walls were painted in pastel colors, and there were motivational pictures all around. The nurses seemed so much happier, too. I felt better just being there, and while I had intuitively understood before, I now understand firsthand why Nightingale underscored the importance of the environment for healing. I felt an immense relief immediately upon arriving on that unit.

The following afternoon I was discharged from the hospital. What did I learn from this experience? I learned that the environment can make all the difference when it comes to healing and that it absolutely is not enough to have the best surgeon; one has to have compassionate, competent nurses to assist in the healing process. I experienced firsthand that disenchantment and dispassionate care go together and comprise key manifestations of the "ugly." The nurses who worked on the neurological unit were clearly unhappy, and it showed in the way they provided care for me. It almost seemed as if the nurse had disappeared entirely, and in her place was an unthinking, uncaring—inhuman—thing. A robot.

THE CONSEQUENCES OF BURNOUT

At this point, no one has to tell you what is at stake; still, I would like to stress that all of what is at risk begins with *our* own health and well-being. Very often the professional literature available to nurses—staff, leaders, and educators—focuses on issues of care performance, quality, safety, productivity, outcomes, and so forth. Yes, that is all important and it is all one; however, at its center is *us*. We are the most important piece of the healthcare system. In fact, as I have already noted elsewhere (and will continue to do), we are so darn important that without *us*, the healthcare system will cease to exist. We must care for ourselves before we can be in an optimal place to care for others. We need to tend to us, personally, professionally, and wholly.

As mentioned, the refined model for Magnet® hospitals includes five key components: transformational leadership; structural empowerment; exemplary professional nursing practice; new knowledge innovations and improvements; and empirical outcomes (Wolf, Triolo, Reid-Ponte, Drenkard, & Moran, 2011). Notably, the model emphasizes the importance of the relational aspects of the work environment in a number of ways. Both patient and nursing satisfaction are given equal attention in addition to clinical outcome measures. The message is clear. It is just not enough to aspire to have great clinical outcomes; people satisfaction (people being both the cared for and the carers) is important too, and without addressing this, we may not be able to attain positive outcomes at all.

Economically, it is not savvy to ignore the needs of the carers, especially nurse carers. By 2025, there will be an increased demand for, and at least in some geographic areas, a significantly reduced supply of, nurses. The 2017 annual report on RN staffing indicates that while nurse retention has improved a little, the vacancy rate has increased and the anticipated shortage of nurses is returning (Nursing Solutions, Inc. [NSI], 2017). We know that job satisfaction is the biggest predictor of whether or not one will stay in a position (Böckerman & Ilmakunnas, 2008), and while we often may not know which comes first, the dissatisfaction or the burnout, we do know that they are linked to one another (Maslach et al., 2001).

Replacing just one unhappy nurse who leaves her job can cost an organization between $38,900 and $59,700 and according to the most recent survey on RN staffing, results in the average hospital losing $5.13M to $7.86M annually (NSI, 2017). And unhappy nurses who stay on the job probably cost their workplaces even more. Absenteeism, lateness, and poor job performance/productivity are all associated with burnout, not to mention that a lack of commitment to the workplace results in a domino effect: it is contagious. So here we have just a few miserable burnt-out nurses on a unit; they call in sick, show up late, do not do their jobs well, and they are not nice to their coworkers. What happens? Everyone on the unit is affected, and ultimately the domino effect results in an ugly transformation of the quality of care rendered to people, people who are depending on and trusting us to care for them. Why am I referring to a domino effect here and not a butterfly effect? Because the transformation that occurs really is not subtle at all (and because butterflies are nice and this is so ugly!).

Nurses repeatedly say stress is interfering with patient care. In one Canadian study, it was found that medication errors were linked to inadequate staffing and resources, feelings of exhaustion or overload, working overtime, poor nurse–physician relations, low coworker support, and low job security (Wilkins & Shields, 2008). All things that contribute to burnout. The dynamics of the whole must be acknowledged.

Complaisance Does Not Fit With Compassionate Care

Working with inadequate resources or in an unhealthy environment, and having an administration that does not hear the voice of nurses when we assert ourselves on behalf of our patients, can result in complaisance. It should not happen, but it does. Complaisance is one form of silence. Being acquiescent, not speaking up about things that affect your practice, for example, consistently working with a lack of basic resources, is passive unhealthy behavior. It is injurious because being silent about things that should matter leads to moral distress, moral residue, and, eventually, burnout. When a nurse is burned out, the apathy results in silence. Remaining silent about one's unhappiness extends to being silent about practice issues—issues the nurse no longer seems to care about. This can include bearing witness to all kinds of negative influences—both covert and overt. The burnt-out nurse becomes a "silent voice" and a "silent witness."

One story comes to mind where a nurse told me that she had worked on a unit with no call bell system for over a year's time after the system had been destroyed due to a storm. All the nurses had repeatedly documented that it was unsafe to work in that environment. They were rightfully distraught about it. Unbelievably, the nurse told me that they were given *ding dongs* (little silver bells) to pass out to all the patients. I am sure that when she told me, my eyes bulged. I was freaked out. I am still freaked out, writing about it now. Imagine. . . those little silver bells getting lost in the linen, or being dropped on the floor. Perhaps a patient fracturing a hip trying to climb out of bed to get the bell to call someone for help? Despite the very real moral distress and fear for their own safety, the nurses continued to show up to work in that environment as if they had no choice in the matter. The fact is, they had a choice, but for varied reasons, chose not to act. Fear of retaliation, in this case, loss of work and benefits, makes some go along to get along, doing everyone a disservice. Still, think about this: If those nurses all banded together and chose not to work in that environment until the call bell system had been fixed, could they all have been fired together? Well, maybe…but heck, I really doubt it. Cause then the media would have told the story and ultimately, it would have been a win-win for the nurses, the patients, and the public at large.

APPLYING *ART* FOR HEALING BURNOUT

Remember when you first went into nursing? More than likely you were excited at the thought that you would make a difference in the lives of those you cared for. You looked forward to contributing to human health and healing and to learning the "how to's" of nursing. This was not because the things you learned were at the heart of nursing, but because learning the "how to's" got you closer to the essence of nursing: to care for, to assist with healing. Are you still eager? Recall the nurse who shared how she had changed from being outgoing and sociable while working with her patients to preferring to float to the emergency department where she could just "do her work" and not have to spend time interacting with her patients. Do you feel similarly disenchanted? You can apply the *ART*© model (Todaro-Franceschi, 2008, 2013, 2015) once again, as follows.

Step 1: Acknowledge a Feeling or Wound That Needs Healing

The first question you need to ask yourself (or if you are a nurse leader or educator ask your staff or students) is the one I offered at the beginning of the book. Do you look forward to going to work? If the answer is no, then you must ask why.

Are you working with people who do nothing but complain and who seem cynical, complaisant, and perhaps callous? Are you one of those people? Do you work with patients who are suffering and no longer feel any anguish on their behalf? Do you walk into a room with loved ones surrounding the bed of one of your acutely ill patients and shut a switch or block any exchange of feelings with your methodical actions to provide care?

As you go about your work, make an effort to be mindfully aware of the things that you dislike or things that you *used* to dislike and no longer notice. You may be surprised to find that there is a lot that used to bother you and no longer does. Such is the case with burned-out carers. At some point, you will want to recapture those feelings related to the things that used to bother you. You want to acknowledge them because they hold the key not only to healing but also to evading compassion fatigue and burnout in the future. It might be helpful to draw two columns and label them as shown in Table 8.2.

Table 8.2 Reasons For and Against Going to Work

Reasons Why I Do Not Want to Go to Work	Reasons Why I Go to Work
1. _____	1. _____
2. _____	2. _____
3. _____	3. _____
4. _____	4. _____

Warning! If you are really unhappy, you might need more room for that column on the left, and if that is the case, take out your notebook or journal. You might also want to pick up the newspaper to begin looking for a new position!

Complete the burnout part of the questionnaire in Stamm's (2010) ProQOL survey in Appendix A. Are you manifesting any of the negative behaviors, feelings, and physical ailments related to burnout? Carefully reflect upon the reasons why you do not want to go to work. What seem to be the most outstanding things on your list? What is the deal breaker for you . . . is it your relationship with coworkers or other members on the healthcare team, workload, a lack of resources, or perhaps even the patient population you are working with? It could be anything—it is your responsibility to identify and acknowledge it. Once you do, you are ready to proceed to the next step. Since burnout develops over time and there are usually a lot of things contributing to it, your healing from it will not happen overnight. Be kind and patient with yourself.

Step 2: *Recognize Choices and Take Purposeful Action*

Once you have identified the reasons why you (or your staff or students) do not want to go to work, you are ready to explore how you might be able to change or facilitate changes in your workplace to enable you (or staff/students) to reaffirm purpose in your work. Are the reasons relational? In other words, is your unhappiness predominantly due to relationships with your leaders, coworkers, or others? Are you lacking a sense of communality—connectedness? Or is it related more to the physical environment?

Things such as chronic short staffing, high acuity, lack of resources such as linens, medications, and so forth, all make for a crummy physical environment, but there are other things that can contribute to an unhealthy workplace. A case in point was a story I heard at a conference a number of years back about a pediatric emergency room where there was no quiet place for families to go and be with their loved ones when a child died. The staff nurses were unhappy, to say the least. One day they got a great idea. There was a little closet off to the side, not much used. They asked for and received administrative permission to move everything out and went on to create a beautiful quiet space. It made a world of difference to the staff to be able to do that for those grieving families and alleviated a lot of additional suffering. Imagine the difference it made for the loved ones of the children who died.

Do you have things on your unit that are making you dislike your work? Can you make changes in your practice or the work environment that can help you to reaffirm your purpose? What choices do you have that might make things better for you and for your patients? List them. Can you approach your administrative staff alone or do you need the support of coworkers? Who might listen to your concerns and support you in making the necessary changes in practice?

Are you suffering with physical or mental health issues as a consequence of your work? If so, you need to make choices that will help you to regain your well-being. A first step is to meet with your primary care provider and talk about it. If you are feeling depressed or are self-medicating with food, alcohol, pills, or some other form of drug, now is the time to seek appropriate help for it. Remember, as knowing participants there are always choices we can make (please see Appendix C, Resources).

With burnout, it is important to recognize that even though you do have many choices, you may not be able to make things better enough to be able to stay in the work environment that you are currently in and be happy or healthy. It may be impossible to regain your well-being and a sense of purpose working in the same place. It might be time for you to change positions. Some things can be fixed and some cannot. It is not a failure to acknowledge it is time to move on—it is a choice—and it may be the best one for you. Keep in mind the often-used quote of Coco Chanel's famous words, "Don't spend time beating on a wall, hoping to transform it into a door."

Step 3: *Turn Outward Toward Self and Other*

In order to heal from burnout once you have identified it, you must make a real effort to be mindfully aware of how you are acting and how others are acting in the workplace. In the literature on relational practices in organizations and systems, when important things like compassion and connection are overlooked, it is frequently referred to as "disappeared," because these important things are not "celebrated, valued or reinforced in any systematic way" (Frost, 1999, p. 130). To undo the harm of long-standing toxicity, we need to make these important things *reappear*. The way to do that is by turning outward—being mindfully aware that this is a process of relearning ourselves by noting patterns of negativity and replacing those patterns with attentive listening and presencing for both ourselves and others.

Reconnecting with our spiritual selves and perhaps one's religiosity is helpful, not only for finding meaning and purpose in life but in the seeming absence of it; our awareness of the interrelatedness of everything can help us to *make* meaning in our lives. Look for things you do not normally notice (or no longer notice). Remember the reconnect contention!

PREVENTION: "BURNIN" AND BRIGHTLY BURNING

Prevention strategies for us as a profession need to begin in nursing education and then continue in practice environments. In one article written on the topic, nurse Kathleen Magill (1982) outlined a process that she called *burnin* to help future nurses develop the necessary coping skills that would enable them to become effective change agents. Burnin includes learning self-care strategies as well as conflict resolution and assertiveness skills.

Magill (1982) also wrote about what she called "the brightly burning," those nurses who were, despite everything, able to cope with stress and avert burnout. She suggested that it would be in our best interests to study those brightly burning nurses to identify their strengths, support systems, and change agency abilities. She noted that, "Most agencies seem to have some professional nursing personnel who manage to humanize and upgrade professional nursing practice in spite of conditions that burn out many other nurses" (p. 20). She went on to note: "If we focus exclusively on the burnout phenomenon in our nursing research, we may unwittingly build in a self-fulfilling prophecy that suggests that nurses tend to burn out" (p. 20).

When working as an upper-level manager, Magill (1982) performed an informal survey of nurses who she considered to be "burning brightly," and while it was a small study ($N = 35$), with an admittedly biased sample, the results were quite interesting. Strong professional self-image, commitment to patients, risk-taking ability, and change agency skills were all apparent and fostered work satisfaction for these nurses. All of these things enhance compassion contentment and are in line with findings from various Magnet studies (Drenkard, Wolf, & Morgan, 2011).

Perhaps the most important prevention strategy is to always hold first and foremost a sense of the meaning and purpose of our nursing work as carers. That has to come from within, but with mindful awareness we can keep it front and center to guide us in our day-to-day practice.

KEY POINTS

- Burnout is a result of interacting in negative ways with one's work environment.

- Burnout in nurses is an ugly transformation in which compassionate care is often replaced with dispassionate care.

- Many things contribute to the development of nurse burnout, including unresolved compassion fatigue, buildup of moral residue, the way one has been educated (or lack thereof), devaluing the art of nursing (the caring aspects of nursing) while stressing the science, inequity in treatment, lack of respect, unrealistic expectations (related to heavy workload, lack of resources, etc.), incivility and bullying in the workplace (and the list goes on and on and on . . .).

- Healing can occur with (a) recognition of the problem and attentive self-reflection upon turning points and experiences that have led up to its development, (b) exploring the choices one has and then choosing purposeful actions to take in order to heal, and (c) a conscious effort to turn outward to reconnect with yourself and others.

- It may not be possible to continue to work in the same place and heal from burnout. It might be necessary to change positions or workplace, in order to achieve a state of well-being and to reaffirm purpose in your work life.

- Remaining in a job or workplace when one is burnt out without seeking help to heal from the syndrome does a serious disservice to everyone—yourself, those you care for, those you work with, your loved ones, and the profession, collectively.

- Prevention strategies include reminding ourselves of the importance, meaning, and purpose of our work.

NOTE

1. CNL is a registered trademark of the American Association of Colleges of Nursing, which created this new nursing role—the first new role in nursing in close to 40 years.

REFERENCES

Benson, J., & Magraith, K. (2005). Compassion fatigue and burnout: The role of Balint groups. *Australian Family Physician*, 34(6), 497–498.

Böckerman, P., & Ilmakunnas, P. (2008). Interaction of working conditions, job satisfaction, and sickness absences: Evidence from a representative sample of employees. *Social Science Medicine*, 67(4), 520–528. doi:10.1016/j.socscimed.2008.04.008

Chenevert, M. (1985). *Pro-nurse handbook: Designed for the nurse who wants to survive/ thrive professionally.* St. Louis, MO: C.V. Mosby.

Chenevert, M. (1988). *STAT: Special techniques in assertiveness training for women in the health professions.* St. Louis, MO: C.V. Mosby.

Drenkard, K., Wolf, G., & Morgan, S. H. (Eds.). (2011). *Magnet®: The next generation—Nurses making the difference*. Silver Spring, MD: American Nurses Credentialing Center.

Freudenberger, H. J. (1975). The staff burnout syndrome in alternative institutions. *Psychotherapy, Theory, Research and Practice, 12*, 72–83. doi:10.1037/h0086411

Freudenberger, H. J., & North, G. (1985). *Women's burnout: How to spot it, how to reverse it, and how to prevent it*. Garden City, NY: Doubleday & Company.

Frost, P. J. (1999). Why compassion counts. *Journal of Management Inquiry, 8*(2), 127–133. doi:10.1177/105649269982004

Kraft, U. (2006, June/July). Burned out. *Scientific American Mind*, 29–33. Retrieved from http://jb-schnittstelle.de/wp-content/uploads/2014/08/Burned-Out.pdf

Langle, A. (2003). Burnout—Existential meaning and possibilities of prevention. *European Psychotherapy, 4*, 107–121.

Leiter, M., & Maslach, C. (2009). Nurse turnover: The mediating role of burnout. *Journal of Nursing Management, 17*, 331–339. doi:10.1111/j.1365-2834.2009.01004.x

Magill, K. A. (1982). Burnin, burnout and the brightly burning. *Nursing Management, 13*, 17–21. doi:10.1097/00006247-198207000-00005

Maslach, C. (1976). Burned-out. *Human Behavior, 5*, 16–22.

Maslach, C. (1982). *Burnout: The cost of caring*. Englewood Cliffs, NJ: Prentice-Hall.

Maslach, C. (1993). Burnout: A multidimensional perspective. In W. B. Schaufeli, C. Maslach, & T. Marek (Eds.), *Professional burnout: Recent developments in theory and research* (pp. 19–32). Washington, DC: Taylor & Francis.

Maslach, C., Jackson, S. E., & Leiter, M. P. (1997). Maslach burnout inventory. In C. P. Zalaquett & R. J. Wood (Eds.), *Evaluating stress: A book of resources* (3rd ed., pp. 191–218). Lanham, MD: The Scarecrow Press.

Maslach, C., & Leiter, M. P. (1999). Take this job and love it! Six ways to beat burnout. *Psychology Today, 32*(5), 50–53.

Maslach, C., & Leiter, M. P. (2017). New insights into burnout and health care: Strategies for improving civility and alleviating burnout. *Medical Teacher, 39*(2), 160–163. doi:10.1080/0142159X.2016.1248918

Maslach, C., Schaufeli, W. B., & Leiter, M. P. (2001). Job burnout. *Annual Review Psychology, 52*, 397–422. doi:10.1146/annurev.psych.52.1.397

Muench, U., Sindelar, J., Busch, S. H., & Buerhaus, P. I. (2015). Salary differences between male and female registered nurses in the United States. *JAMA, 313*(12), 1265–1267. doi:10.1001/jama.2015.1487

NSI Nursing Solutions, Inc. (2017). *National health care retention and RN staffing report*. Retrieved from https://www.emergingrnleader.com/wp-content/uploads/2017/09/NationalHealthcareRNRetentionReport2017.pdf

Pettigrew, J. (1990). Intensive nursing care: The ministry of presence. *Critical Care Nursing Clinics of North America, 2*, 503–508. doi:10.1016/S0899-5885(18)30810-4

Pfifferling, J. H., & Gilley, K. (2000). Overcoming compassion fatigue. *Family Practice Management*, 7(4), 39–44.

Pross, C. (2006). Burnout, vicarious traumatization and its prevention. *Torture, 16*(1), 1–9.

Schaufeli, W. B., Leiter, M. P., & Maslach, C. (2009). Burnout: 35 years of research and practice. *Career Development International, 14*(3), 204–220. doi:10.1108/13620430910966406

Stamm, B. H. (2010). *The ProQOL (Professional Quality of Life Scale: Compassion Satisfaction and Compassion Fatigue)*. Pocatello, ID: ProQOL.org. Retrieved from www.proqol.org

Todaro-Franceschi, V. (2007). Imagining nursing practice in the year 2050: Looking through a Rogerian looking glass. *Nursing Science Quarterly, 20,* 229–231. doi:10.1177/0894318407303441

Todaro-Franceschi, V. (2008). Preventing compassion fatigue and reaffirming purpose in nursing. *Proceedings on the 3rd European Federation of Critical Care Nursing Congress and 27th Aniarti Conference, Influencing Critical Care Nursing in Europe*, Florence, Italy (October).

Todaro-Franceschi, V. (2013). *Compassion fatigue and burnout in nursing: Enhancing professional quality of life*. New York, NY: Springer Publishing.

Todaro-Franceschi, V. (2015). The ART of maintaining the "care" in healthcare. *Nursing Management, 46*(6), 53–55. doi:10.1097/01.numa.0000465407.76450.ab

Valent, P. (2002). Diagnosis and treatment of helper stresses, traumas and illnesses. In C. R. Figley (Ed.), *Treating compassion fatigue* (pp. 17–37). New York, NY: Brunner-Routledge.

Valian, V. (2006). Women at the top in science—and elsewhere. In S. Ceci & W. Williams (Eds.), *Why aren't more women in science?* (pp. 27–37). Washington, DC: American Psychological Association Press.

Weber, M. (1958). *Max Weber: Essays in sociology* (H. H. Gerth & C. W. Mills, Eds. & Trans.). New York, NY: Oxford University Press.

Wilkins, K., & Shields, M. (2008). Correlates of medication error in hospitals. *Health Reports, 19*(2), 7–18.

Wolf, G., Triolo, P., Reid-Ponte, P., Drenkard, K., & Moran, J. (2011). The next generation. In K. Drenkard, G. Wolf, & S. H. Morgan (Eds.), *Magnet®: The next generation—Nurses making the difference* (pp. 23–30). Silver Spring, MD: American Nurses Credentialing Center.

9

Bullying and Incivility in Nursing: An Oxymoron

Not all forms of abuse leave bruises.
—Danielle Steele

For giving voice to open secrets, for moving whisper networks onto social networks, for pushing us all to stop accepting the unacceptable, the Silence Breakers are the 2017 Person of the Year.
—Time Magazine

KEY TOPICS

- Workplace violence and its impact on individual and collective well-being
- Defining incivility, bullying, mobbing, cronyism, and moral muteness
- Silent voices, silent witnesses, and silence breakers
- *ART©* for workplace violence

INTRODUCTION

Incivility, bullying, and mobbing in the workplace directly impact professional quality of life and, for this second edition, I was inspired by many things to give this topic more space. Of late I have started to think of these forms of violence, for violence they are, as "uglier." So, in addition to the

© Springer Publishing Company DOI: 10.1891/9780826155214.0009

good, the bad, the ugly, I have added the uglier and one more, "the ugliest" aspects of nursing professional quality of life. The uglier things unfortunately lead to the very *ugliest* of things; the harming of innocent people because when incivility and bullying occur in healthcare settings, the people who get hurt are not just those who are being bullied. Ultimately, their loved ones, coworkers, and the patients who are being cared for along with their families are also harmed. The point I am stressing is that ultimately, *it is never just one person who gets hurt.*

INCIVILITY AND BULLYING IN HEALTHCARE, REALLY?

Several years back, the 1199 union nursing leadership chose to focus on workforce health for their annual conference. It was a very proactive move on their part and I was pleased to be invited to do a talk on professional quality of life, and an afternoon workshop on the prevention and healing of compassion fatigue. The following year they invited me back to do the opening keynote; this time the day-long conference was focused on bullying and incivility.

The title I chose for my talk was "Incivility and Bullying in Healthcare: Isn't that an Oxymoron?" I reiterate that rhetorical question here. To have incivility, bullying, mobbing, and the like going on in healthcare is utterly antithetical to its purpose, which is to help and care for people. Yet, not only does it exist, it is rampant, and it occurs across the entire spectrum—not just in healthcare organizations, but also in educational settings where we are supposed to be teaching people to care for others.

Nurses Eat Their Young and Their Old, Too

In one of my recent undergraduate RN to BSN classes while we were discussing workplace environment, a new nurse made a comment that eloquently captured the feelings of frustration I have heard so often voiced by new nurses. She said, "they are trying to take the 'me' out of me." Full of enthusiasm for nursing, caring, bright, and appropriately anxious about doing things right, many new nurses are told by their more seasoned coworkers that they are too energetic, too chatty, too friendly, too slow, too, too whatever... As a result, many new nurses' expectations of what it means to be a nurse conflict with the harsh reality of *being a nurse* and working with people who are downright mean to each other.

When you are in a new job as a new nurse, with a significant learning curve to enable you to go from the ideal to the real, it is unconscionable to think that senior nurses would be cruel and uncaring. Yet, the literature shows that nurses frequently do not treat their coworkers nicely. What is more, far too often, students and new nurses are the targeted victims of bullying in the workplace (McKenna, Smith, Poole, & Coverdale, 2003; Thomas & Burk, 2009). In the exemplar with the new graduate nurse who chose to resign from her position (see Chapter 6), the subtle and not-so-subtle negative influences that were portrayed by the behavior of the nurses on the unit can also be explored from the position of those nurses themselves. Some of the questions to ponder include asking why they were criticizing, insulting, and devaluing the new nurse for her meticulous attention to her patients. What made them that way? Is their behavior a means of distancing themselves from their own unhappiness? I cannot imagine that seasoned nurses who are cruel to new nurses are happy people.

Then there are all the baby boomer nurses, who are still very much evident in the workplace. Some of these nurses have developed chronic ailments and as a consequence, might need to move a little bit slower. Some, too, might for whatever reason learn a little slower, or they may have difficulty with the newer electronic equipment. And not everyone was born with a cell phone in their hand or taught at the age of two to use a computer. As an aside, I am a baby boomer nurse, and yes, I definitely move more slowly these days and sometimes my concentration is less than what it used to be . . .but heck, I am not ready to throw in the towel just yet!

I have heard nasty stories from seasoned nurses about newer nurses making fun of their seeming difficulties. A nurse rounds the corner of the unit and several newer (dare I say younger?) nurses are standing together, talking. They immediately become silent, and then one says, "You are slow today" and they all snicker. . . Another dedicated nurse of almost 30 years came up to speak with me after one of my talks and told me that ostensibly innocent comments were made on a regular basis, like, "Why don't you retire?" or "Aren't you ready to retire yet?" Often these comments were followed by the laughter of nearby coworkers, and this nurse was feeling that maybe it was time for her to retire. She prefaced that comment with the fact that she was only 52 years old. Far too young, by most accounts (and definitely mine!), to consider retirement. Apparently, the old adage that *nurses eat their young* is no longer entirely true. *Nurses eat their old, too* (Todaro-Franceschi, 2014).

Making Sense of the Terms: Violence Comes in Different Forms

Not all violence is physical but all violence is harmful. I am intentionally using the term violence here to reiterate that any form of harassment or abuse, even if nonphysical in nature, is an act of violence against another. There are two basic types of workplace bullying: (a) horizontal or lateral violence (also known as peer-to-peer aggression, because the bully and the bullied are equal in stature or employment level) and (b) hierarchical or vertical violence, where the bully is superordinate, for example, a head nurse or supervisor (Broome & Williams-Evans, 2011; Longo, 2007; Thomas & Burk, 2009). It seems that many bullies in the workplace are in management, where by virtue of their positions of power, they are able to control the victims (Cleary, Hunt, & Horsfall, 2010). Both types of bullying behavior foster a hostile work environment. In cases where nurses observe a coworker being repeatedly bullied, although they themselves are not the recipients, they, too, suffer from bearing witness. And because of the antagonistic environment, the witnesses of bullying behavior may join in and take part, even if they do not want to do so—they might go along to get along—and what is known as "mobbing" can occur.

"Mobbing" is a term used by ethologist Konrad Lorenz to describe the predatory actions of some birds and other animal species toward one another. It was later adopted by Heinz Leymann, a Swedish psychologist, to describe abusive behavior in the workplace. Most sources use the term for when more than one person is targeting or ganging up on someone to hurt him or her. Usually, the mob has a leader, or instigator, although it might be difficult to ascertain who is leading who, because many of the actions of mobbers in a workplace are insidious.

Leymann and others have used the term psychological terror and terrorism to denote the severe, albeit nonphysical effects that mobbing can have on human beings. On occasion, I have heard of workplace mobbing being referred to as a civilized form of terrorism because it is nonphysical in nature. However, as someone who has been a victim of mobbing in the workplace, I can tell you that there is nothing civilized about it. And when it occurs in healthcare, it is uglier than ugly.

Researcher and expert on the subject of mobbing, Kenneth Westhues (2003), gives one of the best descriptions:

> Mobbing can be understood as the stressor to beat all stressors. It is an impassioned, collective campaign by co-workers to exclude, punish, and humiliate a targeted worker. Initiated most often by a person in a position of power or influence, mobbing is a desperate urge to crush and eliminate the target. The urge travels through the workplace like a virus, infecting one person after another.

In situations where incivility, bullying, and mobbing occur in the workplace, some degree of cronyism is often apparent as well. The term *cronyism* refers to specific favoritism toward friends and/or associates, and since bullies are often people in positions of power, they can easily and in many ways favor some over others, thereby fortifying relationships with "cronies" while at the same time eroding other relationships and ostracizing the target. The cronies who are being favored often remain silent, becoming in essence, moral mutes.

The term *moral mute* is not one I am especially fond of; however, when I wondered why I was not a fan of it, I realized that it was because, being the compassionate person I am, throughout my life I have tried to understand the other person's story. Indeed, throughout this book I emphasize that we should try to put ourselves in the other person's place. I reflected that using such a term might seem counterintuitive to the idea that there could be a valid reason for a person's actions. The thing is, anyone who knows that what is taking place is wrong is not acting with moral comportment if they stand by and do nothing. Thus, I feel compelled to stress that people who *witness* incivility, bullying, and mobbing, although not active participants in the process, *are nevertheless participating* if they remain silent. Doing nothing is still a choice and in this instance, harmful to others (as well as the witnesses themselves).

The Harm Done

Incivility or bullying in the workplace can be both a symptom of compassion fatigue and burnout and also a contributing factor in the development of compassion fatigue and burnout. It plays a large part in work dissatisfaction overall and can be devastating for the recipients, with physical, psychological, and spiritual ramifications. What has been given little attention is the fact that it is also devastating for the perpetrators, because in a very real sense these nurses have completely lost their sense of purpose as carers. *The pendulum has swung completely the other way.*

The bullied (suffering from primary trauma) and the witnesses, who feel helpless to do anything (cosuffering—secondary trauma), are at increased risk of compassion fatigue, which eventually results in a collective wound. The workplace becomes unhealthy for just about everyone. Victims of bullying have been found to manifest various patterns of mental and/or physical distress, and, in fact, several studies have shown a distinct similarity between the symptoms arising from bullying and posttraumatic stress disorder (PTSD) (Bilgel, Aytac, & Bayram, 2006; Ramos, 2006); see Chapter 11 for a further discussion of PTSD. Recipients of bullying may suffer from anxiety, depression, low self-esteem, eating disorders, weight loss, high blood pressure, and angina, among many other things (Broome & Williams-Evans, 2011).

Toxic work environments where bullying regularly takes place lead to nurse absenteeism and poor staff retention, which then result in financial losses for the institution. Attempts to get a handle on just how much of an economic impact incivility/bullying has on the workplace settings where it takes place have yielded different data; however, we know that it is substantial. Poor work relationships impact not only staff satisfaction but also performance, contributing to emotional exhaustion, the purportedly cardinal manifestation of burnout (Cleveland Clinic, 2011). Ultimately, the care rendered to those who are in need of our caring is negatively affected and, thus, attaining and maintaining a culture of safety for *both* the cared for and the carers becomes impossible:

> Intimidating and disruptive behaviors can foster medical errors, contribute to poor patient satisfaction and preventable adverse outcomes, increase the cost of care, and cause qualified clinicians and managers to seek new positions in more professional environments. (Governance Institute, 2009, p. 22)

As incivility/bullying in healthcare work environments has become an increasing concern, many of the organizations associated with nursing and healthcare in general have strongly advocated for the abolishment of it in the workplace, and preventive strategies have been identified such as the development of codes of acceptable behavior in organizations, increased education, and zero-tolerance policies (see for example, Joint Commission, 2008, 2016, 2018). Since the first edition of this book was published, the American Nurses Association (ANA) has created a number of professional issue panels to address various aspects of the nurse's workplace environment. One such panel focused specifically on the topic herein, and as a result, a new position statement was written in 2015. Entitled "Incivility, Bullying and Workplace Violence" (ANA, 2015b), it leans heavily on the ANA Code of Ethics, and nurses are charged with creating "an ethical environment and culture of civility and kindness, treating colleagues, coworkers, employees, students, and others with dignity and respect" (ANA, 2015a, p.4). The position statement includes acts of violence from patients and family as well as coworkers. It emphasizes that we have a moral and legal responsibility to ensure a healthy and safe work environment. Naturally, most, if not all, nurses emphatically concur. However, most nurses will also agree that position statements, policies, and procedures simply are not enough. It is crucial that we try to understand what is behind the acts of incivility. I see it as another glaring indication of a wounded workforce. Without an understanding and focus on the removal of potential causes, I doubt that we can eradicate it from the workplace.

There is a twofold, and to me, quite glaring, related problem that needs to be addressed. First, there are people in positions of power who are abusive and do not belong there, and second, some people allow themselves to be intimidated, not realizing the power that is their own. As I have noted elsewhere, we nurses do have an inordinate amount of power, individually and collectively, but for various reasons we may not feel able to exercise it.

In the seminal edition of this book, I shared, in the chapter on burnout, a brief synopsis of a true story about a patient who acquired an occipital bed sore while hospitalized. I was not completely transparent at the time, and have in this second edition rectified that by providing a more detailed account in this chapter where it more aptly belongs. The irreversible suffering that was caused was in part related to the complaisance of staff who had apparently become accustomed to not having adequate resources. But there is much more to the story.

At the time, I was not ready to divulge the full story in the first person. However, as a nurse for 37 years, an educator, and most important, the wife of a man who was needlessly and irreversibly physically and psychologically harmed in a hospital by people who are supposed to care, I have since then chosen to share the story in more complete form in various talks and other ways (Todaro-Franceschi, 2013, 2017). In what follows, I share some of the key events from our horrible experience, which reflect and bring together many of the points made thus far about professional quality of life and its relation to quality caring.

NO ONE IS SAFE HERE

My husband Michael is a veteran of the Vietnam War era with long-standing aortic insufficiency, which started when he was on active military service in the U.S. Navy. His condition was closely monitored over the years and aside from an occasional bump here and there, he had done okay. In the winter of 2010, Michael went into heart failure and was admitted to a hospital where they did several diagnostic procedures. He was stabilized and sent home on a number of medications with a somewhat urgent recommendation to go for surgery. We were ill-prepared insurance-wise when this occurred so we did not feel that we had much choice about where he could go for the surgery. But we knew that the regional Department of Veterans Affairs (VA) hospitals have excellent surgeons affiliated with them.

Calling All Angels

Open heart surgery was performed in only one VA hospital in the region where we lived. I called and requested an appointment with the surgeon, but before I did that, I shot off an email to the chief nursing officer (CNO), who I had known for many years and with whom I shared mutual acquaintances. As a nurse educator, I had also collaborated with the nursing department of this particular facility. When we were told how sick his heart had become and that he needed surgery as soon as possible, we knew it was not going to be in the best of circumstances. Indeed, one physician told my husband that it was a flip of the coin as to whether or not he would survive the surgery. So, I sat down and wrote the following email to the CNO:

> *I hope this email finds you doing well and having 'fun' like usual.*
>
> *I think I had told you that my husband is a vet? Anyway, he landed in an MICU near us a few weeks back—in heart failure. . . Long story short; he is home now and doing much better. But he will probably be having surgery to replace his aortic valve in the not too distant future. I have just gotten off the phone with your CT department to schedule his angiogram. . . .*
>
> *I have to tell you, Michael went back into the VA system about 1 1/2 years ago (after many years of being covered by my insurance), and I have been so impressed with everything at the outpatient clinic near us. Most recently, it is an understatement to say I was impressed with the care he received at a nearby VA center from the ER through the ICU and everything in between, they had me literally in tears, I was so grateful!*
>
> *I have had my share of being in the bed since 2003 (with cancer) and then in 2007 (with gallbladder surgery) and I can tell you the care my husband received was hands over heels higher quality than the care I received at purportedly number 1 hospitals. The nurses, physicians, housekeepers, receptionists. . .I just cannot get over it. If what I have seen thus far is the norm throughout the VA system now, the model for the VA should be the norm everywhere. . .*
>
> *I am contacting you right now because you will likely be seeing me on site at some point in the not too distant future since your VA is where the surgery will be done and I didn't want you to wonder why I was there.*
>
> *Of course, there is another motive. . .having had a few "horrific" experiences in health care in recent years, I have been reminded by friends and colleagues to "call on all angels. . . ." I never thought to do that over the years; I didn't think there was a need to call on anyone in order to receive quality care. These days, I am scared, and not so sure. And you are without a doubt one of the Archangels. . .so just a heads up.*

She responded back to me:

Hi—great to hear from you but sorry to hear of your recent "events." Glad you found the care great—give me a heads up when you know that the two of you will be coming and I'll roll out the red carpet. Not that it's necessary because the program is great but just so you feel more at home.

And she sure did roll out the red carpet, right *over the both of us.*

The day before surgery Michael was admitted for routine tests, although we had been told that he would get to spend most of the day with us. We spent a significant portion of the morning in the preadmitting ambulatory clinic area, where he was shuffled around from place to place; none of the people who worked there even introduced themselves to him. There was a complete, and overt, *disconnect* between the people working there and the patients. There were veterans who were getting quite upset about things in that ambulatory care area. In retrospect, I wonder why all those patients were so angry? Might it have been related to the more current day news of long waiting times? I was too anxious to pay much attention at the time and can only remember feeling unsafe there with my husband. So much so that at one point I put in a call to administration to inform them that patients were acting out, clearly angry and upset.

Eventually we were told that Michael was to be admitted to the surgical intensive care unit (SICU). He was put in a private room in the SICU and we—daughters and I—were relegated to the "waiting room," which was not quite that but rather was just a hallway outside the main doors of the unit. Picture 14 or so chairs in a hallway leading up to the unit entrance; the chairs were terribly uncomfortable, and each one had wooden arm rests. The make-believe "waiting room" was the place where, we quickly discovered, housekeeping staff often congealed to watch TV and eat their meals, while other people were there praying for their critically ill family and friends. Loved ones were often seen sleeping on those uncomfortable chairs, awaiting news of both life and death.

We waited for several hours to be allowed into his room, while the healthcare team did the many things they decided to do, a lot of which actually could have been done the next morning presurgery. We had been sitting there for quite a while when I looked over by the doors to the unit and spotted the CNO (the "Archangel"). She was speaking with the unit nurse coordinator (head nurse)—who coincidentally happened to have been a graduate nursing student of mine in a class I created, "Transforming Death in Health Care." I thought to myself—the CNO must have walked right past me, why hadn't she stopped to speak with me? Well, never mind, I thought, perhaps she didn't recognize me. So, I walked over to them and the CNO looked at me as she said—"you need to get a good night's sleep tonight." I recall thinking that her comment was a pretty bizarre thing to say upon first seeing me. I had been with my husband since we were both 15, together almost 40 years at the time —how well would you sleep the night before your other half goes for major surgery, particularly after being told his chances were 50–50 of surviving it? Still, I thanked her for her concern and assured her I would try.

Visiting Hours

When my husband was finally settled in we were allowed into his room. Almost immediately thereafter, the head nurse came in and asked if I would like to come sit in her office to talk a bit. Although I did not want to leave my husband's bedside, I figured perhaps I should. Accordingly, I followed my old graduate student into her office, and as she closed the door she proceeded to tell me that visiting hours were from 11 a.m. to 8 p.m. She emphasized that *it—the care*—was going to be *all* about my husband. There he was, *in a private room*, the day before having surgery that some suspected he might not survive, and I was being told that he would not be allowed to have any of us with him from 8 p.m. until 11 a.m. And this, she claimed, was best for and "all about him?" I was flabbergasted. Like, really?

Frankly, with all the things that had occurred up until this point (several of which I have not shared here), I should have gotten up and taken my husband home but I did not. I was too scared; frightened enough to believe that if he did not have the surgery soon he might die. Fear is a powerful motivator, and, honestly, I had seen this kind of behavior before. Healthcare professionals are human after all, and they obviously felt a bit intimidated by me. I rationalized to myself that they did, after all, want to give him the best care. Nonetheless, I could not help thinking there was something wrong with this picture. When later in the day the surgeon stopped by and told us that we could come back at 6 a.m. the following morning to "say goodbye," my husband and our daughters got really upset. I tried to console them by explaining that he would be in good hands during the night. It was hard to do, especially when I was terribly upset myself.

By the end of the day, Michael had a Swan–Ganz catheter, an arterial line, a femoral line, a peripheral line, and a Foley catheter. I could share a few related stories about other problems that occurred due to the insertion of some of these things, but the technicalities of what occurred are not as important as the fact that most, if not all, of these invasive procedures could have and should have been done the morning of surgery. Instead, the healthcare team chose to do them all the day before surgery; keeping his

family in the waiting room for several hours while he was poked and prod-
ded. Of course, it all quite effectively limited both his mobility and comfort.

Did I sleep in the hotel room I had gotten so I didn't have to drive
over two hours back and forth to the hospital? Hell no. Six a.m. found us
all kissing Michael "goodbye" and then we hunkered down in that make-
believe waiting room–hallway to wait. Many hours went by without a word
and finally, late in the afternoon the surgeon stopped in the hallway to say
it went as expected and that Michael would be coming back to his room in
a little while. He told us the next 24 hours were critical. Postoperatively, in
addition to all the lines he went into surgery with, as was typical he came
out with more: several chest tubes and a nasogastric tube. Naturally, he also
had a cracked chest wound, was intubated on a respirator, and was receiving
several intravenous (IV) medications.

When they let us in to see him, the nurse told us that they were having
difficulty recovering him—they could not get him to wake up. We were told
to stimulate him to wake up and that after we did, they would sedate him for
the night and keep him on the respirator until morning. Then, if everything
went well, they would extubate him. Hence, we talked to him, as we gently
touched his hands. Thankfully Michael started to awaken, but as is the case
with most patients who wake up intubated, he became agitated. His nurse
was going to sedate him as was planned, but before she was able to do so,
another nurse, hearing the alarm from the respirator, came into his room
and literally yelled at us that we were being disruptive and had to leave.

How inappropriate, how distressful. I sit here reminiscing as I write
this account of the events that took place, and I am repeatedly struck by
the wrongness of it, the dispassionate inattentiveness to the whole. We left
his room, but that second night two of our daughters absolutely refused to
leave the "waiting area." All during the night every time they heard an alarm,
they could not help running to their father's room...Amazingly, they were
allowed to go in and see their father, while I sat in a hotel room praying.

At four or so in the morning, the phone rang and when I answered
it, with heart pounding, my daughter proceeded to tell me that "daddy is
'bucking the vent' and he needs a breathing coach." I knew it had to have
been the nurse who told her that; I also knew that the staff did not want *me*
there. I told our daughter that her father would be okay and that I would
be there shortly. Writing this, I cannot help but think of all the possible
scenarios that might have played out. What if something bad had happened
after I told our daughter, who wanted me to go to her father's bedside and
coach his breathing, that I couldn't be there and that he would be okay? She
told me later that she had informed the nurses that I was the only one her
father ever listened to and that if they needed a breathing coach in order
for him to be calm, I should have been allowed to be there.

I arrived at the hospital early to see Michael. I was let in to see him around 7:30 in the morning, after he had been extubated. I stood near the foot of the bed, reaching over to hold his hand because there was so much equipment in the way, and the first thing Michael said to me was: "What is behind my head?" I could not get very close to look but I could see there was a folded sheet behind his head. Before I could investigate further, the head nurse walked in and asked him about his pain. He told her there wasn't much pain as he gestured to his chest, and then said his head was bothering him. Instead of responding to him, she turned to me and said, "You need to leave now. You can come back at 11 a.m., during visiting hours." My husband, grasping my hand, got visibly upset, his hand squeezing mine, as he incredulously repeated, "11 a.m.?" He was staring at a clock on the wall directly in front of him indicating that the time was only 7:45 a.m. I was distressed, too, but I smiled, told him it was okay, and that I would be back soon, once again assuring him (and myself) that he was in good hands.

Before I left, I asked the nurse who was caring for him to please get a pillow for his head. The nurse told me they had no pillows, but the nurse coming on duty piped in saying, "Oh, come on, you can get a pillow!" To which the nurse laughingly replied, "I will go to jail!" I responded with "no, you will go to heaven" and after being told that they would have to "steal" one from another unit, I waited out in the make-believe waiting room, watching the nurse leave and then return to the unit with a pillow for my husband. I thanked the nurse and left.

When I returned to the hospital at 11 a.m., the room had been cleaned up, and when Michael asked me again what was in the back of his head, I was able to take a close look. What I found was no small thing—an open, already draining, occipital decubitus, across the entire back portion of his head, about 5 inches long by 2 inches wide. My husband had wounds all over the place; a Swan–Ganz, central lines, arterial line, chest tubes, Foley catheter, and a cracked chest from open heart surgery. But it was the bed sore that was troubling him. He could not get comfortable.

I went out to a surgical store and bought all kinds of things trying to alleviate the pressure off the back of his head; nothing seemed to work. *Every single time someone came in the room he complained about his head.* The response to his complaints from most of the carers—physicians and nurses alike—was truly apathetic, it was almost as if they did not hear him or see it. . . . It was absolutely frightening. This was NOT a small, inconsequential thing. It was a large, open, angry, draining, painful wound.

In addition, he was pouring sweat and all of his dressings were falling off.[1] The thermostat in the room indicated that it was 86 degrees even though it was only mid-May and not really warm outside. I asked the nurse to please call engineering to do something about it. We all knew it was not just a matter of comfort; it was a matter of the risk for infection as well. A diaphoretic body with multiple wounds and dressings, in a warm place, was ideal for bacterial growth. Yet, the nurse responded by telling me that it was always like this, and that nothing could be done about it. Adding insult to injury, the nurse pointed out how hard it was for them to work in the heat, touching his scrub shirt while saying, "imagine how we feel." Was I supposed to empathize because I am a nurse, too? Instead, I told him my recollection of the experience I had in a hospital where I worked as a clinical supervisor one summer when the air conditioning broke down in the ICU. The staff reported it to administration, and when they did not address the problem quickly enough, the staff called in the State Department of Health. Do you know how quickly the AC was fixed, I asked him? I wish I could say that the nurse then acted empowered, advocating for the AC to get fixed, but he did not.

The next day my husband spiked a high temperature; all of his lines needed to be discontinued and replaced. As per protocol, the lines were sent for culture/sensitivity tests for fear of sepsis and he was placed on vancomycin. And I thought to myself, but didn't say it out loud, I cannot empathize with you that it is too hot for you to work in this room with my husband while your silence, your complaisance about it, endangers the life of my mate. How dare you close your eyes to the very real risk? I could never have done so, when I was in practice. I was not asking for better treatment for my husband because I was a nurse, but I started to wonder why we should be made to settle for any less better treatment.

Apathy and Abusive Power

A few days postoperatively, after he already had a ragingly angry bed sore on the back of his head, was running a temperature, and had to have all his tubes pulled and reinserted, the head nurse tells me how she had thought he'd have *at the minimum* come out of surgery on an intra-aortic balloon pump. All I could think of was how she had insisted that I abide by visiting hour rules and all the things that had happened thus far. Accordingly, I said to her, "You thought he was going to do badly, that he might die, and you made me leave him in a private room ALONE the night before surgery? I guess I failed you." And she replied, "No, I got an A in your class." Again I said to her, "No, I failed you. . .for had you gotten the message I was teaching in that class on dying and death, you would *never ever* have insisted I abide by those 11 a.m. to 8 p.m. 'visiting hour rules.'" I told her then that had my husband died during surgery I would never have forgiven her, nor would I ever have forgiven myself. I was so upset with the care he was receiving, and I was shocked by the total, complete, disconnect displayed by the carers. They just did not seem to recognize that there was anything whatsoever wrong with the way they were acting.

I could go on here about the many other awful things that took place in that facility, which put my loved one in repeated danger and eventually led to my intervening on numerous occasions. Instead, I want to share a few related things to bring all of the preceding into clear perspective. About 5 days postoperatively, the CNO stopped by my husband's room. I will never forget how she walked in, stood by the foot of his bed, and said "Mr. Franceschi, I just wanted to stop in and tell you that you are *one strong man.*" She didn't make eye contact with me, not even a nod in my direction, and frankly I would have been very surprised if she had. For, you see, when I found that bed sore on the back of his head I called her and left a message—and she *never* called me back. I also put calls in to several of the in-service nurse educators whom I knew (one had been another graduate student of mine). I left each of them messages, and they did not call me back either. So, when she stopped in and said how strong my hubby was, I speculated, what exactly did that mean? That you all tried to kill him and it didn't work yet? Seeing her in the lobby later that same day, she glanced over at me and quite literally jogged out the door. *I simply could not believe it.*

It was only after Michael was discharged home that he shared with me how the day before surgery the CNO had come into his room while I was sitting in the waiting area and introduced herself as my colleague. He went on to tell me that right after she left he had overheard her speaking with the head nurse directly in the hallway outside his door. She basically told the head nurse to keep me on a short leash or she would find someone who could. During his hospitalization, he also heard the head nurse on several occasions voice similar kinds of comments to the staff. Everything clicked into place for me then. The behavior of all the nurses, the visiting hours, *all of it.* Apathy and abusive power frequently go hand in hand.

Headaches have become a new norm for Michael. This is a man who never complained of a headache over the many years (46, to be exact) I have been with him. After several months, it was clear that neither of us were going to easily bounce back from our experience with the VA. He was sleeping in a recliner in the living room, constantly complaining of a bad headache, and when he spoke with me about the experience he said things like: "I couldn't believe that they would want me to spend what they thought was going to be my last night alive in a room alone. What kind of people do you work with in nursing?" He told me on several occasions that he had felt I left him hung out to dry—and truthfully, that is how I felt, too.

I might have been going to bed at night, but I, too, was not sleeping well. I pondered how I could have kept quiet, allowing them to keep me away from his bedside, and what, if anything, I could have done, to ensure that he received quality caring.

The physiological and psychological trauma congealed to negatively affect the quality of life for both of us. When months later he still had pain, scabbing, and scarring, we initiated a lawsuit. I cannot tell you how dreadful that process was; we experienced bullying and incivility that was taken to another, even higher, level. For instance (only one of many experiences I could share here) a few months after the lawsuit was initiated, I received an email on a Friday afternoon from the acting dean at my college, indicating that she had gotten a call from the hospital and she needed to meet with me the following week to discuss things. I responded to that email asking what it was in reference to but did not hear back from her until the following week when she walked into my office unannounced, closed the door, and sat down.

I had been multitasking and I often work with a recorder on, especially when I have many projects, in order to capture thoughts I might otherwise lose. As soon as she left, I realized I must have caught our brief talk on tape, during which time she told me that the CNO of the hospital had called and told her that I was not to step foot inside any VA facility. The CNO would not tell her why, she only told her to make sure that I did not. So here was the acting dean in my office fishing for the reason why. I looked at her as she said, this doesn't have anything to do with our students, does it? And I answered no. She said, "I didn't think so" and then asked, "Your husband is a vet, isn't he?" I said yes, and then as she tried to solicit more information I told her I couldn't speak about it and that I didn't mix my personal life with my professional life. I share it *here* because it served to negatively affect *my* professional work life on many levels, and because it was an overt intimidation tactic, one of many that occurred, over time.

We eventually dropped the suit, mostly for reasons definitely related to the topics in this chapter—covert and overt bullying/mobbing occurred in many ways that further affected our overall quality of life. All of what went on is indicative of an abuse of power that is pervasive in many parts of society, and somehow, some way, we need to put a stop to it. I can tell you that in many ways the psychological trauma is far worse than the physiological trauma—we both no longer feel safe in the healthcare system. Michael cannot get over the fact that with my having known people, and some of those people are in *powerful* leadership roles—they treated him (and me) the way they did. He tells me regularly that with colleagues like this you don't need enemies. I wholeheartedly agree.

SILENT VOICES, SILENT WITNESSES, AND SILENCE BREAKERS

Healthcare professionals witness and sometimes participate in things that should not happen in healthcare. Yet, it is well-documented that there is a pervasive "wall of silence" that prevents honest and open discussion (Gibson & Singh, 2003). How can things get better if they are repeatedly hushed up? To err is human; to remain silent about it to the detriment of others, unethical.

As a bedside nurse for years, I had always been an incredible advocate for my patients. As a clinical specialist and when I worked in leadership positions, I was a formidable voice for both nurses and patients. As a nurse educator, I prided myself on teaching students never to take "orders" and to always act in the best interests of their patients. And yet, when it came to my husband, I had been completely paralyzed with fear and anxiety. In essence, I had become a silent voice. In retrospect I was, and continue to be, appalled by my own inaction, but still, I understood it. Fear was the guiding force. We are all vulnerable; more so when we are scared.

I cannot begin to share all the stories I have heard since the first edition of this book was written, while teaching, leading workshops, and doing various talks. Everyone has a related story or two (or more!); stories much worse than ours. What I can tell you is that there are too many "silent voices" and "silent witnesses" working in healthcare. We need to change that.

Cultivating a Culture of Unsafety

There are an inordinate number of poor managers who create a culture of incivility, bullying, and yes, mobbing, and, as a consequence, they cultivate a *culture of unsafety* rather than safety. The things, many not shared here, that my family experienced are only one example of this *culture of unsafety*. The staff, led by the head nurse, who had been told what to do by the CNO, participated in bullying/mobbing activity, geared to control and intimidate us. My husband was given substandard, mediocre care by many, if not all, involved, and his needs were not adequately met. He was also bullied about various aspects of his care, which was completely inappropriate, uncalled for, and caused further detriment. I finally found my voice and intervened numerous times; had I not, he might well have died in that facility. What still haunts me and I absolutely cannot let go of, was the apathy displayed by so many of the nurses and other carers. The complete disconnect from the meaning and purpose of their work was substantial and alarming.

If much of the preceding has not struck a blaringly loud chord with most, if not all, readers, I would be very surprised. Because, every single time I have shared this story in talks and lectures, people from the audience have come to me to share their own terrible stories or sometimes, just to apologize. Whenever I have gotten an apology from a teary-eyed attendee after a talk, I have noted that there is no need for anyone to apologize for another's bad behavior. But, I get it. No compassionate person wants to hear about others suffering needlessly. I myself cringe when I hear bad stories about poor nursing care or the lack of care in health "care." The *heart* of the matter is that no one who works in healthcare should have to be apologizing for this kind of thing because it should not exist.

Time to Be Silent No More

The time has come to no longer pay lip service to the very real, very tangible issues we have in nursing, and healthcare, in general. The cost to everyone is too great, and what we have done to date to fix things, is not working. Having codes, position statements, and policies and procedures maintaining there is zero tolerance to workplace violence of any kind is not enough. Teaching nurses and other healthcare professionals is not enough. We need to *change the culture* and for that, radical change is needed (see also Chapters 12–13 for additional details related to education and leadership).

Speaking of collective actions, in nursing we could take a lesson or two from the global Me Too, and more recently started, Time's Up, movements. Civil rights activist Tarana Burke, an African American who has dedicated her life to helping youths, especially girls and young women of color, started the Me Too movement over a decade ago to help survivors of sexual violence heal. What she began as a local endeavor has become an extraordinary global communal effort to not only support and assist victims of sexual violence in their healing, but to eradicate this kind of violence by "disrupting all systems that allow sexual violence to flourish" (see metoomvmt.org for information on this important movement).

Burke founded an organization called Just Be Inc., and their mission is to empower young women between the ages of 12 and 18. In addition to the Me Too movement, they have another program called JEWELS, which incorporates "Just Be isms" geared to guide young women to be whatever they want to be. I love their "isms" and the JEWELS program; in fact, I can see the value of having a similar kind of program for nurses (check out justbeinc.wixsite.com/justbeinc/just-be-isms).

The Me Too undertaking has gained momentum since 2017 due to a Tweet by actress Alyssa Milano, who initially was not aware of Burke's "Me Too" movement. In her Tweet, Milano asked her many followers to reply to her Tweet with a "me too" if they had ever been sexually harassed or assaulted. Hence, a new hashtag was born. . . . Thousands of women have come out with "me too" stories since, and as the numbers have increased, so, too, has the strength of the advocacy for prevention. Some variation of the hashtag has sprung up in countries all around the world.

Following on the heels of women from all over coming forward to share their experiences, a group of women in Hollywood who have experienced sexual harassment, assault, or discrimination in their work environments started another movement called Time's Up. The goal of this group is to create change that will lead to safety and equity in the workplace (see www. timesupnow.com). They are raising millions of dollars for a legal defense fund that helps victims of sexual violence in the workplace.

I'm thinking we need some kind of a "MeTooinHealthcare" hashtag *and* a movement for all the people who have been harmed due to the bullying and mobbing going on in healthcare organizations (staff as well as patients and families). *Time* magazine chooses a Person of the Year annually, an individual who has influenced the world in some significant way (Zacharek, Dockterman, & Edwards, 2017). For 2017 they did not choose one person, rather, they chose a group of courageous, passionate women who came forward to publicly share their stories and speak up against sexual violence. They dubbed them "The Silence Breakers." We need silence breakers in nursing to stop the bullying, incivility, and mobbing that are causing everyone harm. Unless we individually and collectively are safe from psychological and physical harm in our workplace we will not find joy in our work, nor will we meet the goal of quality caring for all. In a nutshell:

> Workplace preconditions of respect and safety, in which the well-being of every person is a priority, create the conditions for the workforce to habitually pursue excellence. Meaningfully engaged members of the workforce deliver more effective and safer care, are more satisfied, are less likely to experience burnout, and are less likely to leave the organization or the profession. (Lucian Leape Institute, 2013, p. 18)

APPLYING *ART* FOR WORKPLACE VIOLENCE

The ART model (Todaro-Franceschi, 2008, 2013, 2015) is applicable here as well.

Step 1: *Acknowledge* There Is a Problem

Individuals who are being bullied or who might be bullies themselves, first need to concede that there is a problem. Whenever I have done talks on this subject, at least one person in the audience, and oftentimes many, will either acknowledge having been a victim of workplace violence, or conversely being a part of its occurrence.

Some questions to ask yourself: Have you been the brunt of unnecessary jokes or ridicule? Do you feel excluded or marginalized at work? Have you yourself been abrupt or sarcastic with others? Do you become easily irritated by coworkers, staff, or patients? Have you noticed behavior changes over time in coworkers or staff? I can hear some of you going "hmm, sounds familiar." Don't be surprised, after you've done a self-assessment to think, "Oh my, I've become a bully!" or "WOW! I've been a victim of workplace violence for years and never realized it."

You might also use the Clark *Workplace Civility Index* to do a self-assessment. (Please see Clark, 2014, for more information on this tool.)

Step 2: Recognize Choices and Take Purposeful Action

Perhaps it is that you have a coworker (or manager) who has been particularly nasty, bullying just about everyone on the unit, including yourself. Think about your options for handling the situation. The following are some suggestions of choices you can make (not meant to be all-inclusive; there are likely other possibilities unique to your situation):

- You can reach out and try to determine the underlying reason for your coworker's behavior.
- If you are not the only recipient of the bullying, you can choose to get everyone involved, by setting up a group meeting to discuss possible actions to take.
- You can choose to go to your superiors and inform them of the situation. (In taking the problem up the ladder, remember there is power in numbers!)
- You can choose to live and work with your coworker's bullying behavior. (Note, this is *not* a good choice!)
- You can choose to find an alternate place to work.

With the exception of the last choice listed, you actually have more than one choice. For example, you can reach out and try to get at the underlying reason for your coworker's behavior, and if that does not help to improve the situation, you can then go to your supervisor. If you are a nurse leader, you can explore each problem in the same manner (also see Chapter 13).

Step 3: *Turn Outward Toward Self and Other*

If you are a victim of any kind of workplace violence, you cannot accept it as a normal occurrence and should not allow it to continue. Remind yourself that you *are* important! Your life and your happiness are important. Take time out to rejuvenate yourself and enjoy the things that make you happy. Seek out and speak with those you feel comfortable with: your coworkers, family, friends, or a counselor. Counselors can be wonderful impartial listeners. Tell your story and, in the telling, you will gain clarity. Support others at work who might be feeling or experiencing the same or similar things that you are experiencing; support and advocate for one another; remember there is power in numbers!

Psychologists Gary and Ruth Namie founded the first and, to date, only organization in the United States that focuses on all aspects related to incivility and bullying in the workplace. They have developed a three-step "action plan" (see also Appendix C, Resources), for individuals experiencing workplace violence, which fits nicely with the *ART* model (Todaro-Franceschi, 2008, 2013, 2015):

- Step 1: Name it! Legitimize yourself.
- Step 2: Take time off to heal and launch a counterattack.
- Step 3: Expose the bully.

These are steps for individuals to take, but could easily be applied to the collective as well.

Nurse expert on civility and incivility Cynthia Clark (2014) notes a number of things that can be done to foster civility in nursing, including professional role modeling; self-reflection; stress relief and self-care; improved communication and conflict negotiation skills; enlisting leadership support; cocreating norms of decorum; and celebrating successes. She stresses that we can create a positive work environment for everyone.

KEY POINTS

- "Bullying and incivility in healthcare" *is* an oxymoron.
- No one is safe in a broken healthcare system where abusive power is allowed to prevail.
- Witnessing incivility and bullying and doing nothing about it is still a choice of participating and contributing to it.
- It takes courage to act with compassion.
- We owe it to ourselves and to those we serve to be "silence breakers."

NOTE

1. In the original text (Chapter 7), I used a fictitious name "Mrs. Frank" in a narrative; it was in fact, my husband.

REFERENCES

American Nurses Association. (2015a). *Code of ethics for nurses with interpretive statements.* Silver Spring, MD: Author.

American Nurses Association. (2015b). *Position Statement: Incivility, bullying and workplace violence.* Silver Spring, MD: Author.

Bilgel, N., Aytac, S., & Bayram, N. (2006). Bullying in Turkish white-collar workers. *Occupational Medicine, 56,* 226–231. doi:10.1093/occmed/kqj041

Broome, B. A., & Williams-Evans, S. (2011). Bullying in a caring profession: Reasons, results and recommendations. *Journal of Psychosocial Nursing, 49,* 30–35. doi:10.3928/02793695-20110831-02

Clark, C. M. (2014). Seeking civility. *American Nurse Today, 9*(7), 1–6.

Cleary, M., Hunt, G. E., & Horsfall, J. (2010). Identifying and addressing bullying in nursing. *Issues in Mental Health Nursing, 31,* 331–335. doi:10.3109/01612840903308531

Cleveland Clinic. (2011, Spring). Nurse researchers examine relationships and bullying in the workplace. *Notable Nursing, 13.* Retrieved from http://my .clevelandclinic.org/Documents/nursing/notableNursingSpring2011.pdf

Gibson, R., & Singh, J. P. (2003). *Wall of silence: The untold story of the medical mistakes that kill and injure millions of Americans.* Washington, DC: Life Line Press.

Governance Institute. (2009). *Leadership in healthcare organizations: A guide to Joint Commission leadership standards.* Retrieved from http://www.jointcommission. org/assets/1/18/WP_leadership_standards.pdf

Joint Commission. (2008). *Sentinel event alert: Behaviors that undermine a culture of safety.* Retrieved from http://www.jointcommission.org/assets/1/18/SEA_40.pdf

Joint Commission. (2016, June). Bullying has no place in health care. *Quick Safety, 24,* 1–4.

Joint Commission. (2018, April 17). Physical and verbal violence against health care workers. *Sentinel Event Alert, 59,* 1–9.

Longo, J. (2007). Horizontal violence among nursing students. *Archives of Psychiatric Nursing, 21,* 177–178. doi:10.1016/j.apnu.2007.02.005

Lucian Leape Institute. (2013). *Through the eyes of the workforce: Creating joy, meaning, and safer health care.* Boston, MA: National Patient Safety Foundation.

McKenna, B. G., Smith, N. A., Poole, S. J., & Coverdale, J. H. (2003). Horizontal violence: Experiences of registered nurses in their first year of practice. *Journal of Advanced Nursing, 42,* 90–93. doi:10.1046/j.1365-2648.2003.02583.x

Ramos, M. C. (2006). Eliminate destructive behaviors through example and evidence. *Nursing Management, 37*(9), 34–41. doi:10.1097/00006247-200609000-00010

Thomas, S. P., & Burk, R. (2009). Junior nursing students' experiences of vertical violence during clinical rotations. *Nursing Outlook, 57*(4), 226–231. doi:10.1016/j. outlook.2008.08.004

Todaro-Franceschi, V. (2008). Preventing compassion fatigue and reaffirming purpose in nursing. *Proceedings on the 3rd European Federation of Critical Care Nursing Congress and 27th Aniarti Conference, Influencing Critical Care Nursing in Europe,* Florence, Italy (October).

Todaro-Franceschi, V. (2013). *Compassion fatigue and burnout in nursing: Enhancing professional quality of life.* New York, NY: Springer Publishing.

Todaro-Franceschi, V. (2014). Are you being bullied or are you a bully? *New Jersey Nurse & Institute for Nursing Newsletter,* p. 6.

Todaro-Franceschi, V. (2015). The ART of maintaining the "care" in healthcare. *Nursing Management, 46*(6), 53–55. doi:10.1097/01.numa.0000465407.76450.ab

Todaro-Franceschi, V. (2017). *Visiting hours and waiting rooms [A digital story].* Jackson, NJ: Author.

Westhues, K. (2003). At the mercy of the mob. *OHS Canada, Canada's Occupational Health & Safety Magazine, 18*(8), 30–36. Retrieved from http://www.kwesthues.com/ohs-canada.htm

Zacharek, S., Dockterman, E., & Edwards, H. S. (2017, December 18). The silence breakers. *Time.* Retrieved from http://time.com/time-person-of-the-year-2017-silence-breakers/

V

Facing Death

*These special functionaries . . . may not always feel
prepared for the serious and difficult problems that they
face in their daily work. As I see it, the problems are of
two kinds: (1) those that confront each practitioner as an
individual and (2) those that involve the collectivity of
practitioners—whether they be the staff on a hospital ward,
the members of a cancer research team, or the workers in
a nursing home. Both types of problems have their origins
in certain paradoxical characteristics of the work expected
of persons in the health-sickness and helping occupations.
There is the dilemma of coming to terms with the two
somewhat conflicting goals of practice: (1) the maintenance
of life as manifest in recovery-focused activity and (2) the
relief of suffering through effective utilization of comfort
measures and palliation. The work centers around choices.
These choices involve keeping someone alive or letting him
go, remaining objective and detached or becoming subjective
and involved, encouraging independency or allowing
dependency. Finally, in this work there is the high stress of
being in constant or frequent contact with life-threatening
disease and its psychosocial concomitants.*

           —Jeanne Quint Benoliel

10

Being Prepared to Care for the Dying

. . . The practitioner cannot avoid a confrontation with death. He needs to face and come to terms with two realities: the anxiety associated with thoughts of his own forthcoming death and the tremendous power to influence other people's lives inherent in his own work. Stated somewhat differently, the practitioner who experiences the shadow of his own death learns to approach the choices and decisions affecting other people's lives with humility and with respect for the fragile and tragic nature of the human condition.

—Jeanne Quint Benoliel

KEY TOPICS

- Death education and its importance for nurses
- Medical futility and moral distress

INTRODUCTION

Nurses who regularly work with people who are dying know that there is always a last dose, a last meal, a last word, a last breath. Knowing that does

© Springer Publishing Company DOI: 10.1891/9780826155214.0010

not make it easier, especially when the loved ones are there bearing witness to the last everythings. Yet, there is something immensely sacrosanct about it. The memories of those last days will live forever in the hearts and minds of all those involved. Facing death with patients and their loved ones is an opportunity for us in nursing to make all the difference.

Although caring for dying patients and their loved ones offers us a chance to develop and provide sustaining memories at the most vulnerable times in people's lives, many nurses are not equipped with the necessary skills to deal with dying and death. I faced death on a regular basis when I was in nursing practice and, in retrospect, I can admit I was not always very good at it. Having never been educated in how to care for the dying, it was not something I thought much about when I entered into the profession, although soon enough I learned that it was going to be a part of my practice, whether or not I wanted it to be.

CODE 99, AGAIN?

I recall my first patient who died on a medical–surgical unit; she was 93 years old, emaciated, and unresponsive, and we coded her, four times. I am certain ribs were cracked, and I distinctly remember my extreme worry when some of the interns and residents began talking about doing a "slow code" the next go-round if she was revived that last time. I was grateful that she did die and I did not have to witness or participate in any slow codes for her. Still, I did not sleep for days afterward. I just never thought anyone would die on my watch. I remember thinking, no one prepared me for this part of nursing. I was told that "slow codes" were illegal, for heaven's sake! I did not sign up to be a felon, did I?

I never thought kids die, too . . . . But a year or so later, having been floated for the evening tour into the pediatric emergency room, I was forced to deal with the reality that no one is exempt from death. A 5-year-old with asthma coded, twice. She died a few weeks later in the pediatric intensive care unit (PICU), although technically she was considered "brain dead" after that first night. She was an only child in an Italian family, and the parents, grandparents, aunts, and uncles were present 24/7 at the hospital.

I was floated to the PICU twice during the time the child was on that unit and I remember staying clear of the visiting area where all of the family members were. I recollect being grateful that I only floated to these areas and did not have to work in them regularly. I also recall floating years later into the PICU at another hospital and being assigned to work with an 18-month-old with full-blown AIDS. I held him all night, both of us crying for much of it. Another time I floated to the neonatal intensive care unit (NICU) where there were so many babies teetering on the brink of death, and thankfully I was assigned to work with a preemie who suffered from sleep apnea. All I had to do during my time with him, aside from the normal bathing, feeding, and changing, was to flick the bottom of his foot with my finger every now and then to remind him to breathe. And breathe he did, at least for that shift. I do not know if he made it out of the NICU; when tours like that ended, I tended to book out of the hospital like my tail was on fire, without looking back lest something pull me back in there. You know how they say, do not take your work home with you? Those were the mornings when I was tempted to join coworkers as they pulled into the convenience store to buy their wine coolers or beer. I rarely did, but I was tempted, *a lot.*

As a cardiac clinical nurse specialist, I was once called upon to work with a woman with severe cardiomyopathy who had chosen to get pregnant despite the risk. Postdelivery she died and her newborn child lived. Going back to those idioms—do not take your work home with you, shut the switch, leave your work at work—well, that might be possible with papers, numbers, and other things. Rarely is it possible when you are dealing with human beings who are suffering and/or coworkers who are either suffering or, conversely, causing others to suffer. It is pretty hard to shake that kind of work off when you leave to go home at the end of the day, evening, or night.

No one ever talked about the possibility of these death experiences when I was a nursing student. We were taught Kübler-Ross's (1969) five stages of death in psychology, but that was really the extent of our education in this area. We were taught basic postmortem care—how to clean and wrap a body after death. We were never taught how to make eye contact with the patient who was dying, or his loved ones who asked, "Is he dying?" We were never taught how to talk, or listen, for that matter, to patients nearing the end of life. And we were certainly never taught how to comfort those who were left behind after their loved ones died.

Unfortunately, that still seems to be the norm in many schools of nursing; the emphasis is on health, and the prevention and cure of disease (Todaro-Franceschi, 2011b, 2013a, 2013b; Todaro-Franceschi & Lobelo, 2014). Nowadays we emphasize healthy aging. It amazes me how we can focus on the maintenance and restoration of health, without acknowledging that, at some point, no matter what we have done or will do, death is going to occur.

TEACHING ABOUT DEATH

Since going into academia full time in 1997, I have made teaching about death, dying, and bereavement a prominent priority and focus for scholarship.

I have suffered the sometimes slow, and sometimes far too quick, inevitable death of dear loved ones, and I joined the prestigious group called "cancer survivors" in 2003. Up until then, I thought I knew everything one could know about dying and death; however, I found that dwelling with cancer on such a personal basis gave me an even more tangible sense of the fragility of life and living. In any case, I would say I am pretty well rounded with respect to end-of-life care issues.

Today, I am considered a "death educator," not in nursing but in my own transdisciplinary circle of thanatology scholars. Nursing, medicine, psychology, and social work have yet to embrace the idea of "death education," and this is really dismaying because death, like birth, is integral with health and healing. Indeed, many healthcare professionals believe that associating the terms *dying* and *death* with any kind of healthcare is destined to turn people away, rather than turn them toward seeking care. This is especially so with palliative care, where it is often erroneously believed that palliative care is something we only provide at the end of life. Thus, many of the folks working in palliative care make an effort not to talk about "end-of-life care" for fear it will taint the picture and prevent people from seeking care altogether.

What people fail to understand is that palliative care is holistic care aimed at preserving quality of life—and it need not be associated with dying and death. But, and this is a *big* but, at no other time is palliative care more fitting than when people are known to be approaching death. For it is when we acknowledge that we are approaching death and that life is indeed finite that many of us will value ever more readily what living is all about, and, thus, will want to be able to appreciate every single moment we have left. Palliative care is the means to that end.

I could fill another book with my experiences as an educator trying to teach this content over the years, and perhaps one day I will. But for now I will focus on the key points related to the topic at hand, which is our individual and collective professional quality of life. From my perspective, I see this as irrevocably connected with our ability to deal with death, to be able to face it—perhaps, on a daily basis—and work with it permeating our own lives, point blank, plain and simple.

As a nurse educator, it troubles me that we can expect nurses to work in all areas of healthcare with so many people and, yet, we continue *not* to prepare nurses to deal with dying and death, and loss in general. Repeatedly I hear from students who would be nurses that they do not *expect* to work with dying patients. I hear even more from nurses who come back to school for their BS or MS degrees that they were *never* taught how to work with dying patients and how uncomfortable they are doing so, and this is sometimes decades after they have been in practice! How unfair this is to them, the nurses, and how unfair it is to those who receive care *from* them.

My research exploring critical care nurses' perceptions of preparedness to care for the dying and its relationship to their professional quality of life gave me a fair amount of data that indicates there is a significant relationship (Todaro-Franceschi, 2013b). Over 500 nurses from around the country answered the onetime request to participate in the study (final $N = 473$ due to incomplete surveys). To me, that high response rate signified the importance of exploring the subject of how dying and death in the ICU might be affecting our workforce. The majority of nurses, when asked where they had learned to provide end-of-life care, answered "at the bedside." One nurse said, "I feel like I am in a chronic state of PTSD," and she probably is (see Chapter 11 for further information on posttraumatic stress disorder [PTSD]).

In my elective class, "Changing the Face of Death" (the class from which come many of the AHAs!), countless RN to BSN nurses passed through. Some enrolled in the course just because it fit their schedule or they needed an elective. More often, it was because they acknowledged a lack of preparedness to care for the dying. Other times, it was because they either were anticipating or had experienced the death of a loved one. It never ceased to amaze me how great the attendance was in this class, even when it was offered late in the evening. The student engagement was so palpable and I was always humbled by their stories and their AHAs. The following is one from an ED nurse.

Mid-December I found out that a dear colleague and friend whom I've worked beside in the ED and known for 4 years was diagnosed with end-stage pancreatic cancer. He was 50 years old. His name was Brian . . . . Brian taught me how to put a 14 Gauge in a critical patient, and was always the first to start ordering late night pasta deliveries for all of us stuck in the ED at 3 a.m. He was a source of knowledge and laughter for us all. I attended to Brian's bedside several nights a week for about 5 weeks. He went home on hospice on Friday, January 22nd, led out of the ED from the ambulance bay with a standing ovation from all the ED staff and the EMS crews. It was a priceless moment I, and his family, will cherish forever.

I spent the next few nights at Brian's home with his family and our other colleagues from the ED. We had hot tea in the snowstorm, we recanted humorous stories about him from triage, and we looked through his photo books with his Mom. On Wednesday, January 27, Brian was in respiratory distress and was breathing at approximately 50 respirations a minute. He was holding on and holding on, like he was scared to let go.

Myself and three other nurses, along with his mom and dad, turned on some instrumental music I had on my iPhone, gathered round his bed, touched him, and I began to recite poetry and prayer. We all spoke to him and told him that it was OK to go. We gave him a dose of pain medication, and 8 minutes later he took his last breath.

It was finally over. The streets were silent and covered with 2 feet of snow. Outside the midtown apartment in Manhattan, it was so peaceful. He chose the most beautiful night in New York City to die.

My AHA moment was the very first class meeting when Dr. Todaro-Franceschi explained the purpose of this course and the mission of her teachings. I recall sitting in the back, on the highest row of chairs and I cried for the first time since I had found out Brian was ill. I had my moment because I realized that it is okay to grieve—even when you are a nurse in the ED. I am not just supposed to be a stone cold body expected to deal with it all as it comes at me. I can grieve as a friend, as a nurse, and as a person. I never realized why I hadn't shed a tear over Brian and that moment in class it all made sense.

I had been desensitized over the years I have been an ED nurse. I had always practiced the art of "dealing with it and getting over it and moving on"—and fast. Get that body out of that room; I've got 30 patients waiting for a stretcher. My AHA was a special moment for me because I finally realized that not only am I an ED nurse, but I am also an individual filled with emotion. Simply by me expressing that emotion does not take away from my Hard Core Emergency Room Edge and Attitude—it enlightens it.

It does not surprise me that the RN who shared her story had suppressed her feelings time and time again while working in the ED and facing death. Some might think, as she noted, that it is due to being desensitized over the years. It is more likely a combination of things that contributed to her behavior, and I am certain that part of it is the education (or lack thereof) that she received. If we are not taught how to face death during our education, most of us learn how to do it while working, at the bedside. That does not mean we learn how to do it well. For some, facing death means evading it, denying it, and fighting it. For some, it means not showing one's emotion, fragility, or humanness.

Occasionally I have had a hospice or palliative care nurse register for and attend my classes. More often than not, these nurses have such a good handle on caring for the dying that they become cofacilitators in our class discussions. These are also the nurses who seem less likely to burn out—they really love what they do. In recent years there have been a number of studies done to try to identify the prevalence of burnout in palliative care with conflicting results.

Kamal et al. (2016) identified a 62% incidence of burnout in palliative care clinicians, mostly physicians, which they attributed primarily to emotional exhaustion. However, a systematic review of the literature done by a group of palliative care nurses led them to surmise that burnout is less evident in palliative care than it is in other fields (Parola et al., 2017). This finding is in keeping with a prior review of the literature on the occurrence of burnout in palliative care, which indicated that there was *not* a higher incidence of burnout (Pereira, Fonseca, & Carvalho, 2011). In fact, some earlier studies performed in the United Kingdom with physicians indicate that the incidence of burnout may be lower in palliative care than in other healthcare areas (Baumrucker, 2002). It makes enormous sense to me; these folks know how to face death, and because of it, they also know how to appreciate life.

What is clear is that working in hospice and palliative care settings is a choice that some nurses and physicians make; accordingly, these individuals also make a point of developing the skills needed in this area of practice. That includes being able to connect with and talk to others about dying and death—communicating with the dying and their loved ones—as well as facing death on a regular basis. However, many carers do not choose to work (or think that they will never work), in areas where people are suffering. Unfortunately, there are also many educators of carers who lack the skillset (to care for the dying and their loved ones) themselves and thus are ill-equipped to teach anything related to end of life. I am reminded of a student who stopped me in the lobby of our campus building and asked if I had office hours. I did not know her, but I said sure, as I sat down next to her. She told me she was a senior in our generic program and that she had, along with another 125 students, recently attended two of the mandatory end-of-life care seminars I taught.

The student proceeded to tell me about a patient who had died during one of her clinical experiences:

The patient died right in front of me. She was a 70-year-old woman, who had been admitted some time before in heart failure with a bunch of other problems, including several infections that couldn't be controlled. She was unresponsive. I felt a bit anxious during the day; the woman was DNR and was desaturating as the day went on, but I continued to stay in the room and provide care for her. She started to have a change in her breathing, and then she died. I was upset and afterwards I cried even though I felt good that I was able to care for her. It was sad.

When the staff saw me crying, they were cold and seemed so uncaring, but I was really upset by the instructor who said, "Why are you crying? You didn't know her; there is no need to cry." I was actually more upset about the reactions of the nurses and my instructor than the death of the patient.

She told me that by the nurses and the instructor denying her the right to feel sad and to cry, she felt they were invalidating both the woman's life and her emotions.

As the student was telling me this story, she was visibly upset. She asked me if it was wrong for her to have felt sad and to have cried the way she had. She said, "There was nothing I could do for this woman." To that I said, "It sounds like you did a lot. What did you do for her as she lay there in her final moments dying?" She responded, "I sat there beside her and held her hand," and with that, she burst into tears and, heck, so did I. My response to her was that there is nothing wrong with crying and showing human emotion. I told her that it is the nurse who *doesn't* cry that worries me.

Jeanne Quint Benoliel (Benoliel, 1973; Quint, 1967) documented the issues related to us caring for the dying patient—the need for better preparation in nursing education, both didactic and clinical—over 50 years ago. Yet here we are still trying to deny its import—in both education and practice. It is time for us to take Jeanne Quint Benoliel's work to heart and get end-of-life care education to be mandatory and consistently taught in nursing programs. It is time to pull those MDs, social workers, psychologists, and chaplains into it, too.

DISTANCING AND DISCONNECTING: DEATH DENYING PERSISTS

One would think that, by now, human beings would have come to terms with death and what has been referred to since the 1400s as the *ars moriendi*—the art of dying. Since ancient times, humans have philosophized and reflected upon dying and death. Yet, the thought of our death and that of loved ones evokes fear in most, if not all people, and consequently we choose not to think about it—not to go there. It is one of those places that really scares us.

We live in a death denying society; just take a look at some of the headlines, even in the professional healthcare literature. For instance, did you know that "drinking coffee reduces the risk of mortality?" I did not and somehow my dad did not get that message either. He drank more coffee than anyone I know; sadly, he died at the age of 67. How about the headline "can weekend exercise reduce the risk of death?" Okay, let us all go out there and exercise A LOT and we will live forever. Come on now; we need to get real!

Most nurses work in areas where we fight off death every day. However, there does come a point where fighting death will not prevent it from occurring. We know this but many still manage to bypass its reality, most of the time.

In her decisive work, *On Death and Dying*, Kübler-Ross (1969) noted that patients who are dying need to be afforded opportunities to share their concerns:

> . . . It is evident that the terminally ill patient has very special needs which can be fulfilled if we take the time to sit and listen and find out what they are. The most important communication, perhaps, is the fact that we let him know that we are ready and willing to share some of his concerns. (p. 269)

Yet, what is the first thing many of us in healthcare do when we enter the room of someone who is dying? We blatantly ignore or try to deny the reality that death is at the door. Many refuse to talk about it with the patient or family, acting as if everything is normal. We maintain the status quo. In essence, many of us go about providing care, as if the patient is going to go home, resume previous activities, and live forever. Like Morrie said, in *Tuesdays with Morrie* (Albom, 1997), we fill the air, talking about things of little or no importance.

Two decades ago, I wrote:

> Dying, for many, has become a cold, isolated process—cold in the sense that it is hard-core machinery touching the patient, rather than the gentle grasp of a familiar loving hand; isolated in the sense that strangers rather than family and friends often surround patients in their last living moments, strangers who are valiantly trying to prolong life. . . . It is the rare person who would consciously choose to die among strangers and yet in many areas of healthcare today we, in essence, force those who are dying to do so. (Todaro-Franceschi, 1999, p. 130)

Have things changed much since then? I do not think so.

Surveys indicate that most people would prefer to die at home; however, only about a third of patients who are considered to be terminally ill enroll in hospice programs. About a third of the approximately 2.5 million annual deaths in the United States take place in a hospital (Hall, Levant & DeFrances, 2013), and in most European countries, the majority of people continue to die in hospitals (Davies, 2004). What is more, over a fifth of all deaths in the United States take place in an ICU or shortly after discharge from an ICU (Feeley, 2016).

In a retrospective study of people with cancer across seven countries—Belgium, Canada, England, Norway, Germany, Netherlands, and the United States in which researchers explored where people died and healthcare utilization/expenditures, it was found that while the United States had the second lowest hospitalization rate they also had the highest use of ICU; over 40% of the patients with cancer were admitted to an ICU during their last 180 days of life (Bekelman et al., 2016).

The most recent study performed by Teno and colleagues (Teno et al., 2018) indicates a decrease in the number of fee-for-service Medicare beneficiary patient deaths in acute care hospitals, going from 29% in 2000 to 19% in 2015. This is good news; however, use of intensive care during the last 30 days of life among Medicare fee-for-service decedents is still at 29% (it has not changed since 2009), which means that many patients with advanced-stage illness are likely being treated aggressively until they die.

Medically futile (or nonbeneficial) treatment is an issue, the outcome of which is tortuous death for many patients (Zhang et al., 2009). I continually hear from nurses who are morally distressed about patients who are nearing the end of life and receiving care that they believe is causing more harm than good. Cap off this knowledge with the abysmal fact that pain and symptom management in those with serious and/or end-stage illness is frequently substandard, and many places are still not making use of available palliative care services (Center to Advance Palliative Care and the National Palliative Care Research Center, 2015; Institute of Medicine, 2014). We are indeed given a moral imperative to find a way to do things better.

The Institute of Medicine (1997, 2014) has published significant reports on end-of-life care, the first of which in 1997 made it quite clear that there were deficiencies in all healthcare areas regarding dying and death. The report was instrumental for the development of new initiatives in both medicine (Education in Palliative and End-of-Life Care [EPEC] project) and nursing (End-of-Life Nursing Education Consortium [ELNEC]) to improve educational preparation of physicians and nurses. In nursing, the American Association of Colleges of Nursing (AACN) coupled with the City of Hope National Medical Center (COH) to formulate ELNEC to address the lack of end-of-life care curricular content in nursing education across the country (AACN & COH, 1999; COH & AACN, 2017). This ongoing effort, led by palliative care nurse pioneer Betty Ferrell, was initially funded by the Robert Wood Johnson Foundation in 1997 and has expanded into an incredible global effort.

Despite the work being done to rectify deficiencies in end-of-life care education for nurses, a study (Todaro-Franceschi & Lobelo, 2014), in which we surveyed nurse educators in schools of nursing around the country indicated that there continue to be obstacles with getting end-of-life care into nursing curricula. According to those who returned surveys ($N = 233$; participants represented all states with the exception of Alaska, Hawaii, Maryland, Utah, and Wyoming), the biggest obstacles appear to be faculty and administrative resistance. Even in schools where there are death educators, end-of-life care is not always taught. I can attest to that firsthand since it took me 17 years of advocating in the college where I worked before they finally added a required course on end-of-life care into the generic baccalaureate program.

I recently chose to move from one university to another, where there are plans to revise the nursing curriculum. On my broaching the subject of needing mandatory death education in nursing curricula, a colleague said that end-of-life care is taught in an elective course, and that anyone who is interested could take it. I thought to myself, here we go again. . .and then I quickly retorted that everyone does die and we are doing a disservice if we do not teach nurses about it. My colleague then concurred that maybe I was right. Given the fact that it is, most of the time, us—the nurses—who are the strangers surrounding dying patients and their loved ones during their final days of life, it really is up to us to help the transition from life to death, for both patients and their loved ones. Thus, the continued omission of death education in nursing is actually socially unjust for everyone (Todaro-Franceschi, 2011b, 2011c).

Kübler-Ross (1969) wondered if our actions (our denial of death as carers) might really be defense mechanisms—our way of coping with and repressing the anxieties that an acutely or terminally ill patient evokes in us. She pointed out that the dying patient is suffering more today, not less, and asked, are we becoming more or less human? It does often seem that many who work in the various healthcare fields entirely forget that they are dealing with fellow human beings, not only those working in practice but also those in education teaching others to engage in practice. Take, for example, all the people going for these risky surgeries and procedures who are forced to spend days (and nights) beforehand, alone or with strangers who are poking and prodding them, rather than with loved ones during what might well be, and often enough turns out to be, their final hours.

In an exploratory study of seven individuals with advanced cancer, Coyle (2006) noted that it is hard work to *live* in the face of death. Ferrell and Coyle (2008) expand upon this in their book on suffering, emphasizing the fact that *working* in the face of death is also incredibly hard work; nurses have to be prepared to do it and to do it well.

A dear friend of mine, a perinatal clinical nurse specialist, used to care for women who were at high risk during their pregnancies. These were women who had gestational diabetes, hypertension, or HIV, among other things. Invariably (and far too often it seemed), the babies of some of her patients would die (*in utero* or immediately after birth). She would bathe and dress those babies and sit with the parents and loved ones, giving them time to grieve. I always said that if she did that once a year she would be earning her salary tenfold and that I could never do it. Her response to me was why ever not? She always believed it was a gift to be present during both birthing and dying; she said you cannot get closer to God than at those times. To embrace the living–dying process transforms us and those we care for. The rewards are life and death altering for everyone involved.

IS IT NECESSARY OR NOT?

Prolonging or sustaining life with little expectation that it will result in survival, or, if one does survive, a quality life, is considered medical futility. What is and is not considered medically futile care is a complex issue, and it is well-debated in the literature. Renowned bioethicist Dan Callahan (1991) outlined the debate in his discussion of "the-problem-without-a-name," as he described what is considered medical necessity versus what is medically futile. How does one identify what is and is not necessary medical care?

Narrowed down to quantitative and qualitative roots, it has been noted that if a treatment is not expected to succeed, it is *quantitatively* futile, whereas if a treatment is expected to prolong life, but the quality of life is subsequently diminished, it is *qualitatively* futile (Schneiderman, Jecker, & Jonsen, 1990). Obviously this is problematic because none of us have a crystal ball that can predict for sure whether our actions will benefit or harm others. Thus, Schneiderman and colleagues advocated that we think in terms of probability. However, Callahan (1991) argued that this may well not be sufficient because, in healthcare, there is a distinct difference between how we approach the individual versus the collective.

What may likely be good for most is not necessarily good for all, and while we know this to be so, we still value "evidence-based practice" and emphasize predictability. However, evidence-based practice cannot ensure an outcome will be what we want or expect it to be. Nurses who are at the bedside of critically ill patients know how suddenly a patient can turn around. Many oncology nurses will tell you that prognosis means little in the day-to-day scheme of things. It is all about the quality of living–dying. So how do we know we are doing the right thing? Can we ever know?

Before healthcare became so technologically savvy, people got acutely ill and died in a short space of time. Now we get acutely ill and die slowly over time. The entire problem of medical futility stems not just from technologic advances that can lead to cure, but societal expectations of those techno-cures. No one is talking about the risks associated with them. No one really says, well, at the age of 80, having surgery for some slow-growing cancer might kill you or result in a prolonged hospital stay with all kinds of nasty complications, whereas you could possibly live quite a while with cancer and have a great quality of life for much of that time. That is why, when the Patient Self-Determination Act came into being in the early 1990s, it was great in principle but failed in actuality. No one wants to have *the* talk.

Nurses are caring for people who are receiving nonbeneficial care— this is traumatizing, in and of itself. In one survey of nurses across a wide range of settings including emergency rooms, ICU, hospice, and long-term care, significant moral distress was reported related to aggressive care and denying the need for palliative care (Ferrell, 2006). In critical care areas and EDs, many nurses are dealing with moral distress related to medical futility every single day, and some studies indicate that nurses working in these areas may be at increased risk for the development of both compassion fatigue and burnout (Hooper, Craig, Janvrin, Wetsel, & Reimels, 2010; Meltzer & Huckabay, 2004). It should not be surprising that there are reports of higher rates of burnout in areas where carers frequently grapple with difficult choices related to treatment. For example, Pereira, Teixeira, Carvalho, and Hernández-Marrero (2016) performed a nationwide multicenter quantitative comparative survey in Portugal and found that the level of burnout in intensive care participants was double that of those working in palliative care.

We recognize when care is most likely medically futile, but without adequate preparation during professional education, how can we advocate for these patients? Not having been taught how to communicate with patients and their loved ones about their living–dying choices, not knowing how to assert ourselves in order to make our voices heard, we wind up being a wounded workforce—morally distressed—all the while continuing to provide care that we know may not make much, if any, appreciable difference, and that may well be causing more harm than good.

My observations, both formal and informal, indicate that those who feel unprepared to care for the dying and their loved ones are at greater risk for compassion fatigue. Some of my research data also suggests that those who do feel well prepared to care for the dying may be at risk for burnout over time. Intuitively to me it makes sense, because the healthcare system as a whole does not acknowledge the acuity of the dying patient or the acuity of loved ones as recipients of care. Oh, we talk a good talk. Administration and those in charge may say that the family members are our patients, too, but seldom, if ever, are they counted in acuity for staffing needs.

The patient whose life we are trying to save, even if futile, the one with all of the life-saving and life-preserving procedures, equipment, and medication, is perceived to be higher acuity than the patient who we have accepted is in his or her final hours or days transitioning from life to death. In advanced labor and during delivery, a patient usually has a one-to-one carer; for people who are known to be dying, this is rarely the case. This logic has spilled over into our educational programs for nurses (and for physicians and other healthcare professionals). Or perhaps the logic we apply in practice stems from our education (or lack thereof). The question of which came first might be very relevant, but it is a topic for another time. The point is, rare is the nursing program that requires a full-term course on the topic, and, in fact, there sometimes seems to be a hidden curriculum in healthcare professional education that devalues the learning of thanatology topics entirely (Billings, Engelberg, Curtis, Block, & Sullivan, 2010; Todaro-Franceschi & Lobelo, 2014).

WHY IS IT IMPORTANT FOR US TO BE PREPARED TO FACE DEATH?

After years of difficulty getting end-of-life care education to be a permanent fixture in the undergraduate program of the college where I was working, I set out to do an alumni study. I wanted to document what I intuited from both my practice and my experiences teaching. The results of that study are reported in another publication, so I only offer a brief synopsis here (Todaro-Franceschi, 2011a, b). Students were surveyed to ascertain whether they perceived that the education they received at our school had adequately prepared them to care for the dying. They were also asked if they thought that their end-of-life care education has had an impact on their practice and their way of being in the world. "Changes in one's way of being in the world" was defined as an enhanced appreciation of people, places, and/or things; being more appreciative of life, generally speaking. Comparisons were sought between those who had taken the elective course ("Changing the Face of Death") and those who had not.

Findings revealed statistically significant differences among groups in their perceptions of preparedness to care for the dying as well as perceived changes in both practice and ways of being in the world (total $N =$ 154 both generic and RN to BSN students), with those who had taken the elective reporting feeling better prepared and also more appreciative of life (Todaro-Franceschi, 2011a, b). A salient number of the RN participants who had chosen to take the elective offering in end-of-life care reported working in critical care (29%) and EDs (13%; over 42% of RN respondents), which suggests that nurses working in these areas feel more of a need to be prepared to face death. We should take note of the fact that accumulating research data on compassion fatigue and burnout in nursing suggests that in the ED, intensive care, and oncology there is a high incidence of these syndromes. These are areas where nurses face death all the time.

Many folks, nurse faculty colleagues and students among them, have asked me over the years why I think it is so important for us to learn how to face death. The following is my answer:

- Because death is 100% guaranteed for every one of us
- Because we ALL will have to face death, personally and professionally
- Because doing it poorly hurts us
- Because doing it well, while difficult, can infuse us with appreciation for life and living and help us live our moments joyfully and heartfully
- Because our patients need us to help them face it
- Because our patients' loved ones need us to help them through it
- Because the cost of aggressive healthcare at the end of life is astronomical and does not usually result in enhancing the quality of living while dying

APPLYING *ART* IN PREPARATION OF CARING FOR THE DYING

Coming to terms with the possibility that you (or your colleagues and staff) may have a problem with facing death and are ill-prepared to care for the dying is important—again, you cannot fix what you do not recognize or acknowledge as broken. There are many purposeful actions that can be taken to help one feel more prepared to care for the dying and their loved ones. We can become more comfortable with it, and although it will never be an easy thing to do, we can find meaning and purpose in the experiences we have with the dying. Of course, it is a choice you have to make. Some people cannot, or do not want, to face death at all, and that is okay. What is not okay is that we deny another's experience of it by flicking that shutoff switch. If you are regularly facing death and decide that you do not want to deal with it, it will be far better for everyone if you go work in a different area entirely. Applying the *ART©* model (Todaro-Franceschi, 2008, 2013a, 2015) can assist those who are having difficulty facing death.

Step 1: Acknowledge a Feeling or Wound That Needs Healing

Ask yourself if you avoid speaking about dying and death with others, personally and professionally. Is the topic of death "taboo" in your culture? Generally speaking, do you feel able to provide quality care to the dying and their loved ones? You may wish to complete the questionnaire about perceptions of preparedness located in Appendix B.

Sometimes our previous experiences with death "set us up" for how we act in similar situations. Realize that "similar" in this instance simply (or not so simply) means occurrences where dying and death happen—*dying (usually) leads to death*—all have that in common, although every single event of death is unique. You may have had personal or professional experiences that have set you up to be uncomfortable with dying and death. For instance, the student who shared with me how the staff and her instructor ridiculed her for crying and being sad—that might have discouraged her from sharing her feelings in the future, were it not for the fact that she chose to approach me to discuss what had happened. I am hopeful that she will remember my saying that it is the nurse who does not cry that worries me.

Do you ever cry for those who are dying or have died? Did you used to cry easily but no longer do? If you answer in the affirmative, it may be time to go back to Chapter 8 on burnout. Then again it might not; only you can assess whether or not you are distancing yourself from experiences that may be painful. Only you can say for sure if you are evading the places that scare you.

If you work in an area where patients frequently die, and your staff or coworkers seem to be uncaring or dispassionate, encourage them to explore their feelings regarding dying and death. A focused group discussion on the topic can be very useful to identify areas where more staff preparation may be needed.

Step 2: *Recognize Choices and Take Purposeful Action*

First, ask yourself if you want to learn to be more comfortable with dying and death. If so, please see Appendix C, Resources, for end-of-life care education. There are many courses available on the subject. If you are in the New York City area, stop in on one of mine! If you are not interested in becoming more comfortable with dying and death, it might be that you need to do some self-reflection related to experiences you may have had with dying, death, and bereavement. Once you have identified areas that may be contributing to your discomfort with dying and death, the following are some choices you might consider:

- Taking an ELNEC course (please see Appendix C, Resources)
- Enrolling in a university course on dying and death (check your local college)
- Speaking with a spiritual advisor (e.g., your rabbi, priest, pastor)
- Speaking with friends and loved ones about it
- Doing some grief work with a counselor or support group

Depending upon your unique situation, there will be other choices and actions that you can think about. Once again, you may decide that facing death is not something you can do or want to do. If that is the case, list alternative choices and strategies such as changing your area of practice or even changing your nursing role entirely. What you must not do is continue to work in an area where you feel compelled to deny death, although you are forced to deal with it. This choice and concurrent action will lead to turning away from the problem—flicking that shutoff switch, which is unhealthy for you and definitely not helpful for others.

Step 3: *Turn Outward Toward Self and Other*

At no other time is it more imperative for us as carers to turn outward toward ourselves and others than when we face death. Of course, some of my colleagues say I am biased, since I am so passionate about death education. I do not think that is it at all. Turning outward toward ourselves and others is so important when facing death, because having an appreciation of ourselves and our connectedness to all else enables us to live more fully. Recognition that life is fleeting, and seeing, really seeing the things we take for granted every day can help make us feel *heartful*.

If we are able to face the fact that death happens to everyone and as a result can appreciate our moments as we live them, we will be in a better position to help those who are living their final days and moments. We will be more able to go to the places that scare us and them, *with* them. Facing death with them, we bear witness to their suffering, and are able to put ourselves in the person's place because we understand that one day we and our loved ones will be in that same place. As Morrie said, "Learn how to die, and you learn how to live" (Albom, 1997, p. 83). We have to be able to turn outward in order to appreciate living and dying. If we are *really* enjoying life, it is because we are turning outward toward ourselves and others, in most, if not all, of our moments. Morrie

> . . . nodded toward the window with the sunshine streaming in. [He said] "You see that? You can go out there, outside anytime. You can run up and down the block and go crazy. I can't do that. I can't go out. I can't run . . . . But you know what? I *appreciate* that window more than you do . . . . I look out that window every day. I notice the change in the trees, how strong the wind is blowing. It's as if I can see time actually passing through that window. Because I know my time is almost done, I am drawn to nature like I am seeing it for the first time. (Albom, 1997, p. 84)

Without self-reflection and forcing ourselves to face this most complex and, for many, terrifying subject, we never come to face the finite nature of life. We go through our days never realizing that this moment, this *right now*, is the only *right now*, and it may be the *last right now* there is for us, our loved ones, our patients, and their families.

KEY POINTS

- Death happens; it is 100% guaranteed.

- Everyone is going to face death, whether prepared for it or not.

- Nurses who work in areas with people who are dying are especially vulnerable to compassion fatigue and moral distress because they are the ones at the bedside bearing witness to suffering, both from medically futile care and from the "failure to cure."

- Nurses need to learn how to be more comfortable facing death and to develop the concomitant skills necessary to care for the dying and their loved ones.

- Being unable to face death results in flicking the shutoff switch (denying and defying death), which is unhealthy for us and does a disservice to the patient who is dying and his or her loved ones.

- Learning how to face death can teach us how to appreciate life.

REFERENCES

Albom, M. (1997). *Tuesdays with Morrie: An old man, a young man, and life's greatest lesson.* New York, NY: Doubleday.

American Association of Colleges of Nursing (AACN) & City of Hope National Medical Center (COH). (1999). *End-of-Life Nursing Education Consortium Project (ELNEC).* Washington, DC: Author.

Baumrucker, S. J. (2002). Palliative care, burnout, and the pursuit of happiness. *American Journal of Hospice and Palliative Care, 19,* 154–156. doi:10.1177/104990910201900303

Bekelman, J. E., Halpern, S. D., Blankart, C. R., Bynum, J. P., Cohen, J., Fowler, R., . . . for the International Consortium for End-of-Life Research (ICELR). (2016). Comparison of site of death, health care utilization, and hospital expenditures for patients dying with cancer in 7 developed countries. *JAMA, 315*(3), 272–283. doi:10.1001/jama.2015.18603

Benoliel, J. Q. (1973). The practitioner's dilemma: Problems and priorities. In J. Q. Benoliel, H. Feifel, E. S. Shneidman, C. W. Wahl, & E. H. Waechter (Eds.), *Dealing with death* (pp. 33–45). Los Angeles, CA: University of Southern California.

Billings, M. E., Engelberg, R., Curtis, J. R., Block, S., & Sullivan, A. M. (2010). Determinants of medical students' perceived preparation to perform end of life care, quality of end of life care education, and attitudes toward end of life care. *Journal of Palliative Medicine, 13*(3), 319–326. doi:10.1089/jpm.2009.0293

Callahan, D. (1991). Medical futility, medical necessity: The problem-without-a-name. *Hastings Center Report*, *21*(4), 30–35. doi:10.2307/3562999

Center to Advance Palliative Care and the National Palliative Care Research Center. (2015). *America's care of serious illness: A state-by-state report card on access to palliative care in our nation's hospitals*. Retrieved from http://www.capc.org/reportcard

City of Hope (COH) and American Association of Colleges of Nursing (AACN). (2017). *ELNEC core curriculum*. Washington, DC: Authors.

Coyle, N. (2006). The hard work of living in the face of death. *Journal of Pain and Symptom Management*, *32*(3), 266–274. doi:10.1016/j.jpainsymman.2006.04.003

Davies, E. (2004). *What are the palliative care needs of older people and how might they be met? A health evidence network synthesis report*. World Health Organization: Regional Office for Europe. Retrieved from http://www.euro.who.int/__data/assets/pdf_file/0006/74688/E83747.pdf

Feeley, T. W. (2016). The value of ICU care at the end of life. *NEJM Catalyst*. Retrieved from https://catalyst.nejm.org/value-icu-care-end-of-life

Ferrell, B. (2006). Understanding the moral distress of nurses witnessing medically futile care. *Oncology Nursing Forum*, *33*, 922–930. doi:10.1188/06.ONF.922-930

Ferrell, B., & Coyle, N. (2008). *The nature of suffering and the goals of nursing*. New York, NY: Oxford University Press.

Hall, M. J., Levant, S., & De Frances, C. J. (2013). Trends in inpatient hospital deaths: National hospital discharge survey, 2000–2010. U.S. Department of Health and Human Services, Centers for Disease Control and Prevention National Center for Health Statistics. Retrieved from https://www.cdc.gov/nchs/data/databriefs/db118.pdf

Hooper, C., Craig, J., Janvrin, D. R., Wetsel, M. A., & Reimels, E. (2010). Compassion satisfaction, burnout, and compassion fatigue among emergency nurses compared with nurses in other selected inpatient specialties. *Journal of Emergency Nursing*, *36*(5), 420–427. doi:10.1016/j.jen.2009.11.027

Institute of Medicine. (1997). *Approaching death: Improving care at the end of life*. Washington, DC: Author.

Institute of Medicine. (2014). *Dying in America: Improving quality and honoring individual preferences near the end of life*. Washington, DC: The National Academies Press.

Kamal, A. H., Bull, J. H., Wolf, S. P., Swetz, K. M., Shanafelt, T. D., Ast, K., Kavalieratos, D., . . . Abernethy, A. P. (2016). Prevalence and predictors of burnout among hospice and palliative care clinicians in the U.S. *Journal of Pain and Symptom Management*, *51*(4), 690–696. doi:10.1016/j.jpainsymman.2015.10.020

Kübler-Ross, E. (1969). *On death and dying*. New York, NY: Simon & Schuster.

Meltzer, L. S., & Huckabay, L. M. (2004). Critical care nurses' perceptions of futile care and its effect on burnout. *American Journal of Critical Care*, *13*(3), 202–207.

Parola, V., Coelho, A., Cardoso, D., Sandgren, A., & Apostolo, J. (2017). Burnout in palliative care settings compared with other settings: A systematic review. *Journal of Hospice & Palliative Nursing*, *19*(5), 442–451. doi:10.1097/NJH.0000000000000370

Pereira, S. M., Fonseca, A. M., & Carvalho, A. S. (2011). Burnout in palliative care: A systematic review. *Nursing Ethics*, *18*, 317–326. doi:10.1177/0969733011398092

Pereira, S. M., Teixeira, C. M., Carvalho, A. S., & Hernández-Marrero, P. (2016). Compared to palliative care, working in intensive care more than doubles the chances of burnout: Results from a nationwide comparative study. *Plos One*, *11*(9), e0162340. doi:10.1371/journal.pone.0162340

Quint, J. (1967). *The nurse and the dying patient.* New York, NY: Macmillan.

Schneiderman, L. J., Jecker, N. S., & Jonsen, A. R. (1990). Medical futility: Its meaning and ethical implications. *Annals of Internal Medicine*, *112*(12), 949–954.

Teno, J. M., Gozalo, P. L., Trivedi, A. N., Bunker, J., Lima, J., Ogarek, J., & Mor, V. (2018). Site of death, place of care, and health care transitions among US Medicare beneficiaries, 2000-2015. *JAMA*, *320*(3), 264. doi:10.1001/jama.2018.8981

Todaro-Franceschi, V. (1999). *The enigma of energy: Where science and religion converge.* New York, NY: Crossroad.

Todaro-Franceschi, V. (2008). Preventing compassion fatigue and reaffirming purpose in nursing. *Proceedings on the 3rd European Federation of Critical Care Nursing Congress and 27th Aniarti Conference, Influencing Critical Care Nursing in Europe*, Florence, Italy (October).

Todaro-Franceschi, V. (2011a). *Vestiges [A digital story].* Jackson, NJ: Author.

Todaro-Franceschi, V. (2011b). Changing the face of death: A pedagogic intervention. *Journal of Professional Nursing*, *27*(5), 315–319. doi:10.1016/j.profnurs.2011.04.002

Todaro-Franceschi, V. (2011c). Re-patterning health professional death education: A matter of social justice for all. *The Forum: The Quarterly Publication of the Association for Death Education and Counseling*, *37*(3), 26–27.

Todaro-Franceschi, V. (2013a). *Compassion fatigue and burnout in nursing: Enhancing professional quality of life.* New York, NY: Springer Publishing.

Todaro-Franceschi, V. (2013b). Critical care nurse perceptions of preparedness and ability to care for the dying and their professional quality of life. *Dimensions of Critical Care Nursing*, *32*(4), 184–190. doi:10.1097/dcc.0b013e31829980af

Todaro-Franceschi, V., & Lobelo, A. (2014). The voice of nurse educators on teaching end of life care in U.S. schools of nursing. *Journal of Nursing Education and Practice*, *4*(4), 165–171. doi:10.5430/jnep.v4n4p165

Todaro-Franceschi, V. (2015). The ART of maintaining the "care" in healthcare. *Nursing Management*, *46*(6), 53–55. doi:10.1097/01.numa.0000465407.76450.ab

Zhang, B., Wright, A. A., Huskamp, H. A., Nilsson, M. E., Maciejewski, M. L., Earle, C. C., . . . Prigerson, H. G. (2009). Health care costs in the last week of life: Associations with end of life conversations. *Archives of Internal Medicine*, *169*(5), 480–488. doi:10.1001/archinternmed.2008.587

Collective Trauma and Healing in Healthcare: Aching, Breaking Hearts

. . . we could say that most men in a concentration camp believed that the real opportunities of life had passed. Yet, in reality, there was an opportunity and a challenge. One could make a victory of those experiences, turning life into an inner triumph, or one could ignore the challenge and simply vegetate, as did a majority of the prisoners.

—Viktor Frankl

KEY TOPICS

- Collective trauma
- Posttraumatic stress disorder (PTSD)
- Meaning-making and healing

INTRODUCTION

The idea that healthcare professionals, and particularly nurses, might suffer from "death overload," collective trauma, and possibly PTSD has not been

© Springer Publishing Company DOI: 10.1891/9780826155214.0011

given much attention. For nurses who work in areas where death is a frequent occurrence, we would do well to address it. In the larger realm of things, post 9/11 and hurricanes such as Katrina and Sandy in the United States, and globally in the wake of devastating earthquakes, tsunamis, cyclones, and ongoing horrible acts of terrorism, we know that carers must be prepared to face the possibility of collective trauma at any time.

Throughout the world, acts of terror and natural disasters force us to collectively face death and threats of death each day. All of the people involved in every one of these events are personally traumatized, as are all those individuals who may be involved in the rescue efforts. Indeed, as I write this I can hear my mom telling us the story of the airplane that crashed in 1960 in Park Slope. She was an RN working at Methodist Hospital in Brooklyn, where the only survivor of the crash, an 11-year-old boy named Stephen Baltz, was taken, and who a day later succumbed to his injuries. I heard the story on more than one occasion while growing up—clearly indicative of the sustaining memory and horror that the event created for my mom and I am sure all of those who were working at the hospital during that time.

The following account was shared by a nurse in one of our focus group discussions:

This week in our nursing class on death and dying I was reminded of things that I felt were long [gone] from my memory. I was working in my EMS job on a Tuesday morning and I had just picked up my first patient in downtown Manhattan. On my way to the hospital, the Twin Towers were attacked. I remember the events of the day vaguely; what remains vivid is the sound of bodies hitting the ground all around me as people leapt from the burning buildings. I remember the smell of the mixture of burning flesh and jet fuel, and my most vivid memory is that of ashes falling all around. I was asked if I wanted to debrief, I declined . . .

Eight years later I had a bad pediatric trauma. It was a little boy that was pinned between a tree and a car, causing his skull to crack open and his brain matter to spill out. Even now, as I type this, my hands are shaking. I have had hundreds of patients and deaths since then, but this seems to be the one call that still affects me. My supervisor at the time put my partner and I out of service and requested that we debrief. Critical incident stress debriefing (CISD) was readily available for us whenever we needed it, but somehow I never felt I needed it, not even then. I went home and thought I would be okay. . . . I didn't sleep for a few nights.

Years later, whenever I am reminded of the friends and coworkers we lost in 9/11 or of that little boy, tears well up in my eyes. Maybe I should have gone; maybe it would have helped me. I believe now that CISD is important and that it should be offered more often and by all employers,

health related or not. If I had a choice today I would take advantage of
the help offered. I believe that it should be explained that it is alright not
to be okay after any event, whether it is a terrorist attack or a tragic and
sudden death. At the end of the day when we go home, we are no longer
nurses, paramedics, or doctors—we are human beings.

This nurse became aware that she would have benefited from some
treatment for the trauma she suffered. It more than likely was the number
one reason why she took my elective class on death and dying. During our
weekly classes she was able to share her feelings with others who were supportive and were able to bear witness to her anguish. I am sure it not only
facilitated her healing, it helped others who might not otherwise have been
willing to take advantage of CISD when it is needed and offered. Healing
from traumatic experiences begins with the acknowledgment that one is
hurting and it is enhanced by the efforts others make to acknowledge and
support those who are suffering from the trauma.

COLLECTIVE TRAUMA

Collective trauma is when a group of people are traumatized at the same
time by something. Whatever it is, the something is so devastating that
whether or not the trauma is primary in nature does not matter to the
group as a whole. *Everyone* experiences the pain and anguish together. The
suffering is of a palpable nature in an entire group of people. It could be a
small group, a community, or a larger group such as a society or country, or
even of a global magnitude. It does not mean that the trauma is the same
for everyone; some suffer more and others less. What it means, though, is
that everyone is *sharing* in the horror.

For as long as humankind has been in existence, we have had events
that result in collective trauma. Natural disasters and human-made disasters have been many. As a native New Yorker, I have both witnessed and
experienced the devastating feelings arising from collective trauma. The
events of September 11, 2001, will remain forever imprinted in the minds
and hearts of people throughout the world. It was an appalling act of terrorism thrust upon innocent human beings and many people continue to
suffer from PTSD related to it. For those living and working in New York
City (NYC), it constituted both primary and secondary trauma. Working in
the city, I can tell you it was tough stuff to enter the city in the days, weeks,
and months after 9/11. To this day I cannot look at the New York skyline
without welling up with tears (Todaro-Franceschi, 2011d).

In the immediate aftermath of 9/11, nearly half of the American population reported symptoms of PTSD (Schuster et al., 2001), and in the days,

weeks, and months following, many continued to have symptoms of PTSD along with the fear of future terrorist attacks. I worked with one student who had lived in close proximity to the Twin Towers. She watched the events of that day unfold from her apartment window, and she continued to have symptoms of PTSD along with terrible panic attacks for a long time afterward, which affected every single aspect of her life.

Yet, I can also tell you that something occurred in NYC immediately after 9/11 that I wish we could all capture and hold in our hands and hearts and never allow to dissipate. We were *nicer* to one another. There was evidence of unity—connectedness—and purpose, the likes of which I had never seen before in my hometown and have not seen since (Todaro-Franceschi, 2011d). One can attribute it to our sense of vulnerability, but for the grace of God it could have been us or our loved ones. But in actuality, it *was* our loved ones, for we are all one. From that sense of community—the collective nature of the trauma—we were able to continue to function and for a short space of time, we were more acutely aware of our *oneness*, our *we-ness*. This sense of oneness, I believe, is what got us all through that horrible time and it is what contributed to our collective healing, not only in NYC, but throughout the United States and the rest of the world where people suffered because of the 9/11 attacks.

Depending upon the nature of the traumatic event, those who have been collectively traumatized may pull together, such as what happened in the United States and other countries that were affected by 9/11, or the event may completely fracture the social fabric of the group—community, society—because the event causes such widespread devastation that the group can no longer perceive themselves as a group at all, but rather as a bunch of disconnected people who are all trying individually to survive.

A Loss of Communality

The Buffalo Creek disaster is a case in which it has been said that there was a loss of communality due to the nature of the collective trauma (Erikson, 1995). In 1972, a dam burst in a coal mining community, killing 125 people and physically injuring another 1,100. Over 4,000 people were left homeless. Prior to the events of that day, these people who lived in a mountainous community depended upon one another and there was an undeniable kinship. After the flooding, people who had lost everything were scattered in refugee camps, separated from the neighbors they had depended on, and instead were forced to live amid strangers. Consequently, they lost their sense of connectedness and community. An in-depth discussion of collective trauma is outside the purview of this book; however, within the context of compassion fatigue in nursing, I would like to draw attention to the following relationship.

In healthcare settings, whether we acknowledge it or not, collective trauma is, in a very real sense, a regular occurrence. Those who work with individuals and groups of people afflicted by disease and injury are communally traumatized all the time as they work with and bear witness to pain and suffering. In his studies of the Buffalo Creek disaster and how it affected the people, Erikson (1995) wrote about a loss of communality that he deemed was evidenced in various behavioral manifestations. Two in particular are especially noteworthy here: demoralization and loss of connection.

Demoralization was said to have occurred as both a loss of personal morale for those traumatized but also a loss of perceived "morale anchors" (Erikson, 1995):

> The lack of morale is reflected in a profound apathy, a feeling that the world has more or less come to an end and that there are no longer any sound reasons for doing anything. People are drained of energy and conviction, not just because they are still stunned by the savagery of the flood but because activity of any kind seems to have lost much of its direction and purpose in the absence of a confirming community surround. They feel that the ground has been pulled out from under them, that the context in which they had worked, played, and cared for others has more or less disappeared. (p. 409)

It was also demoralizing for the people who suffered this collective trauma in the sense that there had been an earlier disaster related to the same issues and authorities had not fixed the problem, nor were these people ever able to be fully compensated for their terrible losses. Their lives were irrevocably changed.

The second behavioral manifestation related to the loss of communality witnessed in survivors of the Buffalo Creek collective trauma—the loss of connection—was noted to be a sense of being separated from others to the extent that they felt isolated and alone:

> For better or worse, the people of the hollow were deeply enmeshed in the tissues of their community; they drew their very being from them. When those tissues were stripped away by the disaster, people found themselves exposed and alone, suddenly dependent on their personal resources. . . . Many people felt that they had lost meaningful connection with themselves. (Erikson, 1995, p. 412)

I would point out that both of these behavioral manifestations (demoralization and a loss of connection), which were identified to reflect a loss of communality as a result of collective trauma, are also prevalent in people who suffer from burnout. By us not acknowledging the inherently collective traumatic nature of our work and supporting each other along the way, we are contributing to the emotional contagion of burnout.

People who are exposed to collective trauma are at increased risk for anxiety and panic attacks, depression, substance abuse, and the development of PTSD. PTSD poses a particular challenge, since without treatment, it is almost impossible to heal from, but even with prompt treatment it can become chronic in nature.

POSTTRAUMATIC STRESS DISORDER

PTSD is used to describe an anxiety disorder that can emerge in anyone of any age as a response to feelings of fear, helplessness, and horror from a traumatizing event that can be either primary or secondary in nature. It can happen as a result of directly experienced or witnessed, life-threatening traumatic events, such as natural disasters (floods, fires, tornadoes, hurricanes, etc.), war, or terrorist attacks. It can also emerge from experiences of assault, such as domestic violence or rape. Sometimes the sudden death of a loved one can result in PTSD, too.

Veterans of war are at increased risk for PTSD, so much so that there is a Veterans Administration National Center for PTSD. The compassion fatigue and related PTSD experienced by the carers of veterans is widespread as well; the Army has its own term, "provider fatigue," for the people who develop PTSD themselves while caring for traumatized veterans (Conant, 2007). In recent years, it has become evident that family members and loved ones of veterans can also develop PTSD.

Whereas, when one is faced with danger, the normal "fight or flight" response kicks in and is a survival strategy, with those who suffer from PTSD, the response continues to exist after the danger has subsided or the traumatic experience has ended. Studied extensively, it is known to have both psychological and biological aspects—in other words—it is a transformation of the *whole*. Many people do not realize this and think the syndrome is limited to an emotional response. However, studies have shown that there are physiologic changes involved that arise from the failure of the body to respond successfully to the trauma (Yehuda, 2002a, 2002b). PTSD is often noted to be very similar to compassion fatigue, but it has a much greater scope.

It is important to note that it is the unique aspects of each individual (physical, psychological, and spiritual) that contribute to how each of us manifests signs and symptoms of suffering related to traumatic events. The diagnosis of PTSD is made when there are three distinct kinds of symptoms:

reliving the event, avoiding reminders of the event, and hyperarousal (e.g., insomnia and/or impaired concentration) for a minimum of 1 month after the traumatic event (Yehuda, 2002a; see Table 11.1).

As can be seen, there is a similarity between PTSD and compassion fatigue. PTSD is most often, but not always, the direct result of someone experiencing some form of trauma, whereas compassion fatigue is usually a result of witnessing someone else's suffering. Again, what is traumatic for one person may not be for another; however, when the trauma is collective and affects large numbers of people, it is difficult to note whether it is primary or secondary. When NYC was attacked, one could say that every New Yorker was the victim of primary trauma, whether or not they were there that day. Some would not agree and would say that only those who were there suffered primary trauma; for those who were not there, the trauma was secondary in nature. Either way, many people all around the world developed PTSD from the events of 9/11.

Upon close examination, you might note that it is the threat to one's very existence that binds the two syndromes–compassion fatigue and PTSD—together. In cases of compassion fatigue, we cosuffer with those who are ill and/or may be facing the threat of death or are actually dying. With PTSD, be it related to individual or collective trauma, the possibility of death looms before us. Even chronic illness, in a way, threatens one's existence because it often changes one's *way* of life completely. In cases of

Table 11.1 Symptoms of PTSD

Revisiting the Event	Avoiding Reminders of the Event	Hyperarousal
Flashbacks, where one feels as if he or she is reliving the event	Numbness and/or detachment	Trouble concentrating
Nightmares— dreaming of the event	Disconnecting from, things seem surreal	Easily startled, more aware
Repetitive memories or thoughts	Inability to remember aspects of the event	Irritable, easily angered
Reacting to similar events	Avoiding places, people, or things that bring up memories of the event	Difficulty falling or staying asleep

collective trauma, the events threaten many people's ways of living–dying all at once. In all instances, we hurt.

MAKING MEANING FROM TRAUMATIC EVENTS

When horrific events occur, it tests our faith in ourselves and in others. For some, it may test their religious faith as well. Very often, people who are traumatized will seek to understand how and why something has occurred. One may ask, why did it happen to him and not me? Conversely, why did it happen to me and not him? What is the meaning of this? In the larger scheme of things, is there a reason or purpose?

It is a natural human trait to seek meaning in our experiences. But as someone who claims that the universe is so ordered that there must be a purpose and reason for it all, even I have to admit, I have difficulty *finding* meaning in our many shared horrors (Todaro-Franceschi, 1999, 2003). I do not understand how senseless acts of violence can occur. I do not understand why a person must sometimes suffer with incredible pain. I definitely cannot reconcile the enormous suffering I have sometimes witnessed, with any understanding of its purpose.

In 2002, three nursing faculty members at the University of Arizona, Barbara Monroe, Cheryl McGaffic, and Robin Rogers, were killed by a disturbed nursing student who then committed suicide, leaving the entire university in a state of shock and mourning. Understandably, it left the entire profession of nursing reeling, as well. I knew Cheryl and she was one of the most compassionate people I have ever encountered. It made no sense to me that nursing faculty could be killed by a student who believed himself to be so terribly alone that he felt no recourse and no remorse. But I think in instances where we cannot hope to find meaning, it is helpful to try to make meaning.

In a letter to the editor of *Nursing Science Quarterly* after the University of Arizona faculty were killed, I had written, "Yes, we can sit back and shake our heads and say what a tragedy it was. We can try to move on and act as if the whole thing was a senseless act of violence performed by a disturbed person . . . ." I went on to note that "I would like to ensure that those faculty members did not die in a senseless act of violence. I would like to make sense out of this senseless act. There are pearls of wisdom to be found and there is a lesson to be learned" (Todaro-Franceschi, 2003, pp. 184–185). Looking at repeating headlines all over the world, where people are sharing horrors and hearts are aching, I feel compelled to note that by trying to make meaning *together* we can help one another to heal.

There is a large body of literature that suggests that one's search for meaning and those activities geared toward *making* meaning out of bad experiences can help people to heal and overcome feelings of despair from traumatic experiences. The Viennese psychiatrist Viktor E. Frankl (1959), who himself survived years of insurmountable horror in Nazi death camps, went on to create a revolutionary form of psychotherapy called logotherapy, which rests on the premise that our search for meaning is the driving force behind all human endeavor.

In Frankl's (1959) classic work, *Man's Search for Meaning*, he described enormous suffering and, yet, he acknowledged that even in the midst of great anguish, life has meaning and purpose in every moment that we live. He noted that as human beings we have the freedom of will, and that we can will ourselves to seek and move toward making meaning in our lives. Along these lines, in a recently reported longitudinal study of what might facilitate healing for survivors from the collective trauma of the 9/11 terrorist attacks, it was found that the search for meaning helped to predict a higher stress response and incidence of PTSD, whereas *finding* meaning predicted lower PTSD symptoms (Updegraff, Silver, & Holman, 2008). I am not sure that we can always *find* meaning in everything, but I do think we can *make* meaning from anything. In instances of collective trauma it is helpful for us to support each other in the attempt to make meaning.

Collective Healing

When a group shares the horror of a traumatic event and people come together to support one another, healing is facilitated. As healthcare professionals we know this and encourage people who have been traumatized to seek support from their loved ones, support group networks, and so on. Yet, we often do not recognize the need for ourselves to seek the same kind of support. Having compassionate leaders who understand not only the traumatizing nature of our work, but also that we are human beings with unique characteristics is so important because every person will have different ways of dealing with the traumatizing aspects of our work based on personality, culture, and previous experiences, among other things.

In the increasing body of literature on the importance of compassion in organizations, it is repeatedly stressed that it is human beings who make up organizations—it is people who meet the goals and the mission of any workplace. And we *feel*. Noted, "there is always grief somewhere in the room" when you put a bunch of people in it (Dutton, Frost, Worline, Lilius, & Kanov, 2002, p. 60). Experts in organizational behavior who have extensively studied the positive transformation that occurs when compassion is displayed by those in management note that leaders can promote compassion on two levels, by providing:

1. A context for meaning—the leader creates an environment in which people can freely express and discuss the way they feel, which in turn helps them make sense of their pain, seek or provide comfort, and
2. A context for action—the leader creates an environment in which those who experience or witness pain can find ways to alleviate their own and others' suffering (Dutton et al., 2002, p. 56).

A compassionate leader realizes that in the midst of both individual and collective trauma, it is not acceptable to ask folks to come to work and put their thoughts or feelings aside. In cases of collective trauma it is especially unfitting once one realizes that healing will best take place if everyone is offered the opportunity to support and help each other.

Dutton et al. (2002) shared a story from their research on compassion in organizations; they interviewed the employees in a company where a visitor had died suddenly in the firm's hallway, even though employees had heroically tried to revive him. Afterward the company leaders carried on business as usual, never acknowledging what had happened. They noted that it left

> people shocked and demoralized and uncertain about how to respond should such an event occur again. Some employees were wracked with guilt over not being able to save the man's life. Others felt weak and helpless because they had no opportunity to grieve in the presence of their colleagues. They had shared a significant experience and could not console one another—or even recognize people's extraordinary efforts to revive the victim. This one event damaged not just the employees who were directly involved but also the social fabric of the whole company. (p. 57)

Notably, the managers hindered, rather than facilitated, employee healing, which in turn negatively affected the company as a whole.

Years ago, one of my daughters, then a high school student, volunteered to work at an AIDS Memorial quilt event in Washington, DC. I went with her, and the first moment I laid eyes on the quilt, which took up the entire space of the Mall, I was struck by the enormity of the loss—a collective loss like no other. While I had known it before—that young, old, male, and female individuals of every cultural and religious tradition have been lost to this disease, it hit me hard. Having not ever suffered a personal loss from AIDS did not matter. No one viewing that quilt was left unscathed. Anyone who saw that quilt there was traumatized.

Just as compassion fatigue and burnout are contagious, *compassion* is contagious. So why is it that we have few forums in the workplace where we can visibly share the horrors we silently witness and silently share together?

I took care of that 18-month-old child with AIDS during the course of only one 12-hour shift. How many of my coworkers did that and more, and cried all night as I did? Had we the opportunity to share our compassionate caring and cosuffering, we could have consoled one another. Instead, we each carried the pain home with us and, undoubtedly, we carry the sustaining memories forever. I am sure that some of my coworkers developed compassion fatigue and still others over time burnt out.

It would seem that viewing the nature of our work with people who are suffering as a collective traumatic experience could offer us a direction for healing our wounded workforce. Research findings indicate that many people perceive benefits from traumatic experiences and that those who are able to find or make meaning following trauma are more likely to adjust and be able to live well (Poulin, Silver, Gil-Rivas, Holman, & McIntosh, 2009). Making meaning from our experiences with patients who are suffering and their loved ones can be a social benefit for all of us engaged in healthcare practice.

APPLYING *ART* FOR HEALING FROM SHARED HORRORS

The *ART*© model (Todaro-Franceschi, 2008, 2013, 2015) can help to guide those suffering with PTSD. Healing from traumatic events, be they individual or collective in nature, as with anything else, must begin with the *Acknowledgment* that there is a problem. Treatment for PTSD usually entails one-to-one counseling and/or support group therapy and frequently also requires medication for anxiety, depressive symptoms, and/or sleep disturbances. In order to *recognize* and make choices and take purposeful action to heal from PTSD, the afflicted person first has to have an understanding of the nature of the problem. For many people who are suffering with PTSD, there is so much anxiety that medication and counseling are usually the best choices that they can make initially in order to clear the way for other choices and purposeful actions. *Recognize* that PTSD is not something that we create by ourselves. It is physiologically and psychologically instigated and transforms the whole. Thus, a holistic approach is needed in identifying choices and purposeful actions for healing, and, as always, the action plan will need to be finely tailored to each person. *T*urning outward toward self and other is of vital importance because it is difficult to heal from PTSD without therapeutic intervention. Journaling, meditation, and reconnecting with nature and with loved ones can facilitate finding meaning and in instances where it may seem impossible to find meaning, we can make meaning.

ART (acknowledging, recognizing choices of purposeful actions one can take, and turning outward toward self and other) can also be applied in group work to heal from instances of collective trauma. People who suffer from traumatic experiences can be encouraged to appreciate the meaningful connections in their moments together. We can encourage ourselves and each other in making meaning.

When people experience collective trauma, we learn that life is not always fair and that sometimes no matter how hard we try, we cannot control the events leading to changes in our lives. Dying, death, and threats of death are all integral with life and living. Yet there are always choices that we can make to move forward and to heal. Turning toward ourselves and each other, we can explore what choices we have and can make right now to help reaffirm our sense that this moment *right now* is meaningful and filled with purpose.

I have often wondered how it was that so many children imprisoned in concentration camps drew pictures of, and wrote about, butterflies. The very young as well as older children saw in butterflies a way to overcome some of their isolation and terror for a brief time, and they were able to describe the beauty, along with the ugliness, all the meaning and purpose of their lives, in such vivid portrayals (e.g., as have been shared in the drawings and poems from the Terezin concentration camp in 1942–1944; Volavkova, 1993). In some ways, children are smarter than adults; these children knew what no one was saying, that many of them would die. Yet, by their reflections, it is clear that many held hope for their future, while being in the moment.

Nurses can find hope for the future while being in moments where we bear witness to individual and collective trauma. We readily acknowledge when others are traumatized and are suffering. For our own quality of life, both personal and professional, it is perhaps time for us to acknowledge that we have been and continue to be collectively traumatized in our work environments. We can encourage ourselves and each other to make meaning from our collective suffering. We can turn outward toward ourselves and each other.

KEY POINTS

- Collective trauma occurs when a group of people experience a life-threatening event or bear witness to another person (or persons) experiencing a life-threatening event.
- What is traumatic for one person may not be for another.
- Working with people who have life-threatening illness or injury and are suffering can be viewed as a form of collective trauma that all healthcare professionals and others who work in healthcare settings experience together.
- PTSD is an anxiety disorder that has a biological as well as psychological basis and emerges from traumatic life-threatening experiences.
- PTSD and healing from traumatic events require one to first acknowledge that he or she has been traumatized and that an intervention of some sort is necessary.

- Healing from experiences of collective trauma is facilitated by compassionate caring and being supportive of each other.

- Healing from traumatic experiences may be facilitated by finding, or making, meaning.

REFERENCES

Conant, E. (2007, March 19). To share in the horror. *Newsweek, 149*(12), p. 34.

Dutton, J. E., Frost, P. J., Worline, M. C., Lilius, J. M., & Kanov, J. M. (2002). Leading in times of trauma. *Harvard Business Review, 80*(1), pp. 54–61.

Erikson, K. T. (1995). Loss of communality at Buffalo Creek. In J. B. Williamson & E. S. Shneidman (Eds.), *Death: Current perspectives* (4th ed., pp. 407–413). Mountain View, CA: Mayfield Publishing.

Frankl, V. (1959). *Man's search for meaning.* New York, NY: Beacon Press.

Poulin, M. J., Silver, R. C., Gil-Rivas, V., Holman, E. A., & McIntosh, D. N. (2009). Finding social benefits after a collective trauma: Perceiving societal changes and well-being following 9/11. *Journal of Traumatic Stress, 22*(2), 81–90. doi:10.1002/jts.20391

Schuster, M. A., Stein, B. D., Jaycox, L. H., Collins, R. L., Marshall, G. N., Elliott, M. N., . . . Berry, S. H. (2001). A national survey of stress reactions after the September 11, 2001 terrorist attacks. *New England Journal of Medicine, 345*(20), 1507–1512. doi:10.1056/NEJM200111153452024

Todaro-Franceschi, V. (1999). *The enigma of energy: Where science and religion converge.* New York, NY: Crossroad.

Todaro-Franceschi, V. (2003). Letter to the editor. *Nursing Science Quarterly, 16,* 184–185.

Todaro-Franceschi, V. (2008). Preventing compassion fatigue and reaffirming purpose in nursing. *Proceedings on the 3rd European Federation of Critical Care Nursing Congress and 27th Aniarti Conference, Influencing Critical Care Nursing in Europe,* Florence, Italy (October).

Todaro-Franceschi, V. (2011). *Remembering.* A digital story. Retrieved from http://www.youtube.com/watch?v=SB2EATOU0wo&context=C320c904ADOEgsT oPDskK9oh_kCfN3JWP6bHkRZcpi

Todaro-Franceschi, V. (2013). *Compassion fatigue and burnout in nursing: Enhancing professional quality of life.* New York, NY: Springer Publishing.

Todaro-Franceschi, V. (2015). The ART of maintaining the "care" in healthcare. *Nursing Management, 46*(6), 53–55. doi:10.1097/01.numa.0000465407.76450.ab

Updegraff, J. A., Silver, R. C., & Holman, E. A. (2008). Searching for and finding meaning in collective trauma: Results from a national longitudinal study of the 9/11 terrorist attacks. *Journal of Personality and Social Psychology, 95*(3), 709–722. doi:10.1037/0022-3514.95.3.709

Volavkova, H. (Ed.). (1993). *I never saw another butterfly* . . . . New York, NY: Schocken Books.

Yehuda, R. (2002a). Post-traumatic stress disorder. *New England Journal of Medicine, 346*(2), 108–114. doi:10.1056/NEJMra012941

Yehuda, R. (Ed.). (2002b). *Treating trauma: Survivors with PTSD.* Washington, DC: American Psychiatric Publishing.

VI

Beating the Odds

It's up to us. We can spend our lives cultivating our resentments and cravings or we can explore the path of the warrior—nurturing open-mindedness and courage.

—Pema Chodron

12

Changing the Mindset in Nursing Education

Educating the mind without educating the heart is no education at all.

— Aristotle

Intelligence plus character—that is the goal of true education.

— Martin Luther King, Jr.

KEY TOPICS

- Enhancing nursing education and quality caring
- Hidden curriculum
- Delineating and articulating our nurseculture

INTRODUCTION

A decade ago, the Committee on the Robert Wood Johnson Foundation (RWJF) Initiative for the Future of Nursing, at the Institute of Medicine (IOM, 2009), developed a vision for a transformed healthcare

© Springer Publishing Company DOI: 10.1891/9780826155214.0012

system.[1] To summarize the key message of the in-depth report, they noted the following:

1. Nurses should practice to the full extent of their education and training.
2. Nurses should achieve higher levels of education and training through an improved education system that promotes seamless academic progression.
3. Nurses should be full partners, with physicians and other health professionals, in redesigning healthcare in the United States.
4. Effective workforce planning and policy making require better data collection and an improved information infrastructure. (p. 4)

The committee emphasized that, "The education system should provide nurses with the tools needed to evaluate and improve standards of patient care and the quality and safety of care while preserving fundamental elements of nursing education, such as ethics and integrity and holistic, compassionate approaches to care" (IOM, 2009, p. 31).

Thereafter, the RWJF, in conjunction with the AARP initiated a campaign for action to meet the objectives set forth in their landmark report on the future of nursing. According to updates on the campaign, progress has been made in several areas such as increased numbers of baccalaureate and doctorally prepared nurses. Over the past few years in a number of states, advanced practice nurses have finally attained full autonomy over their practice. Finally, the BSN in ten is becoming a reality.

A BIRD'S-EYE VIEW

Although the current status of nursing education has improved in some respects, it has not done so abundantly. Certainly, it has not changed enough during the past decade to transform nursing and healthcare. Over time, the established essentials for nursing education put forward by the American Association of Colleges of Nursing (AACN) have become increasingly more inclusive; however, the emphasis in most nursing programs seems to be on *more* pharmacology, *more* pathophysiology, *more* physical assessment, more, well, *medical* knowledge. I have taught in five different nursing programs, consulted at a number of hospitals, and have done numerous talks/workshops at various organizations and facilities, particularly in the past five or so years. I have heard from nurses working in all sectors of healthcare, including many nurse educators, and from nursing students across undergraduate, graduate, and doctoral nursing programs. All is *not* as it should be in many schools of nursing.

Hidden Curricula, Both Good and Bad

There is quite a bit in the literature about hidden curricula but not enough of a focus on it in nursing. The term *hidden curriculum* usually refers to content that is being taught without intention, but sometimes it is also used to depict something that is being taught covertly with intention. For example, I always have a hidden curriculum; in all of my classes, no matter what content I am teaching, I stress the importance of the nurse and how the choices we make always have a butterfly effect.

In nursing, there is omission of important curricular content, which in part, contributes to a hidden curriculum that is not good for the profession of nursing or the people the profession serves. When we say that we do not have time to teach certain subjects, say, ethics, end of life, or self-care, we are sending a subliminal message to the students whether intended or not. The students do not know that they are essentially being short-changed.

As someone who has advocated (for over two decades) to have bioethics, end-of-life, and professional quality of life issues be part of nursing education, I have repeatedly felt the pushback by faculty and administrators. Resistance to the teaching of this content occurs across undergraduate-, graduate-, and doctoral-level programs. I have gone to and participated in many conferences focused on bioethics and end of life over the years, and spoken with many educators who have faced similar resistance.

A while back, faculty in our PhD nursing program made the decision to downsize a 3-credit full-term–required bioethics course and make two 1-credit courses, one of which focuses specifically on institutional review board (IRB) requirements. The message being sent seemed clear and not at all hidden at the time: bioethics has less value than meeting the minimal requirements for doctoral education and getting the research done. I was the faculty member for the original 3-credit required bioethics course, and I knew there was enormous value in having a full-term course for PhD nursing students.

Most of the nurses in these classes, all of whom had undergraduate and graduate degrees in nursing, had never taken a bioethics course before. But almost all of them came into the course having experienced numerous ethical dilemmas in their practice. Many suffered with moral distress and residue from years of carrying around heavy, heavy baggage. Unsurprisingly to me, a lot of the moral distress was centered on end-of-life issues, although very few of these nurses had chosen to work in practice areas where dying and death regularly occur. Naturally, most of these students had never been adequately prepared to face dying and death during their basic nursing education either.

The classes were illuminating for everyone. Students often disclosed that the stories they were sharing in class had not been shared or discussed with anyone before; truly heart-rending stories of their experiences with patients, families, and coworkers. During these classes, I was regularly informed by students that some of them felt for the *very first time, as if they had a voice, and that what they had to say was important.* They felt empowered to go back to their respective practices and knowingly, actively participate in ways that they felt they had never been able to do before. My faculty colleagues did not know this or if they did, clearly they did not see the value in it. The additional shame of it was that while many of these doctoral students came into the course at the beginning of the term without an identified area for study, many left, upon its completion, with a renewed sense of purpose and a very clear sense of the direction in which they wanted to go.

Nurse Kathleen MacMillan (2016) asks us to explore the hidden curriculum in nursing to see what we are actually teaching about basic nursing care. She reiterates some of what I have noted throughout this book. For example, the use of terminology such as "doctor's orders," the extraordinary emphasis being placed on learning certain clinical skills, and the displacement or inappropriate placement of certain topics all contribute to the notion that some things are more or less important.

Minimizing topics like ethics, end of life, self-care, and so on does not make any sense whatsoever. You cannot expect nurses to love their work without being given the tools that enable them to do it. You cannot ask nurses to lead healthcare transformation if they are led to believe, or are treated as if, they are subordinate or "less than."

Incivility in Nursing Academia

I am worried about our future workforce and I know that many other nurse educators are, too. I have witnessed the denigration of faculty who speak up, trying to make things better, and have myself been a victim of cruel mobbing by other nurse academics. Nurse educators have an impetus to be role models and teach compassion. Yet, the behavior of some nurse educators belies our moral code, sometimes in quite blatant ways but more often than not, surreptitiously. Some of the nurse educators I have encountered over the course of my career as either a student or coworker are so utterly horrid that I would rather not refer to them as nurses. Countless times I have either witnessed firsthand, or heard about, the bad behavior of faculty toward students; indeed, in many instances I have intervened (much to my own detriment).

For years I walked around shaking my head; it felt so surreal. Then I began to read the literature on incivility in nursing academia and I was honestly kind of relieved to read about some of it, especially the phenomenon of "gaslighting," which is an insidious form of emotional abuse where one is manipulated into questioning their own memory, perceptions, judgment, or even sanity. Reading about it helped to validate that what I had experienced was in fact real. It did not make it any less painful, but it did help to know I was not hallucinating all the time.

A non-nurse vice president (VP) in higher education once told me that in her vast, many-year experience working with faculty, she had found that nurse educators were more malicious to each other than people from any other discipline. Is it any wonder why nurses are out there being uncivil to one another? They probably learned the bad behavior in nursing school. This is a topic that requires far more space than I can allocate here, but those who are interested should really take a look at nurse expert Cynthia Clark's extensive work on incivility in nursing academia.

A PEDAGOGIC GOAL: THE WELL-BEING OF THE NURSE

The nursing education literature calls for radical transformation. In their book on the implications of the IOM reports for nursing, nurse authors Anita Finkelman and Carol Kenner (2012) wrote in great detail about how we could use the IOM reports to guide, generate, and sustain positive change in nursing education and practice. The core competencies of providing patient-centered care, participating in interdisciplinary teamwork, employing evidence-based practice, applying quality improvement, and using informatics are quite visible (Finkelman & Kenner, 2012). Their relationship to the forces of magnetism is very clear.

In order to make it all come together, educators (and leaders, who I will come back to in Chapter 13) need to emphasize the importance of putting the oxygen mask on first. In fact, since the first edition of this book was published, in which I repeatedly emphasized the need for the oxygen mask to go on our own faces first, one organization has developed a series of workshops entitled "Oxygen for Caregivers" (see Appendix C, Resources). Around the globe, employers are focusing more effort on workforce health as a whole. But the healthcare sector is still lagging behind, and our profession, which should be leading the effort, cannot do so because we have not actually fixed ourselves yet.

There needs to be inclusion on the development of ways to meet our needs and care for ourselves individually and collectively so that we are prepared to care for others without hurting ourselves in the process. Kenner, Finkelman, Weatherby, Long, and Kupperschmidt (2009) carefully addressed the issues that our profession faces, many of which came out in the wash, so to speak, with Gordon's (2005) book on nursing against the odds. They wrote:

We do not play well together, and this hurts us tremendously in the bigger political arena. We cannot blame all this on physicians and healthcare organizations because they can only take away as much power as we are willing to give up. (p. 255)

That was a decade ago, and unfortunately still holds true.

What has been stressed as important for nursing education in a lot of the literature does not address the needs of the *nurse*. As Kenner et al. (2009) note, only we can do that. We have to come to terms with the fact that we preach self-care to people, but we do not teach, practice, and live what we preach. The many intertwined issues related to the incidence of compassion fatigue, moral distress, burnout, and incivility in nursing detailed throughout this book and in the growing body of literature on these and related subjects mandate that we turn toward ourselves at this juncture. We simply cannot afford not to do so. The health and quality of life for *all of us*—nurses, patients, their loved ones, and, indeed, *our* loved ones—is at stake.

In 2007, when the Carnegie Foundation report on nursing education came out, spearheaded by nurse scholar Pat Benner and colleagues (Benner, Sutphen, Leonard, Day, & Shulman, 2009), a clear emphasis was placed on three apprenticeships, which all seemed to be of equal importance: (a) teaching "nurse think"—the learning of practical reasoning skills; (b) teaching skills through coaching and simulation, where clinical reasoning development goes hand in hand with skill acquisition; and (c) teaching and facilitating the development of social/moral roles and ethical behaviors. The third one seems to consistently get the short end of the stick. While nurse educators, scholars, and leaders have, over the course of nursing's historical development, repeatedly advocated for our selfhood (which includes our inherent ability to compassionately care) and self-recognition, as powerful contributors in healthcare, the very essence of our being continues to be denied by many individuals, in, and out of, nursing.

In addition to the studies that the IOM performed related to nursing, several other key studies were done. Just to mention a few, the Josiah Macy, Jr., Foundation work, *Who Will Provide Primary Care and How Will They Be Trained?* and *Continuing Education in the Health Professions: Improving Healthcare Through Lifelong Learning*, both suggested that nurses are key players in healthcare and that more emphasis needs to be placed on education and lifelong learning (IOM, 2009). The question we need to ask ourselves at this juncture is: Are we *teaching* the things that nurses need to learn during their lifelong learning? Are we teaching the things that will enable them to love what they do and to do it well?

When so many intelligent groups keep stressing the importance of nurses in achieving transformation in healthcare, how is it that this fundamental aspect is so frequently left out of our nursing curricula—that in most programs we do not teach students to appreciate themselves and each other? Without having been taught that they are important (and I reiterate—full partners, with physicians and other health professionals), nurses cannot expect to know that they are. Nurses are, quite frankly, being deprived of the fundamental elements that could help to sustain our individual and collective well-being while working in complex healthcare environments. If, and only if, we change the basic education of our future workforce, can we rise to meet the challenges in healthcare and the expectations of society.

In the seminal work for which Benner (1984) became so well known, *From Novice to Expert: Excellence and Power in Clinical Nursing Practice*, she expounded upon what makes a nurse an expert practitioner. Through her observations and critical analysis of nurses in practice, she offered us a clear path forward. It would be helpful to our profession, if at this time, folks in nursing education and leadership who have this book were to take it down from their bookshelves, dust it off, and reread it. Those who do not have the book should really get a copy to read; it is enlightening, to say the least. I often think that had we all taken this work to heart and mind when she wrote it, we would have transformed nursing education *radically* back then—over 35 years ago.

In her studies, Benner (1984) identified six qualities of power inherent in the caring provided by the expert nurses she observed: transformative, integrative, advocacy, healing, participative/affirmative, and problem solving (p. 210). While space does not permit a discussion on each of them, I want to stress that all of them combined reflect the compassionate caring practices inherent in our work. Throughout her book, Benner repeatedly comes back to caring and knowing participation as foundational elements for expert nursing practice. I offer just a few of her thoughts here to reemphasize what has already been noted. Benner emphatically wrote: ". . . It is *not* true that the best protection against burnout lies in distancing and control strategies—that is, protection against caring" (p. 214). She shared an exemplar of a nurse who provided comfort and presence during a woman's last moments of life and noted that it

> . . . illustrates the best antidote to burnout in the work setting; engagement and involvement . . . . In participating, this nurse was able to use the meanings and resources inherent in this poignant event. In caring, she not only experienced pain, but also strength and affirmation. She learned first-hand about a human possibility that many never experience or witness and she felt affirmed and stronger for it. One could imagine that a detached, avoiding

approach would have offered only frail protection and no positive resources such as the participative and affirmative power of caring that this nurse gained. (p. 214)

Benner (1984) also stated that the emotional component of our caring practices can lead us in meaningful ways that impersonal, disconnected caring will not. Our unique ways of knowing can make all the difference: "A preference for detached, reflective reasoning and formal explicit knowledge overlooks the role of caring with its attendant emotions—vague feelings, hunches, a sense that something is not right—or the creative search and cue sensitivity that occur as a result of caring" (p. 216). Yet, in much of the literature where authors are stressing the changes that need to take place in nursing education, there is little to indicate that any importance is being (or even should be) placed on the development of social/moral roles, ethical behaviors, and unique ways of knowing. There is little that addresses self-care strategies for the nurse—something that is, in our code of ethics, noted to be *central* to the well-being of our profession. There is little or no mention of compassion, or caring practices, and by this I am referring to that human-to-human connection so vital to us in our practice.

In 2014, a national summit on nursing ethics was sponsored by the Johns Hopkins School of Nursing and Johns Hopkins Berman Institute of Bioethics (2014), led by nurse expert and bioethicist Cynda Rushton. A group of nurse leaders came together to discuss and put forward a blueprint for supporting ethical nursing practice in ways that would hopefully culminate in transforming our healthcare culture to more strongly support basic ethical values and principles; this in turn would better enable nurses to provide quality care. The report on this summit stresses the need to make the teaching of nursing ethics foundational for all levels of nursing education and practice. Following on the heels of this summit, the American Nurses Association (ANA) designated 2015 as the "Year of Ethics" and our revised ANA code of ethics was published. Nonetheless, many nursing schools continue to downsize important content across the board in undergraduate, graduate, and doctoral programs. In some places, it has been downsized so much it is nonexistent. The social and caring aspects that are clearly delineated in our code of ethics are visibly *invisible*. The omission sticks out like a sore thumb, and that it is an ominous omission one cannot doubt.

Benner (1984) wrote that, "to abandon the power inherent in caring relationships is to sell out but, worse yet, it is to become alienated from our own identity and to thwart our own excellence . . . . Nursing without caring is powerful and devastating" (p. 216). If we are not selling ourselves out entirely, as Benner suggested, we are definitely selling ourselves *short*. As a result, we have a lot of unhappy nurses, increasing incivility and bullying among ourselves in our workplaces, including in academia, many people leaving nursing who should stay, and, conversely, people not coming into nursing who should. The cost to us individually and collectively as a profession is nothing compared to the cost to those we serve, those whose quality of living–dying is most assuredly in jeopardy.

DELINEATING AND MAKING OUR UNIQUE *NURSECULTURE* VISIBLE

Nurse educators can do much to minimize and prevent the contagion of the syndromes of compassion fatigue and burnout. In order to fix us, we need to have a real emphasis on the development of an inclusive "nurseculture" that includes character building. We already have a kind of nurseculture when it comes to the meaning and purpose of our work—to care with compassion for others puts us in a vulnerable place at times.[2] However, it is not sufficient to be a compassionate carer; one must be fortified to do it well. By this I mean a whole cadre of things, which includes a sense of one's own salience and a sense of our collective importance. It should not be potluck whether our future nurses are taught that they are the most important healthcare constituents and that their voices count.

Fortifying our nurses for lifelong commitment to service means that they must learn assertiveness, advocacy, end of life, and ethics (the code needs to be apparent across nursing curricula). It means that they need to develop mindful awareness of their own needs as well as the needs of others, and be able to apply their compassionate caring in ways that will instill joy in their own lives as well as the lives of others. And before any of you—my colleagues in nursing education—go shaking your heads, think about all the stories I have shared here, and others you may have heard. Think about the potential for harm if we do not change the approach we currently have in nursing education. We keep emphasizing the science, and yes, it is important. But unless nurses do better at caring for ourselves, which means a total mindset reboot for us in nursing, knowing the science will not help. We cannot continue to teach nurses as many of us in nursing have ourselves been taught (i.e., go back to the previous chapters on the idea of gendered labor). The nurse who is taught to "take orders" (to be subservient) and self-sacrificing is not a happy nurse or a healthy nurse.

In one of my classes on communication, I asked students to watch the powerful clip from the film *Wit*, during which the nurse Suzie sits with the patient Vivian, who is visibly frightened and lonely, as they share a popsicle. They talk about prognosis and end-of-life care wishes. Suzie explained the choices Vivian had—to seek aggressive treatment for as long as possible and in the event of cardiopulmonary arrest to resuscitate or conversely to allow natural death (do not resuscitate [DNR]). At the end of the discussion, Vivian opts to allow natural death. When I asked the students, most of whom had already taken the board exams and were registered nurses, to share their thoughts on it, one student actually questioned the legal right of the nurse to talk about treatment and prognosis at all. That same student also seemed concerned that the writers of the film were advocating for people to end their lives earlier. Ask yourself, what was this student taught in basic nursing education? With this kind of mindset, would this student be able to work in the world of nursing for any length of time and be effective or happy?

With assertiveness and advocacy skills we need to include more (or better) communication skill development, along with conflict resolution strategies. The tenets of civility and professional behavior must be a part of basic education in nursing, too. Clark (2014) says, "To me, civility is like handwashing: It needs to be taught, reinforced, and given constant attention and reminders" (p. 1). I say ditto that!

Nursing theory should be introduced at the beginning of nursing school. Not many students seem enthusiastic to take classes on nursing theory and I think it is at least in part because they have been biased against it by the hidden curriculum. Many nursing faculty do not seem to value it. However, whenever I have taught nursing theory, I have witnessed a heightened awareness in many students regarding the meaning and purpose of our nursing work. Many share AHA! moments that occur in their practice, events they actually attribute to the learning of nursing theory. There is an awful lot of affirmative "nodding," in my theory classes, especially when we get to the caring theoretic frameworks. Given that nurses must care for people of all races and religions, it is imperative that we have an understanding of the intricate nature of both healing and suffering from a transcultural perspective. Nursing theory covers all the varied perspectives in language that is unique to our discipline. Shouldn't we be teaching it and using it?

Leadership and the Clinical Nurse Leader (CNL) Role

Nursing leadership is integral to meeting the goal of healthcare transformation, and the creation of the CNL role is an intervention that has enormous potential to help fix significant issues in healthcare. Some might ask why the CNL is considered an intervention with the potential to transform healthcare; a relevant question, but one that to me has an obvious answer and is germane to many of the topics discussed in this book. It is because the CNL student is being educated based on the core values and excellences of the nursing profession with a unique skill set. The CNL has been taught all about quality, safety, change agency, advocacy and assertiveness, professional quality of life and organizational behavior, ethics, and in the program I developed, all of the students were End-of-Life Nursing Education Consortium (ELNEC) trained, too. Thus, the CNL student is learning many of the foundational elements that have been downsized, or, on occasion, completely omitted in the nurse's primary or basic education.

For about 10 years I was the coordinator for the only CNL program in the New York City region. We had developed the program following the AACN template for CNL education; the CNL was the first new role in nursing to be developed in over four decades. When I was asked to take on curriculum development and coordination for this new program in 2007, I was also the coordinator for the adult health medical–surgical clinical nurse specialist (CNS) program. I was not sold on the idea of a new role in nursing. Rather, I was perturbed because it seemed to me that the CNS role had never been adequately defined or established by the profession, and that perhaps we should just market the CNS a little better. However, as I looked more closely at the goals for the CNL versus the goals for the CNS, I realized there were distinct differences between the two roles, and I began to see the value of a new role specifically designed to create change in healthcare. Much needed, as in, desperately needed, change. Yet, here it is over 10 years later, and the program was closed by the university.

The fact of the matter is that at least part of the Northeast has not really embraced the idea of the CNL. Graduates from our program had to leave the area if they wanted to find CNL specific positions, which several of them did over the years, or they sought, and easily found, other kinds of leadership or educator positions. None of the CNL graduates from our program had difficulty finding employment, and I am certain that all of them regularly use the unique skill set that they obtained during their graduate education to the benefit of everyone. I also know that several of the students were inspired during their studies to go on to work in palliative care and quite a few have enrolled in PhD or doctor of nursing practice (DNP) programs.

Now and then I ponder why the CNL has not caught on throughout the country as an intervention for healthcare woes; AACN has surely done a great job of marketing the role as such. The voice of that CNL student keeps reverberating in my head; the one who worked in a Magnet® facility and emphatically shared with me her fear that if she identified any problems at work she would get fired; adding the comment that her employers were too busy hiding the problems to want to solve any of them. So, the CNL *should* be there to support and appreciate the carers—the bedside nurses and all the other staff who are so vitally important to the provision of quality caring. The CNL *could* be uniquely positioned to facilitate the enhancement of quality caring at the bedside. However, even with adequate education, staff nurses and CNLs cannot transform healthcare alone. Especially if there are those in the workplace who do not share the same values or have forgotten the meaning and purpose of their work. We need ALL nurses to have the same basic elements that the CNLs have in their education. The roles may differ, and with it the level of education, but the foundation should be the same.

Educators should not assume that nurses coming into graduate programs already have any of the necessary skill set, for it is likely that many do not. To be blunt, as far as I can see, without all of it, nurses will continue to move along as they have in the past. Some will be much more effective than others; however, with the development of a *nurseculture* that includes learning how important nurses are and how to make our voices heard, the profession of nursing might finally move forward into the driver's seat where it belongs.

End-of-Life and Palliative Care

In prior chapters I have shared some information on the elective course I created and taught for many years. I had written it to meet the university pluralism and diversity requirements; it was writing intensive, and it was the first interprofessional course offering in the school of nursing. Despite the effort I put into making it so lucrative, the course was never offered more than once a year, and for about 8 years *no* seats were allocated to any discipline outside of nursing. Whenever the course was offered, it filled up within days, and then there were numerous requests from students to overtally. It was often offered at horrible times, like from 6 to 9 p.m. (the students frequently made note of the bad timing on their evaluations because it made an incredibly long day for many of them and definitely a horribly long one for me who could not get home until after midnight when the class was offered that late). The cap on the course enrollment went from 40 to 60 to 80 within a few years. Then, shortly after a change in administrative personnel, miraculously, non-nursing majors were allowed to enroll in the course. I had no control over any of this; course scheduling and enrollment was always the domain of the administration. Yet I was thrilled that my 2001 dream of an interdisciplinary course on changing the face of death was finally coming to fruition.

Educators in schools of nursing need to assess their curricula for whether or not end-of-life/palliative care content is in it. If it is only being offered in an elective, why is that the case? If the answer is that there isn't time for it, or that it isn't necessary content, I would ask again, why? Reiterating the main points in Chapter 10: Everyone dies and it is usually a nurse who is at the bedside of patients who are dying, and the nurse who is left to console the families of the dying.

In the fall of 2015, I was pleased to be invited as part of a national group of 25 experts in end-of-life/palliative care to work on the revision of the AACN 1997 document "Peaceful Death," which highlighted the educational preparation nurses needed in order to care for the dying and their families. Generously funded by the Cambria Foundation, we convened for several days in Portland, where the enthusiasm of nurse educators engaged in death and palliative care education was contagious. This endeavor led to the creation of a new document entitled "CARES" (**C**ompetencies **A**nd **R**ecommendations for **E**ducating undergraduate nursing **S**tudents), which provides an in-depth template for teaching nurses essential content in order to care for those with serious illness and their families (AACN, 2016; Ferrell, Malloy, Mazanec, & Virani, 2016). Hopefully, nurse educators will use this document to guide curriculum development.

Compassion Lessons and Reaffirming Purpose

How do we cultivate an atmosphere that will support us to do the work we do, and do it in a way that gets our hearts to stay *full* instead of becoming heavy or empty? We have to readily acknowledge and explore those things that can help us to foster mindful awareness in order to be able to, day after day, go to the places that scare us and still emerge joyful and content at the end of the day. There are many techniques that can help us to reconnect with and reaffirm purpose in our being in the world of nursing. I think collectively it has to begin with compassion lessons. This is not to say that we are not all compassionate people; it is rather to say that we need to develop that part of our personhood in ways that allow us to emulate compassion in our day-to-day living and working. Not just expressing it to others—but also to ourselves.

I have occasionally heard people say that compassion is not something that can be taught. You either have it or you do not. Consequently, I often marvel at how I have managed to teach others to be more compassionate over the course of my long nursing career. For I know that I have changed the way others approach caring. I know because I have been told so repeatedly; and because the actions of others who I have mentored, educated, or led continue to validate it. Yes, nurses and other carers have been called to care—we are compassionate people, but as I have said elsewhere, caring is a double-edged sword; it can harm us if we are not going about it in a mindful manner.

Nussbaum (1996) noted that there are practical strategies that one may use to teach compassion and that this should be one of the goals of public education in order to develop the qualities of good citizenship. She stressed that those engaged in education teach and "cultivate the ability to imagine the experiences of others and to participate in their suffering" (p. 50). She went on to note the following:

This education of the imagination should take a particular form. I have said that a crucial part of the ethical value of pity is its ability to cross boundaries of class, nationality, race, and gender, as the pitier assumes these different positions in imagination, and comes to see the obstacles to flourishing faced by human beings in these many concrete situations. (p. 51)

In nursing, while we teach cultural sensitivity, we do not aim to teach compassion in this manner. It seems to be taken for granted that nurses will place themselves in the position of their patients and try to understand their suffering. It is time to change this and make compassion lessons an integral part of the curriculum. Nurse educators can teach compassionate caring using clinical vignettes and reflective exercises.

During 3 years of research at the Compassion Lab, a joint project of the University of Michigan Business School and the University of British Columbia, researchers explored how stories of compassionate acts could inspire further compassionate acts (Dutton, Frost, Worline, Lilius, & Kanov, 2002). Storytelling is the main pedagogic strategy I use in many of my classes for I have found that it enhances not only teaching and learning, but also student engagement.

One year I found out after the fact that several students had cheated on a pharmacology exam. According to the university policy where I was working, unless you witnessed and/or had documentation from others who had witnessed cheating, there was not much you could do about it. Two students came to me to tell me of the cheating; they did not give me any names and they did not want to document what they had seen. So, I thought about what I could do and came up with an imagery exercise. I walked into class the following week and asked the students to close their eyes and do the following:

> *Picture your loved one coming into the ER in a life-threatening situation. The nurse, who had cheated her way through pharmacology classes, is not all that knowledgeable about the medications that should be administered in this instance, and as a result, she gives the wrong medication or the wrong dose. Consequently, your loved one codes and winds up in a vegetative state.*

I left the rest to their imagination. Noticeably, quite a few students were in tears, and I like to think that imagery exercise created a sustaining memory for many students, which occasionally resurfaces to remind them to always consider that their actions inevitably have consequences for others.

Physician Wiley Souba (2002) wrote that many of his colleagues have become "disenchanted with their ability to serve as advocates for and provide care to their patients" and that their work is ultimately less fulfilling (p. 139). He claimed that medicine needs to build dialogue on meaning and purpose into the medical curricula; I would say that it needs to be part of all health professional curricula and even take it further to suggest that all people should reflect upon the meaning and purpose of their work. Maybe people will be more attentive and happier for it. In nursing, if we take the time to talk about and reflect upon the meaning and purpose of our work, we will never lose sight of the fact that it emerges from and is maintained by our connection with others.

Nurse theorist Myra Levine (1972) shared a poignant story of how her life and nursing career evolved over time. Trained when nursing was still considered gendered labor, she noted the basic technical skills that nurses had to develop and how she excelled at learning and practicing them. She shared how she gave birth to her first child, and when waiting for her newborn son to be brought to her, she realized something must be wrong. She asked and then begged for her son. The nursery supervisor who "had no time" finally came by to tell her there was just a little mucus and he would be brought in later (p. 137). The next time she saw her son, he was dead. She described how the grief (both hers and the staff's) was so palpable:

> I could not see their sorrow from within my own, and they could not reach through to mine. They could not come, in silence, to stand beside me and share my grief. They could not watch the tears, and so I could not weep in my bewildered need not to offend them. They came to me smiling and left hurt and frightened from the mirror of my sorrow. Beyond that door was still the joy they daily lived amidst, and soon they came through it to me only when they had to come. (p. 137)

Levine (1972) went on to share how the death of her newborn son contributed to a change in her nursing practice and her development of compassion:

> Out of my own torn spirit I had learned that I could not offer only a part of what I was to nursing. The cautious selection that allowed me to share only a small part of myself with the patient left us both deprived. Unless my humanity could speak to him, his could never flourish. (p. 137)

With her terrible loss, Levine learned that nursing has to be more than a technical skill set. We need not (and should not!) learn this lesson through horrific personal experiences. We can learn or, in cases where burnout has occurred, *relearn* how to feel and express compassion, and we can teach it by sharing our stories and by taking time to reflect upon them.

Teaching Self-Compassion and *ART*

Psychotherapist Paul Gilbert notes that there are three focal points related to compassion: "the compassion that we feel and express towards others; the compassion that we are open to from others; and self-compassion" (Gilbert, 2013, p. 67). People may have difficulty with receiving compassion from others or being compassionate to self. Learning mindfulness is key to overcoming that difficulty. Research has demonstrated that mindfulness-based stress reduction (MBSR) increases self-compassion significantly, along with overall well-being (Baer, 2010; Kabat-Zinn, 1994).

Many nurses are self-sacrificing and do not take care of themselves; I know, because I was one of them. . . I learned the hard way that shortcutting on one's own self-care eventually catches up in many detrimental ways. Mindfulness, practiced over time, has been found to create positive, and permanent, changes in the way parts of the brain communicate with each other (Ireland, 2014). Changes after an 8-week course in mindfulness include shrinking of the "fight or flight" center (the amygdala) and thickening of the region associated with higher order brain functions such as increased awareness and concentration (the prefrontal cortex). This means that individuals who practice mindfulness regularly overall have less reaction to stress and better ability to focus. Considering the important nature of the work that nurses do, it seems to me that nurse educators have a responsibility to teach our students how to take good care of themselves so that they can take good care of others. Teaching mindfulness is one way to do that.

All students going into nursing (and other caring professions) should learn about professional quality of life; the good, the bad, the ugly, and uglier. Nurses should be taught the relationship between professional quality of life and how it contributes to work performance. Using the *ART*© model (Todaro-Franceschi, 2008, 2013, 2015) as a guide, nurses can learn to regularly evaluate how they feel in relation to their work and how it might be affecting the way they are going about it.

A—Acknowledge: They need to be able to acknowledge when they are in trouble, learning to recognize signs of compassion fatigue, moral distress, death overload, burnout, and bullying/incivility.

R—Recognize choices and take purposeful action: They need to be able to assess not only themselves but also their coworkers for problems. They need to know when they should seek assistance, and when to suggest that someone else seeks help. They need to know that they always have a choice and that they can take actions to be content at work.

T—Turn toward self and other: They need to know how to take care of themselves; that they matter; the importance of supporting one another, and the value of teamwork.

The Bottom Line Needs to Be Moved Up

So to recap, I would like to once again propose that we take all of this downsized and missing curricular material and move it on up to the number one slot in terms of pedagogic importance for nursing. This would include the following regularly omitted or displaced content:

- Development of a sense of the importance of nursing *as a collective body* and as the largest constituents of healthcare professionals involved in ensuring the quality of living–dying for people.
- Development of a sense of one's own salience as a nurse engaged in providing quality caring for people during both living and dying.
- Compassion skill development that encompasses learning first how to apply it to ourselves and each other with self and group care strategies (mentoring and coaching) and then how to apply it in practice (compassion as a value, virtue, and excellence). Herein we need to include civility lessons (and it would be a really good idea to run some workshops with focus group sessions for faculty, too).
- Learning and applying, through knowing participation, assertiveness and advocacy skills—enough of them in order to make sure that our voices are heard! It goes without saying that interpersonal communication skills including conflict resolution belong here.
- The identification of, and prevention strategies for, professional quality of life issues (compassion fatigue, moral distress, burnout, etc., and this includes learning how to face death and care for the dying!).

The best place for nurse educators to begin is probably to explore their own curricula to identify the hidden curriculum and then take it from there.

APPLYING *ART* TO NURSING EDUCATION

It is time for nurse educators to *acknowledge* that we have some significant issues in nursing academia that need our attention. We have to *recognize* that we have choices and can take purposeful actions to improve our work environment and to reboot the mindset in nursing education. To continue things as they are—is in many ways doing a disservice to the profession and to society.

We must improve the sense of communality in many schools of nursing and foster better mutual respect for each other. We need to band together rather than compete with, and isolate, each other. We all have something to contribute and should value each other's expertise. How can we teach the importance of teamwork, if we cannot seem to get it together ourselves? We need to support and protect colleagues from would-be bullies. Faculty who go along to get along need to *stop* doing it and instead speak up, *together*.

We need to explore the hidden curriculum in our respective schools of nursing to evaluate curricula for key content. We should examine how much, and where, in the program all of the necessary elements are being taught for a thorough development of our unique *nurseculture*. Teaching nurses how important they are to the people they serve, and how the buck really does stop with us. . . . These are the things that will help nurses withstand the stress of the difficult work that we do; these are the things we need to emphasize so that compassionate, competent nurses remain in the profession and love what they do. Last, but absolutely not least, we should all be asking ourselves, in our programs are we teaching students and role-modeling how to best emulate compassion?

KEY POINTS

- A hidden curriculum persists in nursing education that needs to be explored in all schools of nursing.

- Nurses need to learn how important they are individually and collectively, to the well-being of society.

- We need to *believe* that we are full partners with physicians and other health professionals in the healthcare system. They need to know that they matter, are respected and heard.

- The oxygen mask has to go on our face first; nurses need to learn how to show compassion to self as well as others.

- All nurses should have foundational knowledge of ethics, assertiveness, advocacy, conflict resolution, leadership, civility, self-care strategies, end-of-life care, and professional quality of life issues. The inclusion of these things in nursing education will help us to develop ways to meet our needs and care for ourselves individually and collectively, so that we are prepared to care for others without hurting ourselves in the process.

- We need to make time for nursing students to talk about and reflect upon the meaning and purpose of nursing work; to look at and reflect upon the whole.

NOTES

1. The IOM is now known as the National Academies of Science, Engineering and Medicine, also known as National Academies.
2. Some might say it is more a female thing. See Carol Gilligan's (1982) classic work, *In A Different Voice*, where she reflects on the way women think and act in relational terms.

REFERENCES

AACN. (2016). *CARES: Competencies and recommendations for educating undergraduate nursing students: Preparing nurses to care for the seriously ill and their families.* Washington, DC: Author.

Baer, R. A. (2010). Self-compassion as a mechanism of change in mindfulness- and acceptance-based treatments. In R. A. Baer (Ed.), *Assessing mindfulness and acceptance processes in clients: Illuminating the theory and practice of change* (pp. 135–153). Oakland, CA: New Harbinger.

Benner, P. (1984). *From novice to expert: Excellence and power in clinical nursing practice.* Menlo Park, CA: Addison-Wesley Publishing.

Benner, P., Sutphen, M., Leonard, V., Day, L., & Shulman, L. (2009). Foreword. In *Educating nurses: A call for radical transformation* (Jossey-Bass/Carnegie Foundation for the Advancement of Teaching). Kindle Edition. Retrieved from www.amazon.com

Clark, C. M. (2014). Seeking civility. *American Nurse Today, 9*(7), 1–6.

Dutton, J. E., Frost, P. J., Worline, M. C., Lilius, J. M., & Kanov, J. M. (2002). Leading in times of trauma. *Harvard Business Review, 80*(1), 54–61.

Ferrell, B., Malloy, P., Mazanec, P., & Virani, R. (2016). CARES: Competencies and recommendations for educating undergraduate nursing students to improve palliative care. *Journal of Professional Nursing, 32*(5), 327–333. doi: 10.1016/j.profnurs.2016.07.002

Finkelman, A., & Kenner, C. (2012). *Teaching IOM: Implications of the Institute of Medicine reports for nursing education* (3rd ed.). Silver Spring, MD: American Nurses Association.

Gilbert, P. (2013). Compassion-focused therapy: Working with arising fears and resistance. In T. Singer & M. Boltz, *Compassion: Bridging practice and science* (pp. 66–80). Munich, Germany: Max Plank Institute.

Gilligan, C. (1982). *In a different voice: Psychological theory and women's development.* Cambridge, MA: Harvard University Press.

Gordon, S. (2005). *Nursing against the odds: How health care cost cutting, media stereotypes, and medical hubris undermine nurses and patient care.* Ithaca, NY: ILR Press (an imprint of Cornell University Press).

Institute of Medicine. (2009). Robert Wood Johnson Initiative on the Future of Nursing, at the Institute of Medicine: The future of nursing: Leading change, advancing health. National Academy of Sciences. Retrieved from http://www.nationalacademies.org/hmd/Reports/2010/The-Future-of-Nursing-Leading-Change-Advancing-Health.aspx

Ireland, T. (2014, June). What does mindfulness meditation do to your brain? *Scientific American,* 1-6. Retrieved from https://blogs.scientificamerican.com/guest-blog/what-does-mindfulness-meditation-do-to-your-brain

John Hopkins School of Nursing and John Hopkins Berman Institute of Bioethics. (2014). *A blueprint for 21st century nursing ethics: Report of the National Nursing Summit.* Retrieved from http://www.bioethicsinstitute.org/wp-content/uploads/2014/09/Executive_summary.pdf

Kabat-Zinn, J. (1994). *Wherever you go, there you are: Mindfulness meditation in everyday life*. New York, NY: Hyperion.

Kenner, C., Finkelman, A., Weatherby, F., Long, L. E., & Kupperschmidt, B. R. (2009). Appendix K: Nursing against whose odds? Commentary on Gordon (2005) an example of teaching to the IOM reports. In A. Finkelman & C. Kenner (Eds.), *Teaching IOM: Implications of the Institute of Medicine reports for nursing education* (2nd ed., pp. 247–256). Silver Spring, MD: American Nurses Association.

Levine, M. (1972). Benoni. In M. H. Browning & E. P. Lewis (Eds.), *The dying patient: A nursing perspective* (pp. 134–138). New York, NY: The American Journal of Nursing Company.

MacMillan, K. (2016). The hidden curriculum: What are we actually teaching about the fundamentals of care? *Nursing Leadership, 29*(1), 37–46. doi:10.12927/cjnl.2016.24644

Nussbaum, M. (1996). Compassion: The basic social emotion. *Social Philosophy and Policy, 13*, 27–58. doi:10.1017/S0265052500001515

Souba, W. W. (2002). Academic medicine and the search for meaning and purpose. *Academic Medicine, 77*, 139–144. doi:10.1097/00001888-200202000-00008

Todaro-Franceschi, V. (2008). Preventing compassion fatigue and reaffirming purpose in nursing. *Proceedings on the 3rd European Federation of Critical Care Nursing Congress and 27th Aniarti Conference, Influencing Critical Care Nursing in Europe*, Florence, Italy (October).

Todaro-Franceschi, V. (2013). *Compassion fatigue and burnout in nursing: Enhancing professional quality of life*. New York, NY: Springer Publishing.

Todaro-Franceschi, V. (2015). The ART of maintaining the "care" in healthcare. *Nursing Management, 46*(6), 53–55. doi:10.1097/01.numa.0000465407.76450.ab

13

Cultivating Collective Mindful Awareness in Nursing: A Leadership Agenda

I think we have to transform the culture, by beginning with a nucleus which makes a new culture. It doesn't begin with a practice. Practice must follow out of something deeper.
—David Bohm

KEY TOPICS

- Fostering collective mindful awareness
- Compassionate, transformational nursing leadership is instrumental for reaffirming our purpose
- Positive workplace culture, employee happiness, and productivity
- Magnets, appreciative inquiry, meaningful recognition, and nursing theory
- Finding joy and burning brightly
- *ART*© in group-focused work can help to address issues of professional quality of life

© Springer Publishing Company DOI: 10.1891/9780826155214.0013

INTRODUCTION

To cultivate collective mindful awareness aimed at healing and preventing compassion fatigue and burnout in nursing, we need to first begin to "think in a vocabulary of oneness" (Myss, 1996, p. 286).

Researchers at the Institute of Noetic Sciences, an organization that focuses predominantly on how human beings actualize their potentials, explore what they refer to as "consciousness transformation," where one has shifts in consciousness, usually through meditative practices, somewhat akin to peak or optimal experiences (Vieten, Amorok, & Schlitz, 2006). They noted that these experiences lead one from an "I to we" way of viewing the world, a broadening of one's sense of self that has a spiritual component where one is aware of something greater than his or her self, something bigger even than "we" or "us"—it is beyond us. This, too, gets at my basic premise in the enigma of energy—we come to see that whatever we do is reflected in the whole; it is all essentially one (Todaro-Franceschi, 1998, 1999). I am reminded of a quote from physicist David Bohm (1998) that I use often: "To see that everybody not merely *depends* on everybody, but actually everybody *is* everybody in a deeper sense" (p. 110).

Scientists can be very philosophical, and unsurprisingly (to me), very spiritual. Thus, I have never understood why many individuals in nursing believe that spirituality is not something we should refer to in our teaching, research, and practice, and that religion is better relegated to a place where it cannot infect objectivity (and science). When those such as Albert Einstein, Stephen Hawking, Paul Davies, and David Bohm, among numerous others, could repeatedly reflect in depth upon, and discuss spirituality and, indeed, religion in their work, it seems almost sacrilegious for us in nursing not to do so.

There is an unquestionably inherent *spiritual* component to nursing, for spirituality is nothing more (or less) than a sense of being connected with everything and everyone else. Nurses who are *heartful*—compassion content—are those who are mindfully aware of their connectedness to others, and it fuels them to be with and do more for their patients.

In a discussion on science and theology, David Steindl-Rast (Capra, Steindl-Rast, & Matus, 1991) talked about how we can walk around feeling lost or orphaned and then suddenly there is a moment where everything clicks and we feel like we belong, where we think:

> "I belong to all other humans." Even if there is nobody around, this is clearly felt. I belong to all the animals, to the plants. And belonging means I am at home with them, I am responsible for them and to them. You see, I belong to them as much as they belong to me. We all belong together in this great cosmic unity. (p. 15)

In nursing, we need to cultivate and foster a collective awareness of our we-ness—our oneness—in order to enhance our professional quality of life.

TRANSFORMING THE WHOLE THROUGH TRANSFORMATIONAL LEADERSHIP AND STAFF DEVELOPMENT

For our current workforce, we must look to our nurse leaders and staff development educators for guidance. The goal for leaders is always to get a group of individuals to work cohesively in attaining the overall mission of the workplace; for those of us in healthcare, the mission is the provision of quality healthcare *and* quality caring to enhance the quality of living–dying for all people. A good leader in any organization knows that in order to meet any end point, one must begin with the community of people who have to do the work, acknowledging that without those people, the work could not get done. Cultivating a communal environment is crucial, and for nurses today, perhaps more essential than ever before. Effective leadership is necessary for this cultivation, hence the need for transformational leaders.

Toxic Leadership and Handlers of Toxicity

Transformational nurse leaders who identify areas where change is needed to enhance quality caring focus on the interaction between *all* of the environment and *all* of the human beings that are a part of it. Notably, to be a leader in healthcare today is extremely stressful at times. Frost and Robinson, in their studies of organizational behavior, identified and described a phenomenon they called *toxic leadership* (Frost, 1999a; Frost & Robinson, 1999). They posited that there are two kinds: (a) "a form of action and practice by leaders and systems that creates pain and suffering in others and in the organizations" and (b) "the compassionate face of leadership and its costs on the individuals who exercise it" (Frost, 1999a, p. 130).

The "toxic leader" is the one who causes pain and suffering in others around them (Frost, 1999a). I would call these people "managers," not leaders. They manage to make everyone miserable, and they usually do it by applying *power as control* (Barrett, 2010). This manager does not capitalize on the strengths of staff; does not recognize, respect, or acknowledge their good qualities, and thus devalues their contributions to the workplace. Everyone encounters at least one of these "toxic leaders" during the course of their work life. I have certainly met more than a few!

The second kind of leader is a "handler" of toxicity in the workplace. Leaders who are *toxin* handlers, through their compassionate caring actions, alleviate the suffering of their staff by dispersing, dissipating, or dissolving the emotional toxins in the environment (Frost, 1999a, 1999b). These are also the leaders who acknowledge and value the contributions their staff makes to the organization and they are the kind of leaders we need in nursing, the ones who lead by *power as knowing participation* and who inspire others to develop their own power (as knowing participation); see Barrett (2010).

Frost pointed out that *toxin* handlers can, and often do, absorb toxicity and consequently are themselves more vulnerable to emotional exhaustion. The thing is, nurse leaders are called upon to do what all *nurses* do: they need to appreciate and cosuffer with their staff as their staff, in turn, are called upon to cosuffer with, and appreciate, patients and their loved ones:

> When toxin handlers help others, they often . . . wrap the other person's suffering in love, though they might not characterize it quite this way. To respond constructively to someone else in pain is an act of compassion, a way of reaching out to a person who is alone and suffering. Efforts to reconnect people to their competence and sense of self-worth are expressions of love. (Frost, 1999b, p. 108)

It is necessary to have higher level administrators who are also transformational in their approach—those who compassionately lead by example. A requisite skill for all exemplary leaders is knowing how to be an effective toxin handler without becoming burned out themselves. One cannot understate the importance of that oxygen mask needing to go on one's own face first!

No, You Cannot Leave Now

The nurse was pregnant with her first child and working full time on a medical–surgical unit in a Magnet® hospital while in her last term of graduate studies; she was happily busy. However, during a shift at work one day she began spotting, and anxiously she went to tell the head nurse that she needed to leave to go see her obstetrician. The head nurse told her that she could not leave because there was no one to cover for her. She thought perhaps the head nurse had misunderstood, so she repeated again that she was pregnant and bleeding, and that she needed to leave. When, for the second time, the head nurse told her that she was not allowed to leave, the nurse proceeded up the next rung of leadership to tell the director of nursing, who not only listened to her, but then went on to procure a wheelchair, wheel her down and out of the building to a taxi, and gave the nurse a hug before she got in the cab to go to her obstetrician.

Soon after that awful day at work, the nurse miscarried. She grappled with the aftermath of profound grief from the loss of her first child, which was compounded severely by the utter lack of compassion on the part of her head nurse. Although the director of nursing had shown her compassion (in essence acting as a toxin handler), the nurse still had to face that head nurse (the toxic leader) every time she went to work. She could not get beyond the fact that the head nurse had minimized her crisis situation and that she had not seemed to care at all. It became impossible for her to continue to work there. Upon graduation, she sought a new position in another state and moved to the new location with her husband, where, when last I heard from her, she was loving her work and life in general.

I will never forget this story; it was one of my graduate students. She was an extraordinary student and nurse. As she shared her experience with me, I noted the suffering on her face and I cried along with her. Honestly, I am teary-eyed right now, recalling it. And I think to myself, how dare that woman manager, who I will not dignify by calling her a nurse, do something like that to another person? This is a drastic account of dispassionate authoritarian management; the outcome of this toxic manager's act was equally drastic; that facility lost an exemplary nurse not only from the unit, but from the hospital as well (and we lost her from the entire geographic region!). I wonder what, if any, follow-up occurred by the administration regarding what had transpired.

A CLEAR PATH FORWARD

In nursing, we talk about and emphasize patient-centered care, patient advocacy, and of late, even patient etiquette. How do we really go about getting it to happen? The first step is for all of us engaged in the multiplicity of nursing roles to look at ourselves and at what is going on *in* nursing. Are *we* happy or content? Do we believe in ourselves individually and collectively as professionals who are important? Does our practice emulate what we emphatically note in our code of ethics, to be the values, virtues, and excellences of our profession? Are we treating ourselves and each other well? Do we support each other, mentor each other, and acknowledge each other as human beings? Are we providing the best care that we possibly can to those who need us? We need to explore these questions individually and collectively in our work environments.

The answer to so many of our woes might best be served by more fully embracing what I have discussed in earlier chapters—Relationship-Based Care (RBC) as a model for patient care across the entire healthcare spectrum (Koloroutis, 2004; Koloroutis & Abelson, 2017). In the clinical nurse leader (CNL) program I coordinated, we used RBC as the foundation for practice. In her groundbreaking work on RBC, nurse consultant Mary Koloroutis (2004) noted, ". . .ultimately, it is the transformation of people that changes an organization" (p. 249). She and her colleagues also provided an extensive field guide for the use of RBC that includes learning to be an RBC leader (Koloroutis, Felgen, Person, & Wessel, 2007). For transformation to occur in healthcare, we need leaders who have people skills!

Using the RBC model to foster better communication can also do much to enhance civility among staff and between disciplines. As Maslach and Leiter (1999) identified, the quality of the relationships among people in the workplace (the sense of community) plays a central role in workplace engagement. Various interventions to improve civility are finding their way into healthcare organizations with the hope that it will contribute to reducing the incidence of burnout (Maslach & Leiter, 2017).

Positive Workplace Culture, Employee Happiness, and Productivity

There has been an exponential increase in the recent literature on the relationship between employee happiness and productivity. In order to have both, you need to have a *positive work culture*, which essentially means that addressing such things as salary, benefits, and even workload just will not get you there. There are other things that count more.

One of the Advisory Board Daily Briefings–News for Health Care Executives (2017) grabbed my interest with the heading, "Money can't buy you happy employees, study finds." The research it referred to was performed by Glassdoor, a company that collects employment data and studies workplace salaries, cultures, and leadership. The nitty-gritty of this particular study was that in exploring thousands of people's reviews of their respective employers, *culture and values* were consistently noted to be the most important aspects of the workplace to employees. Also noteworthy was that *senior leadership* came in second place. Having read this brief, I then spent some time browsing their website and read through a few more Glassdoor reports. In one synopsis, Andrew Chamberlain (2017), the chief economist at Glassdoor, highlighted the findings of six studies that indicate satisfied employees outperform unsatisfied employees, which overall equates with better business (see www.Glassdoor.com for a lot of enlightening research reports).

In their research on workplace culture, experts Emma Seppala and Kim Cameron (2015) have found that fostering social connections in the workplace improves employee well-being and productivity, while a poor work environment leads to social isolation, which negatively affects health and, as a result, overall life expectancy. They identify six characteristics that are essential for positive workplace culture: (a) caring for and being interested in colleagues as friends; (b) providing support for each other (showing kindness and compassion); (c) avoiding blame and forgiving mistakes; (d) inspiring one another; (e) emphasizing the meaningful nature of the work; and (f) treating each other with respect, gratitude, trust, and integrity (p. 4). Seppala and Cameron go on to describe fours steps that leaders can apply to help create and maintain a good work environment: (a) foster social connections; (b) show empathy; (c) go out of your way to help; and (d) encourage people to talk to you—especially about their problems.

What all of this implies is that getting to know your staff on a more personal basis has enormous benefits—for you, your staff, and ultimately to the organization. It is so important to acknowledge that we are all human, that every person has a story to tell, and that everyone suffers at some time or another. Dutton and colleagues (Dutton, Frost, Worline, Lilius, & Kanov, 2002) capture this sentiment well:

> . . .there is always grief somewhere in the room. One person may be feeling personal pain due to a death in the family. Another may find personality conflicts in the workplace unbearable. . . . But you can use your leadership to begin the healing process. Through your presence you can model behaviors that set the stage for the process of making meaning out of terrible events. And through your actions you can empower people to find their own ways to support one another through painful times. This is a kind of leadership we wish we would never have to use, yet it is vital if we are to nourish the very humanity that can make people—and organizations—great.

Knowing how to inspire and lead people is imperative; however, in order to be truly effective, one must lead with compassion. Leading with compassion takes courage as well as skill; hence, assertiveness, ethics, and professional quality of life issues truly are foundational subjects for all nurses, and especially so for our leaders.

Why People Quit

Nurse leaders are vitally important for the overall health of the workplace environment; for employee happiness and well-being, productivity, quality and safety, patient outcomes. . .and the list goes on. It is no small surprise that whenever there is a sentinel event in a healthcare setting, leadership is often scrutinized more closely in the follow-up analysis. The Joint Commission (2008, 2017) stresses the importance of leaders in attaining and maintaining a culture of safety in the workplace. A culture of safety in turn will contribute to healthier and happier staff (see also Chapter 9). In a report on joy, meaning, and safety in the workplace, the

Lucian Leape Institute (2013) at the National Patient Safety Foundation highlights both the emotional and physical harm that carers are exposed to at work, and how it negatively affects patient care. They point out that effective organizations make their workforce well-being and safety the first priority and that unfortunately, in many healthcare organizations that is not what is done.

There is a saying being bandied about on the Internet, something along the lines of "people do not quit their jobs, they quit their bosses."[1] While not 100% the case, leadership does play a part in employee decisions to leave. One can have a nasty boss, and as a consequence, decide to quit, or conversely, one might have a nice boss, and still decide to quit. There are many places where there are nice bosses, and they still cannot retain staff. The reason why? It is a combination of the work itself and the workplace environment. The question then becomes, "who is responsible for the work and workplace environment?" Well, in a report on an engagement study of employees at Facebook, the authors surmised that, "at Facebook people don't quit a boss—they quit a job. And who's responsible for what that job is like? Managers" (Goler, Gale, Harrington, & Grant, 2018, p. 2). Oops, it seems the onus falls on leadership no matter what!

Magnets, Appreciative Inquiry, and Meaningful Recognition

One of the underlying themes throughout the preceding pages has been an emphasis on making opportunities to appreciate ourselves individually and collectively as important contributors in healthcare. Appreciative inquiry is a method of research and a model for organizational change that is based on recognizing the positive strengths or aspects of others and also things in our environment (Cooperrider & Whitney, 2005). Instead of focusing on problems and trying to get to their root cause in order to fix them, with appreciative inquiry, positive change comes about from a focus on the things that we already know work. Looking at what experts in organizational change management refer to as the positive core—the assets, strengths, and resources—of a workplace, the people in a work setting come to appreciate more, and are then better able to actualize the potentials of the organization as a whole in order to meet its mission (Cooperrider & Whitney, 2005).

In healthcare organizations, the heart of the positive core is us—nurses, with our unique ways of knowing and our compassionate caring practices. That is why the Magnet model is so powerful—it acknowledges and builds on our strengths, valuing and capitalizing on the many positive aspects of nursing. I am convinced that many hospitals cannot attain Magnet status because they are still looking for the root causes of problems instead of looking at and building upon what makes things work and work well . . .

WE make things work, and we get it done especially well when we are supported to do it the way we know it should be done, with both clinical competency and compassionate caring.

Appreciative inquiry is noted to make "a space in which people are free to be heard" (Cooperrider & Whitney, 2005, Kindle Location 828–33). Most, if not all leaders in Magnet-designated settings tend to be strong advocates for their staff and foster an environment where nurses practice more autonomously, being given not only the responsibility and accountability for their practice, but also the authority. In these settings, nurses' voices are heard! Undoubtedly, transformational leaders in Magnet-designated hospitals are so successful because they are compassionate carers and their staff feel adequately supported.

Maslach and Leiter (1999) identified recognition for one's contributions at work (reward) as one of six important areas of work life (AW) that can contribute to burnout or conversely, engagement. Data is continuing to accrue on the use of rewards and recognition to reduce the incidence of burnout in the workplace. In healthcare, various physician and nurse groups are using meaningful recognition programs to improve professional quality of life.

Compassion in Organizations, Nursing Theory, and Magnet Status

While the idea of compassion has been around since the ancients, and there has been much discourse about it in various disciplines, up until recently there has been very little focus on the part compassion plays in organizations (Frost et al., 2006). If we reflect on this a bit in nursing, we must come to realize that in this there is an opportunity for the discipline of nursing to move forward and make great strides in healthcare organizations, simply because compassion is an integral part of nursing.

We have many nursing theoretic frameworks that emphasize the good—notions of caring and an ethic of care that meld together and can guide us in practice to provide quality caring while at the same time, foster our personal and professional compassion contentment. Many of these theories rest on the assumption that it is all one—that human beings and their environments are inextricably connected. It is no surprise that hospitals with Magnet status are also those that successfully adopt a nursing theoretic framework to guide their practice. Our nurse theorists have captured the essence of nursing—as both an art and a science.

The Magnet movement came about while trying to address nurse retention during a time when there was a shortage of nurses and when new nurse attrition was high. This is once again the current state of affairs, and it is in large part due to the culture of the institutions where the important stuff—the compassion and human-to-human connection—has either disappeared or is not readily apparent and nurtured.

Magnet designation is achieved through the efforts of nurses and nursing, but as McClure (2011) stresses, nurses cannot do it alone. It is truly an organizational accomplishment that is attained with the full support of all the people who work in it:

> The hospital either embodies the necessary exemplary corporate culture or it does not. It is either a place in which all employees find satisfaction in their work or it is not. It is impossible for hospitals to provide a rich and rewarding environment for nurses alone. Every individual—from the CEO to the entry-level employee—affects, and is affected by, the quality of the workplace environment. (McClure, 2011, p. 6)

Thus far, only 475 hospitals have achieved Magnet designation, approximately 8% of the total number of hospitals in the United States. In order to move toward the ideal, which we recognize Magnet status to be, we need to address the real issues related to our lack of contentment in the workplace. The cultivation of compassionate caring and the acknowledgment that it is a motivating force behind all we do in healthcare is utterly necessary for us to turn things around.

Reports from a 10-year longitudinal study that began in 2006 indicate that nurses perceive work-group cohesion—"the degree to which members of a workgroup are friendly, helpful, and take an interest in each other"—to be a significant factor in the provision of quality care (Djukic, Kovner, Brewer, Fatehi, & Cline, 2011, p. 5). The researchers stressed that while we may not be able to do much about nurse–patient ratios, there is much we can do to change the work environment in order to make it more conducive to the provision of quality care. As in previous studies, nurses noted that their relationships with physicians and procedural justice—where "people involved in implementing decisions have a say in making the decisions" (when our voices are heard!)—were also important factors in patient care (Djukic et al., 2011, p. 5). Even in exploring the direct and indirect influences of physical work environment on job satisfaction (for early career nurses working in hospitals), a recommendation was made to pay attention to the structure of the physical environment when designing new units to enhance work-group cohesion and nurse–physician relations (Djukic, Kovner, Brewer, Fatehi, & Greene, 2014).

Over and over again, research and literature point to the importance of the relational factors—the human-to-human connection—that they can make or break us in our work environment. In Magnet status hospitals, where everyone has paid attention to these factors, nurses and others involved in the care of patients are content and subsequently retained, patients are satisfied, and outcomes are better. In other words, quality of care is quality caring for all.

Finding Joy

Finding joy (or keeping joy) in our work is important on many levels. As I have mentioned previously, being happy has been linked to being healthier and living longer. Happier employees are more productive and in healthcare having happy employees is a win-win for everyone. Conversely, joyless work contributes to the bad, the ugly, the uglier, and ugliest in healthcare, resulting in a lose-lose for everyone.

Recently I picked up a special edition of *Time* magazine entitled *The Science of Happiness: New Discoveries for a More Joyful Life*. The articles in it offer a wealth of information about finding and keeping joy in our lives. Research findings in positive psychology have suggested that about 50% of our ability to be happy is genetically inherited but another 40% of our ability to be happy is attributed to our behavior—which means the choices we make in life—and the remaining approximately 10% is related to our individual circumstances in life (Lyubomirsky, 2007).

In many of the articles, the authors accentuate the positive effects of mindfulness and being consciously present in the moment. Nurses and nursing leaders are multitaskers; we do many things at once and it is impossible while multitasking to be consciously present. This undoubtedly contributes to feeling overwhelmed and inefficacious at times. The more we do, the harder it can get to do things well. So here is a *choice* factor; choosing to be in the moment you are living, instead of multitasking, can make you feel happier.

Seppala (2018) suggests that a great way to bring your mind into the present is to take a technology fast for a half or whole day. Of course no one can shut things completely down while at work, but staff and leadership can practice disconnecting everything for brief periods on days off. Ideally, while disconnecting, you want to relax the mind. What does it take to relax your mind? Everyone is different. For me, getting outside in my garden works wonders. For others, it might be meditation, or swimming, or just plain breathing. Whatever it is, you can increase the joy in your life and encourage others to do the same, simply by *being present in the present*!

Along with meaningful recognition programs, resilience programs are popping up in healthcare (for employees as well as patients). Resilience, or the ability to bounce back from difficult situations or events, also contributes to happiness and well-being. There are physiologic changes in the parts of the brain that govern emotions when a person is faced with stress, and resilient people (or resilient brains!) appear to have the ability to regulate and shut off the stress response more quickly. Research indicates that we can train our minds to bounce back and withstand hard times (Charney & Southwick, 2012; Oaklander, 2018). One of the things that is said to contribute to developing resilience is learning to be focused on what you are doing while you are doing it; in other words, being mindful. Another thing noted to be good for developing resilience is facing rather than running from the things that scare you, which purportedly relaxes the fear circuitry in the brain (Oaklander, 2018). As I read this, I was reminded of Pema Chodron's work about us going to the places that scare us and how she highlighted that it can help us be more compassionate. Other things noted to increase resilience include participating in a regular exercise regimen, having adequate support systems, maintaining a positive outlook, finding meaning and purpose, and holding close your core values/beliefs (Charney & Southwick, 2012). Does this sound familiar? It is all inextricably related.

APPLYING *ART* TO CULTIVATE COLLECTIVE MINDFUL AWARENESS

In collaboration with staff, nurse leaders and staff development educators can identify the positive and negative aspects of professional quality of life and can, through visioning and innovative thinking, facilitate and implement needed changes in the systems that are creating workforce woes. Keith (2003) wrote about finding personal meaning in a chaotic, crazy world. His message is simple; it is not what is external to us that creates our lives and gives us meaning and happiness. Instead, he noted, it depends on how we respond to what is outside ourselves; it is always a matter of choice and we control our inner lives. Then again, I do believe that what exists outside of us is a part of us, a part of the whole, and we never really respond to anything; we change or transform with everything, all together, all the time. The notion that things are separate entities is a leftover idea from Newtonian times and it just is not so. We are the whole—*only we can make things different.*

To reiterate, each step of *ART* (Todaro-Franceschi, 2008, 2013, 2015) can be looked at separately or together. It is all intertwined and all steps need to be ongoing. At this juncture, I hope *ART* has helped to frame a *wholistic* (not *hole*, the *whole*!) picture of what we need to do to heal. We need to acknowledge individual and collective feelings—make known the unknown about ourselves and one another. We need to acknowledge what makes us happy and ensures a sense of meaning and purpose in our work, and then we need to recognize what choices we have that can move us in the direction we need to go. Once we have outlined all the choices, we can develop a purposeful action plan. We can turn toward ourselves and each other and make whatever we want to happen, happen!

Step 1: Acknowledge a Feeling or Wound That Needs Healing

Anyone can make copies of Stamm's ProQOL (2010) tool and pass it around at work (see Appendix A). Identifying and acknowledging how staff feel about their work is key. Leaders can make the time for everyone to reflect on collective wounds in the workplace, knowing that a lack of acknowledgment can transform into poor productivity, job dissatisfaction, and burnout.

With the knowledge that how we feel *cannot* be removed from our workplace, and that our individual and collective feelings count in our efforts to provide care, we must accept the reality that pain and anguish exists everywhere, including in the workplace. If one views civility the way nurse Cynthia Clark (2010) defined it, as "an authentic respect for others that requires time, presence, willingness to engage in genuine discourse and intention to seek common ground," then perhaps a lack of acknowledgment of another's suffering is actually incivility in disguise. Clark went on to note that, "Civility matters because treating one another with respect is requisite to communicating effectively, building community and creating high-functioning teams. Without civility, we miss opportunities to really listen and understand other points of view." Unless we make an effort to know the unknown about others in our environment, we cannot begin to understand why they may act the way they do. Some people might have good cause to be miserable, but no one has good cause to be cruel and uncaring.

Have a Wit Day, a Patch Adams Day, or a Tuesdays with Morrie Day

Check out YouTube for clips from these and other motion pictures that poignantly capture what it means to feel compassion (and what it can do when one tries to flick the shutoff switch). Show one or two short clips at a staff meeting and have a focused group discussion on key points (or, alternatively, ask participants to jot down their feelings about the clip and reflect upon them later).

Leaders should join staff in practice to say "ouch" collectively. Recall the motion picture film *E.T. The Extra-Terrestrial*, where the boy and E.T. are so inextricably connected that whatever one feels, the other feels. Each of them displays compassion for the other—they cannot help but do so. Through their compassionate caring, each is able to facilitate the healing of the other. Being able to say ouch collectively means that you have to see, and encourage others to see, things you might not normally see (or that you have not been acknowledging)—becoming more mindfully aware. It also means that you have to go to places you normally avoid, and perhaps even the places that scare you.

Appreciating Our Moments Exercise

Share, or if you are a nurse leader, have your frontline nurses share, stories of their caring moments (Watson, 1999). Offering opportunities to share these moments not only shows recognition of their value, it also serves as teaching moments for other staff who may be distancing themselves for whatever reason. Whenever and wherever you can, build opportunities for storytelling of caring moments into the work environment.

Step 2: *Recognize Choices and Take Purposeful Action*

Some of the things that can be done to foster a community of caring include having sessions for focused group discussion on feelings concerning the workplace environment. Build in time to make known the unknown about each other. This would include discussions regarding areas of difficulty as well as areas that are conducive to one's well-being. Bitching sessions can be very beneficial; however, they can also be time-wasting. It is far better to focus on the positive aspects of the environment and try to build upon them, than it is to spend too much time discussing the negative.

"Hear you, Hear me" Listening Exercise

I learned the following listening exercise many years ago at a workshop on effective communication, and I use it in classes to teach active listening. When I was in nursing management I also used it with staff. Those who may think that they are great listeners are often quite surprised to find that they are not as good at it as they thought. Listening is a skill that can be taught and learned.

- Choose a partner. For 5 minutes one person should talk—sharing some important experience in his or her life. To also work on the development of compassion skills, you can ask the person to share a loss of some kind—it does not have to be the death of a loved one; it can be any loss. During the 5 minutes one person is speaking, the other person must do nothing but listen. Those who are listening are not allowed to speak at all. At the end of the 5 minutes, have them switch places; the person being listened to becomes the listener and the other person gets to share a meaningful experience or loss. After the second 5 minutes is up, go around the room and have everyone share how they felt when they were listened to, and alternatively, how they felt when they listened. If there is not enough time to go around the room, have everyone reflect upon and later write down the following:

> I felt . . . when I was listened to.
>
> I felt . . . when I listened.

- Post their responses anonymously in the nursing lounge or on the course board. Have a discussion about them at your next meeting (or class).

Caution: Some folks have a *really* hard time with this exercise.

"I see me and I see you" Exercise

This exercise, which I have arbitrarily named here, is an adaption from Melodie Chenevert's (1988) shared gold mine of assertiveness training techniques. In a staff meeting (or a class), have everyone jot down one personal thing about themselves (e.g., I like to garden, and I love butterflies!), one good thing they like about themselves, and then one good thing they like about the person sitting on their left. Afterward, have each person in turn, going around the room, share how they felt when asked to do this and what they wrote about themselves and their colleague.

I have found that this exercise is a real eye-opener. First off, a lot of us have difficulty choosing one personal thing to share about ourselves and we have even more difficulty identifying and articulating things that we think are *good* about ourselves. More often than not, nurses will identify relational things such as "I'm kind," "I care about people," "I'm respectful of others," "I'm sensitive," and so forth. Many of us define ourselves by the way we connect with, and care for, others. It is a nurse thing and it goes back to that *nurseculture* I keep alluding to throughout this book. Much less often you will get someone who says, "I am intelligent," "creative," "resourceful," "objective," and so on. While doing this exercise, some participants will also be surprised to find that they do not know all that much about one another (Chenevert, 1988, noted this, too). So, having your staff or students do this exercise has the added benefit of helping everyone get to know and appreciate one another.

We need to do appreciative inquiries into our "we-ness." Collective work can be done to get to know the unknown about each other and find common ground. The dictate that we cannot bring our home to work and vice versa is baloney. We are human beings and our luggage goes with us. We need to embrace it—carry it along, but at the same time, acknowledge that it need not get so into the moment that it unwinds that moment enough to make it meaningless.

Do a CQI Activity on Compassion Contentment (Employee Happiness Being the Goal)!

When I was in nursing administration, total quality management (TQM) and continuous quality improvement (CQI) first came into being. With

TQM, the organizational systems are explored from a multidisciplinary perspective and issues are supposed to be addressed as a whole, *by the whole*. Blame is not placed (or not supposed to be placed) on any one discipline or system because it is acknowledged that everything feeds into everything else.

The basic premise of TQM fits with my basic philosophy—it is all one. I led many successful CQI team efforts in my time. Perhaps what is needed in our healthcare world today is a systemwide (very big!) CQI, which focuses primarily on compassion for the cared for *and* the carers, a CQI that explores the issues that feed into productivity, recruitment, and retention of the carers, as well as quality and safety of care for the patients—you know, the *whole*, everything together. Things that might be explored would evolve around compassion contentment for everyone, and in this way we could spruce up the quality of care rendered *and* quality of professional life at the same time. Nurse leaders are well positioned for this kind of work, since they are always concerned with workforce productivity and quality of care.

Maslach and Leiter (1999) identified six key areas for employee happiness: (a) a manageable workload, (b) a sense of control, (c) the opportunity for rewards, (d) a feeling of community, (e) faith in the fairness of the workplace, and (f) shared values (p. 50). Taking each in turn, both staff and leaders can reflect upon the work environment and come up with a purposeful action plan to improve any areas that are less than optimal. All are self-explanatory, but I would draw attention to the feeling of community—once again a clear reference to our connectedness.

Encourage Yourself and Others to Burn Brightly

I am always looking for ways to encourage a passion for nursing in students, and when I was in nursing management I looked for ways to empower and encourage staff. I have been known to play songs during classes and staff meetings—like the song sung by Yolanda Adams in *Honey* titled "I Believe . . .," or for laughs, the classic "I Can't Get No Satisfaction," or my favorite inspirational song entitled "What A Wonderful World," sung by "Satchmo"—Louie Armstrong. Role-playing also works. Today there are a slew of games and resources available in cyberspace. Be creative; engage yourself and one another (check out Appendix C, Resources, for more information).

You can brainstorm with coworkers to come up with creative strategies that address the need for both patients and carers to connect. Years ago, for instance, at many places there was an overlap of shift time, like the 3:30 to 11:30 shift had to report at 3:15 for a 15-minute overlap during which time report was given. How about an hour overlap for some of the staff, where the hour would be for the nurse coming on to spend that time sitting with each patient (and or family) while the other nurses wrapped up the shift and then gave report after the first nurse had spent time with the patients?

Step 3: *Turn Outward Toward Self and Other*

After 9/11, I began an initiative to create a butterfly memorial garden on the campus where I worked for many years. People ask me all the time, why butterflies? They ask why I talk so much about them and why my office is full of butterfly paraphernalia. People who come to my home in the spring and summer months might find a caterpillar (or several) climbing up my walls, having escaped their temporary safety pen, and they will surely see many different kinds of butterflies in my gardens.

Butterflies, as I have already mentioned, are a perfect representation of purposeful energy transformation, a sign of renewal, and through their continual metamorphosis, a symbol of everlasting change. Many people of different cultural backgrounds believe that the butterfly is their dead loved one come back to life in another fashion. It is a beautiful creature of nature and, to me, the most magnificent.

In a novel, *The Butterfly's Daughter*, written by Mary Alice Monroe (2011), the protagonist shares a memory of her grandmother—her *Abuela*—taking her to the park. Abuela would say to her, "Look there! Watch them. See how people smile when they see a butterfly? They can't help themselves. Butterflies are joy with wings" (Monroe, 2011, p. 154). I too have observed that when people notice a butterfly they smile. Yet, it has never ceased to amaze me how many people do *not see* butterflies. They are not aware of the fact that they fly about us all the time, occasionally even getting trapped in a car or a home.

Obviously I cannot seem to separate my passion for butterflies from my work life, and getting the students involved in the butterfly memorial garden was a delight for me. I have been known to do an impromptu lesson on raising butterflies now and then in class and would even pass around a milkweed leaf with a caterpillar on it! So, it is unsurprising that my enthusiasm is a bit infectious; for example, one of my students emailed me from the school library during final exam cram time. He said, "Before I had you for a teacher, I never noticed butterflies. Now I see them everywhere. There is a butterfly right now fluttering about in the library; it made me smile."

Do you notice the butterflies? The first time we went to Costa Rica on vacation one of my main goals was to see a blue morpho butterfly in the wild. I had only seen them in man-made conservatories before and I cannot tell you how marvelous it was to see them flying about in their natural habitat. It struck me that there were many natural happenings going on that other tourists and even native Costa Ricans did not seem to notice. Like the white-faced monkeys flitting from tree to tree and the egret I saw communing with a horse in a field, or the poisonous but oh so colorful dart frogs blending in with their surroundings; I could go on and on, but you get the point. We can make the opportunities to see things we normally do not see and, in doing so, reconnect with ourselves and other(s). We can reaffirm our sense of belonging to the universe and each other by *turning toward self and other.*

Individually and collectively we can seek to make meaning. We know what the purpose of our work is; we can be passionate about it together. Maisel (2005) notes that passionately making meaning is a skill that can be learned. He lists a number of things we can do in order to develop it:

> First, you need to decide how you will lead your life. . . . You decide to matter, to live a principled, creative, active life in support of your cherished ideals, to manifest your potential, to do good work, in short, to make your life meaningful. . . . (p. 20)

He goes on to emphasize that we can *intend* to make meaning when we establish what our life purposes are and keep them ever present in our awareness as we go about living. In nursing, we need to hold and maintain the intention to fulfill our purpose as compassionate carers.

KEY POINTS

- Nurse leaders can cultivate and foster a collective awareness of our we-ness—our oneness—in order to enhance nurse professional quality of life.

- Organizational culture is more important for keeping employees happy than their salary.

- Nurses need to be *treated* like we are full partners with physicians and other health professionals in the healthcare system. They need to know that they matter, are respected and heard.

- Having a healthy work environment where one feels valued and respected, leads to living healthier and longer, being happier, and doing more meaningful work!

- There needs to be time for nurses to talk about and reflect upon the meaning and purpose of our work, so that we do not lose sight of the fact that it emerges from and is maintained by our connection with others.

- Making time to see things we do not normally see is healing. Leaving our own pain and suffering behind when we go to work (or when we leave work) is an unrealistic expectation. We need to acknowledge and support ourselves and each other as human beings. Making known the unknown about each other will foster a more healthy work environment.

NOTE

1. I think it might have originated from a book written by Victor Litman (2015). *The Type B Manager: Leading Successfully in a Type A World.* New York, NY: Prentice Hall. In it, he titled a chapter "People Leave Managers, Not Companies."

REFERENCES

Advisory Board Company. (2017). Money can't buy you happy employees, study finds: Company culture is most important across all income levels. *The Daily Briefing: News for Healthcare Executives.* Retrieved from https://www.advisory.com/daily-briefing/2017/02/09/happy-employees

Barrett, E. A. M. (2010). Power as knowing participation in change: What's new and what's next. *Nursing Science Quarterly, 23*(1), 47–54. doi:10.1177/0894318409353797

Bohm, D. (1998). In L. Nichol (Ed.), *On creativity.* New York, NY: Routledge.

Capra, F., Steindl-Rast, D., & Matus, T. (1991). *Belonging to the universe: Explorations on the frontiers of science and spirituality.* San Francisco, CA: Harper & Row.

Chamberlain, A. (2017). 6 studies showing satisfied employees drive business results. Retrieved from https://www.glassdoor.com/research/satisfied-employees-drive-business-results

Charney, S. M., & Southwick, D. S. (2012). *Resilience: The science of mastering life's greatest challenges.* New York, NY: Cambridge University Press.

Chenevert, M. (1988). *STAT: Special techniques in assertiveness training for women in the health professions.* St. Louis, MO: C.V. Mosby.

Clark, C. M. (2010). Why civility matters. *Sigma Theta Tau International Reflections on Leadership, 36*(1). Retrieved from https://www.reflectionsonnursingleadership.org/features/more-features/Vol36_1_why-civility-matters

Cooperrider, D. L., & Whitney, D. (2005). *Appreciative inquiry: A positive revolution in change.* San Francisco, CA: Berrett-Koehler Publishers.

Djukic, M., Kovner, C. T., Brewer, C. S., Fatehi, F. K., & Cline, D. D. (2011). Nurse work environment factors other than staffing associated with nurses' ratings of patient care quality. *Health Care Management Review.* Advance online publication. Retrieved from http://rnworkproject.org/resource_type/published-paper

Djukic, M., Kovner, C. T., Brewer, C. S., Fatehi, F., & Greene, W. H. (2014). Exploring direct and indirect influences of physical work environment on job satisfaction for early-career registered nurses employed in hospitals. *Research in Nursing and Health, 37*(4), 312–325. doi:10.1002/nur.21606

Dutton, J. E., Frost, P. J., Worline, M. C., Lilius, J. M., & Kanov, J. M. (2002). Leading in times of trauma. *Harvard Business Review, 80*(1), 54–61.

Frost, P. J. (1999a). Why compassion counts. *Journal of Management Inquiry, 8*(2), 127–133. doi:10.1177/105649269982004

Frost, P. J. (1999b). *Toxic emotions at work and what you can do about them.* Boston, MA: Harvard Business School Press.

Frost, P. J., Dutton, J. E., Maitlis, S., Lilius, J. M., Kanov, J. M., & Worline, M. C. (2006). Seeing organizations differently: Three lenses on compassion. In C. Hardy, S. Clegg, T. Lawrence, & W. Nord (Eds.), *Handbook of organization studies* (2nd ed., pp. 843–866). London: Sage.

Frost, P., & Robinson, S. (1999). The toxic handler: Organizational hero—and casualty. *Harvard Business Review*, pp. 96–106.

Goler, L., Gale, J., Harrington, B., & Grant, A. (2018). Why people really quit their jobs. *Harvard Business Review*. Retrieved from https://hbr.org/2018/01/why-people-really-quit-their-jobs

Joint Commission. (2008). *Sentinel event alert: Behaviors that undermine a culture of safety*. Retrieved from http://www.jointcommission.org/assets/1/18/SEA_40.pdf

Joint Commission. (2017). *Sentinel event alert: The essential role of leadership in developing a safety culture*. Retrieved from https://www.jointcommission.org/assets/1/18/SEA_57_Safety_Culture_Leadership_0317.pdf

Koloroutis, M. (Ed.). (2004). *Relationship-based care: A model for transforming practice*. Minneapolis, MN: Creative Health Care Management.

Koloroutis, M., & Abelson, D. (Eds.). (2017). *Advancing relationship-based cultures*. Minneapolis, MN. Creative Health Care Management.

Koloroutis, M., Felgen, J. A., Person, C., & Wessel, S. (2007). *Relationship-based care: Visions, strategies, tools, and exemplars for transforming practice*. Minneapolis, MN: Creative Health Care Management.

Lucian Leape Institute. (2013). *Through the eyes of the workforce: Creating joy, meaning, and safer health care*. Boston, MA: National Patient Safety Foundation.

Lyubomirsky, S. (2007). *The how of happiness: A scientific approach to getting the life you want*. New York, NY: Penguin Press.

Maisel, E. (2005). *Coaching the artist within*. Novato, CA: New World Library.

Maslach, C., & Leiter, M. P. (1999). Take this job and love it! Six ways to beat burnout. *Psychology Today*, *32*(5), 50–53.

Maslach, C., & Leiter, M. P. (2017). New insights into burnout and health care: Strategies for improving civility and alleviating burnout. *Medical Teacher*, *39*(2), 160–163. doi:10.1080/0142159x.2016.1248918

McClure, M. L. (2011). The first generation. In K. Drenkard, G. Wolf, & S. H. Morgan (Eds.), *Magnet®: The next generation—Nurses making the difference* (pp. 1–8). Silver Spring, MD: American Nurses Credentialing Center.

Monroe, M. A. (2011). *The butterfly's daughter*. New York, NY: Gallery Books.

Myss, C. (1996). *Anatomy of the spirit: The seven stages of power and healing*. New York, NY: Harmony Books.

Oaklander, M. (2018). How to bounce back. In *Time special edition: The science of happiness: New discoveries for a more joyful life* (pp. 22–29).

Seppala, E. (2018). *The happiness track: How to apply the science of happiness to accelerate your success*. New York, NY: HarperCollins.

Seppala, E., & Cameron, K. (2015). Proof that positive work cultures are more productive. *Harvard Business Review*, pp. 1–8.

Stamm, B. H. (2010). *The ProQOL (Professional Quality of Life Scale: Compassion Satisfaction and Compassion Fatigue)*. Pocatello, ID: ProQOL.org. Retrieved from www.proqol.org

Todaro-Franceschi, V. (1998). *The enigma of energy: A philosophical inquiry.* Doctoral dissertation. New York, NY: New York University (UMI No. 9819881).

Todaro-Franceschi, V. (1999). *The enigma of energy: Where science and religion converge.* New York, NY: Crossroad.

Todaro-Franceschi, V. (2008). Preventing compassion fatigue and reaffirming purpose in nursing. *Proceedings on the 3rd European Federation of Critical Care Nursing Congress and 27th Aniarti Conference, Influencing Critical Care Nursing in Europe,* Florence, Italy (October).

Todaro-Franceschi, V. (2013). *Compassion fatigue and burnout in nursing: Enhancing professional quality of life.* New York, NY: Springer Publishing.

Todaro-Franceschi, V. (2015). The ART of maintaining the "care" in healthcare. *Nursing Management, 46*(6), 53–55. doi:10.1097/01.numa.0000465407.76450.ab

Vieten, C., Amorok, T., & Schlitz, M. M. (2006). I to we: The role of consciousness transformation in compassion and altruism. *Zygon, 41*(4), 915–931. doi:10.1111/j.1467-9744.2006.00788.x

Watson, J. (1999). *Postmodern nursing and beyond.* Edinburgh, UK: Churchill.

14

Imagining and Actualizing the Power of Nursing

"You see that old shack down there?" Lou looked at a mud-chinked, falling-down log cabin . . . "Louisa told me about a story your father wrote when he was a little boy. It was about a family that survived one winter up here in that little house. Without wood, or food."
"How'd they do it?"
"They believed in things."
"Like what? Wishing wells?" she said with scorn.
"No, they believed in each other. And created something of a miracle. Some say truth is stranger than fiction. I think that means that whatever a person can imagine really does exist, somewhere. Isn't that a wonderful possibility?"
— Baldacci, 2000, p. 233

KEY TOPICS

- Imagination as a vehicle for change
- Our importance, our power
- A reiteration of how we can reaffirm our purpose

© Springer Publishing Company DOI: 10.1891/9780826155214.0014 **249**

INTRODUCTION

In the preceding chapters I have highlighted the many things in our chaotic and apparently broken healthcare system that contribute to diminished professional quality of life, and in particular, compassion fatigue and the related syndrome of burnout in nursing. Can the broken healthcare system be fixed? I answer in the affirmative; our healthcare system was created by humans, and it has fallen apart because of us, so we can certainly fix it. But we can only do so by acting in concert, together. Nurses, as the largest constituents in the healthcare system, can lead the effort to fix things, and in places where Magnet® status has been attained, nurses are the ones who have led the efforts to make the ideal become the reality. However, in order to proceed we need to get that oxygen mask on ourselves first.

Our profession as a whole needs healing and it is *ours* to heal. The many, many nurses who are compassion fatigued, morally distressed, and/or burned out, along with the bullied (and the bullies) need to turn toward themselves and one another. It is up to us nurses to turn things around in order to move forward as primary transformers. Remen's (1996) words on the nature of healing are so applicable here:

> The healing of our present woundedness may lie in recognizing and reclaiming the capacity we all have to heal each other, the enormous power in the simplest of human relationships; the strength of a touch, the blessing of forgiveness, the grace of someone else taking you just as you are and finding in you an unexpected goodness. (p. 217)

While I was wrapping up the first edition of this book, I had just read the most recent Medscape news headlines: "One Fourth of ICU Clinicians Report Inappropriate Care" (Hand, 2011). The article highlighted the findings of a survey of ICU nurses and physicians done in Europe and Israel. Of course, it pointed out that many of the clinicians suffered from moral distress; but just how many of them were compassion fatigued and over time would burn out, one can only imagine. At the time, the top three most-read articles (by nurses) on Medscape had to do with bullying, incivility in the workplace, and nursing education. Here it is now 5 years later, and one cannot count the slew of articles published on the incidence of both moral distress and burnout in nursing (McAndrew, Leske, & Schroeter, 2016). Of course, it is not surprising that frequent headlines continue to note that although the majority of people want to die at home, many people continue to die in hospitals after receiving unwanted care. We are still not mandating basic end-of-life care education for healthcare professionals. Perhaps, as Gordon (2005) noted, nurses are working against the odds; yet as I point out, to some extent it appears that *we* are the ones creating the odds (that we are working against).

We need to remember we are all essentially one. We are irrevocably connected in a manner that is often camouflaged in our places of employment, but if we remain cognizant of our inseparable nature, we can still provide caring presence despite a seemingly negative work environment, and in so doing change it for the better (Todaro-Franceschi, 1999). I believe that we are here on purpose; we each chose nursing, a healthcare profession, to make a difference in the lives of others, and that we do this on a day-to-day basis whether we acknowledge it or not, and that we can always strive to do it better, *on purpose.*

IMAGINE "WHAT IF"

In their book, *Imagination First,* authors Eric Liu and Scott Noppe-Brandon (2009) share some ostensibly simple but really quite profound insights regarding the importance of imagining and constructing new realities. They make a case for imagination to come first in any attempt to create change and emphasize how our imagination can fuel creativity and innovation. They define *imagination* as the:

> capacity to conceive of *what is not*—something that, as far as we know, does not exist; or something that may exist but we simply cannot perceive. It is the ability to conjure new realities and possibilities: in John Dewey's words, "to look at things as if they could be otherwise." (p. 19)

Asking "what if" requires courage. Liu and Noppe-Brandon note that it is scary because, "What if encompasses not only the possibility that the world is round and circumnavigable but also the possibility that it is flat and drops off abruptly to Hell" (p. 33).

Taking all of the preceding into consideration, it seems clear that imagination is required to move us forward. We have to imagine a different way from what currently is. We have to, as Dewey noted, *look at things as if they could be otherwise.* With our collective knowledge and our nursing talents and skills, we *can* make things be otherwise. Take, for example, the case of Joe, the patient who might have slept the rest of his life away with a medication patch on, were it not for us questioning "doctor's orders." We can take what is, and what has been, and make it better. With our intelligence and nursing knowledge—our unique ways of knowing—of how it should be, we are extremely well equipped.

We all have the ability to imagine a different way—and the ability to hold a picture in our minds to guide us as we actualize our potential, collectively. Liu and Noppe-Brandon (2009) help us by outlining the following list of capabilities:

- Noticing deeply—identifying and articulating layers of detail through continuous interaction with an object of study
- Embodying—experiencing a work through your senses and emotions, and physically representing that experience
- Questioning—asking "Why?" and "What if?" throughout your explorations
- Identifying patterns—finding relationships among the details you notice, and grouping them into patterns
- Making connections—linking the patterns you notice to prior knowledge and experience (both your own and others')
- Exhibiting empathy—understanding and respecting the experiences of others
- Creating meaning—creating interpretations of what you encounter, and synthesizing them with the perspectives of others
- Taking action—acting on the synthesis through a project or an action that expresses your learning
- Reflecting and assessing—looking back on your learning to identify what challenges remain and to begin learning anew. (p. 38)

WE CAN MAKE IT HAPPEN

What can be imagined *can* become reality. What do you imagine? As an educator, I imagine the day when an elective course offering such as "Changing the Face of Death" will become required for all undergraduate nursing students, when compassion lessons are a main part of the curriculum, and during clinical practicums students will be expected to also practice developing their compassion skills in addition to medication administration, wound care skills, and the like.

I imagine the day when there need be little fear that *my* nurse (or your nurse) will show compassion along with clinical skill competency, because not only does she (or he) have the time for it, having had compassion time built into the acuity level for staffing along with the technical aspects of care, but also because she (or he) *absolutely insists* on doing it—knowing it will be good for her or him as well as the people she (or he) is caring for.

I imagine the day where nurses will stick together and support one another, no longer eating their young or old. And when a bully shows up, I imagine the day when nurses band together to protect and support the bullied, rather than remaining silent about it.

I imagine the day when nurses, and especially advanced practice nurses—nurse practitioners (NPs) and clinical nurse specialists (CNSs)—will *always* feel and be able to say "nope, we are not doing it that way—we are doing it our way, because we know our way works better" (and that day is coming fast!). It will only take consensus among *us*, for as I have noted, it is nursing that makes the healthcare system work (or not work) at all!

What do you imagine? Imagining a rebuilt New Orleans in Antieau's (2008) story, the protagonist Ruby notes:

> People rebuild the houses here to use the sun to power them. There's a whole lot of jobs created just to make these houses. . . . I can see it. Can you? . . . And there's no more poor people. Not because they goes to live somewheres else. No! Everyone has jobs they likes and cares about. They have work that inspires and heals them. They have homes of beauty. . . . I can see it. I can see the parties and the food and the laughter and the love. I loves, loves, loves it. Can you see it? Can you feel it? Can you make it happen? Yes, yes, yes. This will be the Place Where We Renewed the World. I tapped my chest. "Right here." I looked around. "Right in all of us." (p. 195)

Imagine. Right now this can be the place where we—nurses—heal ourselves and reaffirm our purpose, and in doing so, renew the healthcare world. . . . Right here, right in all of us.

Having explored the many facets of compassion fatigue and burnout, it is hoped that readers now recognize their own vulnerability as well as that of their staff and coworkers. Lee Shulman (2009), president emeritus of the Carnegie Foundation for the Advancement of Teaching (Benner, Sutphen, Leonard, Day, & Shulman, 2009), reflected:

> . . . when I think about the preparation of nurses, I see key elements of preparing lawyers and teachers, engineers and ministers, physicians and psychotherapists, social workers and institutional managers. The work is physically grueling and intellectually taxing. It is both routine and filled with the unexpected and the surprising. Nursing education is preparation for remarkably hard work . . . Nursing is indeed a hybrid profession, an interdisciplinary and interprofessional nexus of roles and obligations. At its core, however, remain the expectations for caring and for advocacy, for ministering to the needs of those who are ill. Hybrids are often particularly robust because they combine the strengths of several species into one. But they may also be particularly vulnerable. (p. xi)

We cannot eradicate or overcome our vulnerability; however, by recognizing that we are all one, nurses can work together to transform the quality of living–dying for everyone.

Individually and collectively, we can heal from and/or avert compassion fatigue and the related syndrome of burnout. Nurses are natural warriors. Not warriors in the ways of aggression, but rather warriors of nonaggression—people who bear witness to the suffering of others and try to alleviate it. Chodron (2001) noted that these warriors—the bodhisattvas—are people who "hear the cries of the world" and are willing to train "in the middle of the fire," meeting challenges that take unbelievable courage and perseverance to overcome, and doing so despite sometimes enormous degrees of discomfort to oneself (p. 5).

Caring for a 4-year-old with multiple trauma who is clearly dying, and bearing witness to not only that child's suffering but also that of his family members, takes colossal courage. Sitting with a woman during the night who is in terrible pain with advanced cancer, knowing she will not live to see her children reach adulthood, sharing her life story, her hopes and regrets, or holding an 18-month-old who is dying of AIDS, never having really lived; these are no simple tasks. Standing up to a physician (or anyone for that matter) who does not respect what you bring to the healthcare world—saying no, this is not right, or we can do it better—these are all acts of the warrior, the bodhisattva.

EVERYONE IS A VIP AND HAS THE RIGHT TO BE!

I had the misfortune to need surgery once more, this time for gallbladder disease. I again chose the surgeon carefully. Preadmitting snags the day of surgery almost convinced me to turn around and go home. The nurse who took my vital signs and admitting history was curt, and at times downright rude; it seemed apparent that she hated her job. The nurse who came to start my IV line told me her entire family medical history as she fished around for quite a while in the same puncture site for a vein, until I finally requested she remove the needle and start from scratch.

Postoperatively I was extremely nauseated (this time it was nausea!) and the two nurses I had to depend on during my brief 4-hour sojourn in ambulatory recovery were travel nurses. I made a point of telling them at the onset that I was a nurse, since I had not done this the last time I was in a hospital and I was rather hoping it might make this experience a bit more positive. Though both were efficient, I very clearly overheard one tell the other that she "couldn't stand caring for patients who told her they were nurses or physicians," because, she said, "they want to be treated as VIPs." I thought at the time that she was really saying this for my benefit since she made no attempt not to be overheard. The thing is, I have never believed that any one person is more important or more entitled to quality healthcare (or anything else for that matter) than another. It was my feelings of both fear and vulnerability related to memories of my previous hospitalization experience that had motivated me to speak up about being a nurse.

As an educator, I am always looking for teachable moments that arise in our experiences. I have used this story in classes to get at the fact that we are all vulnerable, even if we are healthcare professionals. One day the majority of us will take at least one turn in a hospital bed. Having thought about her comment no small amount, I have the following rejoinder as both a patient *and* as a nurse. I do not want to be treated as a "very important person," a VIP. I want to be treated as I would treat you. I want to be treated as if I were one of your loved ones, for that is how I would most assuredly treat you, and that has always, always, been my mantra during my entire nursing career.

I do not want to make any excuses for my fellow nurses. Having a tough shift, week, or month just is not a good enough excuse for any of us to provide *dis*passionate and, on occasion, substandard care. In nursing, to *care* must mean to look at the whole, not the parts. Human beings are living things, not inanimate objects; a patient is not an IV, a Foley, a dressing change, or a set of vital signs. I want to reiterate that we have an autonomous practice and that we are never *ordered* to do anything. We provide care, when it is prescribed, because *we* believe it is the *right* care to assist in healing. There is power in numbers and we are many. In concert we *can* ensure that the care provided to people is not only the most knowledgeable but also the most compassionate care we can muster.

In the motion picture *Patch Adams*, there is a line that goes something like this: "I want the knowledgeable prick . . . not the clown." Well, I for one would rather the compassionate clown who is knowledgeable, instead of a dispassionate, albeit knowledgeable professional. I want the person who treats me as a person, not an inert object. I want the person who will advocate for me and who wants to participate in my healing. I want all of this for all people; *we are all VIPs*. To that end I will continue to remind colleagues, nurses, and physicians, alike, to think carefully before acting and to continually ask your selves, "Would I be providing this care, in quite this same manner, if this person were my loved one?" I invite my colleagues to try this line whenever you witness someone providing care dispassionately. Together we might all renew our purpose in healthcare.

Speaking Up

One of the repeating themes throughout this book that I would draw attention to here has been the notion of *speaking up*. About a decade ago the Joint

Commission (2011) began a great initiative called "Speak Up." These days there are signs on the walls in many facilities encouraging recipients of healthcare to *speak up* if they do not see their healthcare providers washing their hands, or if they have concerns about treatments. Folks are being told to pay attention to the care that they are being provided. Patients are given key points to help prevent the occurrence of errors in healthcare as follows:

- Speak up if you have questions or concerns.
- Pay attention to the care you get—make sure the treatments you receive are the right ones.
- Educate yourself about your illness.
- Ask a trusted family member or friend to be your advocate.
- Know what medications you take and why you take them.
- Use healthcare facilities that have been checked out.
- Participate in all decisions about your treatment (Joint Commission, 2011)

If your hospital has adopted a "Speak Up" or another such initiative to help safeguard patients, you need to reflect upon whether or not your facility is really living it or just paying lip service to it. It is ironic that we can have overt signs and guidelines encouraging people to speak up while healthcare providers (not just nurses) often seem to become quite annoyed with patients and/or families who do speak up. Indeed, far too frequently, when colleagues—nurses and physicians—or their loved ones are the recipients of care and they speak up, even they are treated by their healthcare providers—colleagues—as if they are a threat or a nuisance or both. Is not their advocacy for themselves or their loved ones in our best interests, too? Do we not all want the same thing? We are saying we want our patients to speak up, and then when they do so, we take offense.

From the many years of listening to horrible stories from other patients and families, including nurses and physicians, I can tell you that it seems like many places do not want anyone to speak up. People are oftentimes made to feel as if they are burdens; it seems to be a commonly voiced complaint of patients and their loved ones, who, as a result, many times feel that they cannot voice any concerns to their healthcare providers. Yes, family members, and especially those who might seem to "know too much," can appear to get in the way sometimes. Yet, more often than not, what they have to contribute to the care we are rendering can help us to meet the goals of care, if only we would take the time to pay attention and listen to them. In order to fix our healthcare system we need to develop the idea of *speaking up* a little bit better. In today's lingo, we cannot just talk the talk, we need to walk the talk.

Not only should patients and their loved ones speak up; as I have said throughout the preceding pages, nurses must speak up, too. The system does not and will not work well without us; *we* are the superglue that holds it all together, and if we stand firm, we can actualize whatever potentials we can envision. We need not give up our values, our compassion, our goals of care, our ethic. We can say no, this is not right, and this does not work. If we mobilize together as one, while we still may not be able to have a utopia in healthcare, we will be able to work collectively in a state of contentment, at least most of the time. We can work *heartfully* together.

Regaining Our Passion

The 2018 American Nurses Association (ANA) theme was the Year for Advocacy. Advocacy needs to be for all—both carers and cared for. Reaffirming purpose in nursing and healing our wounded workforce will undoubtedly and positively transform healthcare, for "Healing in its essence is about breaking through the fears associated with life—fears that we don't want to face—and finding our own special inspiration, a vision of the future, that we know we're here to help create" (Redfield, 1996, p. 66). If we can regain our passion and become re-enchanted, it will be a win-win for all.

In nursing we have such a vast opportunity; how many people get to participate in the unceasing dance of human life and death on such a large scale? To bear witness to another's suffering, to be with people during both birthing and dying experiences, and everything in between, all of it is such an honor. We have a moral responsibility to do it right. The moral imperative is not just for those entrusted to our professional care, but for ourselves as well!

Maybe the template we need to use is Cinderella. . . she is one of my all-time favorite Disney characters. Recently, after watching Cinderella with my granddaughter, I found a great blog, written by Audrey van Petegem (2015), on the more recent version (with actresses Lily James and Cate Blanchett). This blogger nailed it on many of the life lessons that were shared in this motion picture. I think we should use them in nursing! The first one is the most potent, and classic: "have courage and be kind." The others she notes are as follows: "don't give away your power to anyone"; "no matter how bad things get stay true to yourself"; "there is always something to sing about"; there is nothing wrong with believing in a bit of magic"; "you reap what you sow"; "practice forgiveness"; and "happily ever after is possible." So, there you have it! Be brave and compassionate. Never sell yourself short; you are important. Follow your heart and be true to your authentic self; take care of others the way you would want yourself or a loved one to be cared for. Sing through your days and love what you do; be happy doing it.

Make This Time Our Tipping Point

As I come to the closing, I find myself thinking about tipping points and choices. Gladwell (2000) wrote that:

> There is more than one way to tip an epidemic . . . Epidemics are a function of the people who transmit infectious agents, the infectious agent itself, and the environment in which the infectious agent is operating. And when an epidemic tips, when it is jolted out of equilibrium, it tips because something has happened, some change has occurred in one (or two or three) of those areas. (pp. 18–19)

It is up to us, individually and collectively, to turn this epidemic around. It is our choice.

We can choose to overlook rather than acknowledge that there is a problem and we can continue to allow it to get increasingly out of control. Or we can accept that there is a problem and do something about it. We can allow our admirable profession to have a reputation for bullying and incivility, and we can discourage all the "would-be" wonderful nurses right out of it. Or we can get to the crux of the matter and stop this behavior, getting help for the bullied *and* the bullies. We can support and encourage our young so that the "would-be nurses" know that they will be supported to become the wonderful nurses we know they can be. I think we all would rather that our profession does not have a reputation for bullying and incivility. It is far better for us to remain pictured beside those physicians and kittens as the epitome of compassion. Far better, too, for us to remain at the top of the Gallup poll, where we have been for many years and where we rightfully belong.

In a formula for leading change with Relationship-Based Care (RBC) models, Koloroutis (2004) notes that we need to understand five key conditions—"the 5 Cs"—that support our ability to participate in change: clarity, competency, confidence, collaboration, and commitment (pp. 9–10). While compassionate caring is notably evident everywhere in RBC models of care and thus one may think it is subsumed into any depiction of competency in the profession of nursing, for the purpose of understanding and emphasizing its importance, we could make it a stand-alone sixth "C."

Each of us has butterfly power. As we work, we *can* ditch the robot-like action and reconnect with ourselves and others. We can mind our moments and make them meaningful. For as the saying goes, we will not pass this way again—the moments with patients and their loved ones, just as those we spend with colleagues and loved ones, count and can be joyful, *heartful* moments. We *can* speak the mantra, "I will not die an unlived life." *Live* the mantra as Dawna Markova (2000), renowned inspirational writer and speaker, encourages in her poem and book of wisdom. She beseeches us to live on purpose, to explore ways to make contributions to our world that fulfill and renew us.

A few years back, while talking about butterfly effects and butterfly power, I decided we needed a word to reflect and remind us of the purposeful acts that we should strive to do as we go about our living and working. Naturally, it had to be a term associated with butterflies! I coined the term "flutterbying" and defined it as, "enhancing and transforming the quality of living-dying for all—through mindful awareness of our butterfly power and its effects" (Todaro-Franceschi, 2013). It has not made it into the modern dictionary yet; but I remain hopeful. Ask yourself on occasion: Are you flutterbying?

There is power in numbers. It is really all about having "power with" rather than "power over." It is about actualizing our potential assertively and collectively through knowing participation rather than aggressively, in acts of power as control (Barrett, 2010). We need to teach it, preach it, and live it. The time to do so is now.

Eugene Peterson (1994), a Presbyterian pastor, professor, and author, shared some insightful thoughts concerning why there is a crisis in care: "Instead of being cared for people find themselves abused, exploited, organized, bullied, condescended to, and ripped off" (pp. 66–67). It is noted that the crisis of care we find ourselves in seems to have developed from:

> Something . . . subtle and pervasive, and far more likely to involve the well-intentioned rather than the ill-willed. In order to do something about it, it is not enough to get rid of a few bad eggs in our respective professions. Something like a renovation of the imagination is required—a re-visioning of who we are and what we are doing that recovers the essential sacredness of all vocational caring . . . (p. 67)

We have to first begin by re-visioning and appreciating ourselves and each other. Society most truly should know the value of the nurse as a healing presence, the person who, with knowledge and competence, *compassionately* and *passionately* cares and advocates for the healing and well-being of all. Begin with being compassionate to yourself and passionate about yourself. Then reconnect with others.

The most potent nursing intervention we have at our disposal is not technological in nature, nor is it directly related to our knowledge and skills. It is related more to our humanness and the ability to provide true presence, in whatever capacity we can offer it. Nurses have a responsibility, a personal and professional ethic, and the *power* to knowingly engage in healthcare practices that benefit *us* and *others*. We bring gifts to our community of patients every day; it is our calling to do so. Yet, as author Dan Millman (2000) notes: "If we wait until we have permission, until we feel more motivated, until it gets easier, until fear vanishes, or hell freezes over, we may miss the chance to act at all" (p. 74). Do not let a lifetime of precious moments go by. As I tell senior students getting ready to go out into the world of nursing: Robots are not wanted here!

The end result of a windfall or snowball effect is transformational change; nothing less is called for in this era where there is a critical shortage of nurses and recruitment and retention of experienced staff is an ever-increasing problem. Combined with enormous challenges in the provision of quality care related to economic burdens, it is more than time to build a community of self and other care. It is time to heal ourselves and each other.

Whether you are currently in practice or in school, look carefully at the prospects before you. Is there ample opportunity for you to round out your skills to enable you to be all that you can be? You do not need to learn more about that barnyard of chickens that Chenevert (1988) wrote about. You want to learn how to fly! Maybe you are an eagle, or perhaps you are a butterfly. . . .

> Above them were thousands and thousands of monarchs riding a current across the sky. It was impossible to guess exactly how many there were. She felt humbled watching them. These fragile, heroic voyagers, each following an age-old instinct, formed a magnificent river of purpose flowing across the sky. (Monroe, 2011, p. 321)

Imagine. Millions of nurses all working *together in harmony*. Transformers of living–dying, engaged in the most important work there is—for what could be more important than assisting people to actualize their potentials to live well and die well? Nurses are just like butterflies; we make people smile and we transform, for the better, those whose lives we touch. We are fragile, and we are heroic. We *are* a magnificent river of purpose flowing through healthcare.

REFERENCES

Antieau, K. (2008). *Ruby's imagine*. Boston, MA: Houghton Mifflin.

Baldacci, D. (2000). *Wish you well*. New York, NY: Hachette.

Barrett, E. A. M. (2010). Power as knowing participation in change: What's new and what's next. *Nursing Science Quarterly, 23*(1), 47–54. doi:10.1177/0894318409353797

Benner, P., Sutphen, M., Leonard, V., Day, L., & Shulman, L. (2009). Foreword. In *Educating nurses: A call for radical transformation* (Jossey-Bass/Carnegie Foundation for the Advancement of Teaching). Kindle Edition. Retrieved from www.amazon.com

Chenevert, M. (1988). *STAT: Special techniques in assertiveness training for women in the health professions.* St. Louis, MO: C.V. Mosby.

Chodron, P. (2001). *The places that scare you: A guide to fearlessness in difficult times.* Boston, MA: Shambala.

Gladwell, M. (2000). *The tipping point: How little things can make a big difference.* New York, NY: Little Brown.

Gordon, S. (2005). *Nursing against the odds: How health care cost cutting, media stereotypes, and medical hubris undermine nurses and patient care.* Ithaca, NY: ILR Press (an imprint of Cornell University Press).

Hand, L. (2011). *One fourth of ICU clinicians report inappropriate care.* Retrieved from http://www.medscape.com/viewarticle/756089_print

Joint Commission. (2011). *Speak up.* Retrieved from Joint Commission: http://www.jointcommission.org/assets/1/6/speakup.pdf

Koloroutis, M. (Ed.). (2004). *Relationship-based care: A model for transforming practice.* Minneapolis, MN: Creative Health Care Management.

Liu, E., & Noppe-Brandon, S. (2009). *Imagination first: Unlocking the power of possibility.* Kindle version. San Francisco, CA: Jossey-Bass.

Markova, D. (2000). *I will not die an unlived life: Reclaiming purpose and passion.* San Francisco, CA: Conari Press.

McAndrew, N. S., Leske, J., & Schroeter, K. (2016). Moral distress in critical care: The state of the science. *Nursing Ethics, 25,* 1–19 (e-published ahead of print). doi:10.1177/0969733016664975

Millman, D. (2000). *Living on purpose: Straight answers to life's tough questions.* Novato, CA: New World Library.

Monroe, M. A. (2011). *The butterfly's daughter.* New York, NY: Gallery Books.

Peterson, E. H. (1994). Teaching us to care and not to care. In S. S. Phillips & P. Benner (Eds.), *The crisis of care: Affirming and restoring caring practices in the helping professions* (pp. 66–79). Washington, DC: Georgetown University Press.

Redfield, J. (1996). *The tenth insight: Holding the vision.* New York, NY: Warner Books.

Remen, E. N. (1996). *Kitchen table wisdom: Stories that heal.* New York, NY: Riverhead Books.

Shulman, L. S. (2009). Foreword. In P. Benner, M. Sutphen, V. Leonard, & L. Day (Eds.), *Educating nurses: A call for radical transformation.* Kindle version (Location 112–193). San Francisco, CA: Jossey-Bass/Carnegie Foundation for the Advancement of Teaching. Kindle Edition. Retrieved from www.amazon.com

Todaro-Franceschi, V. (1999). *The enigma of energy: Where science and religion converge.* New York, NY: Crossroad.

Todaro-Franceschi, V. (2013). *Are you flutterbying?* Retrieved from http://www.qualitycaring.org/blog/2013/11/02/are-you-flutterbying

van Petegem, A. (2015). Have courage and always be kind and 7 other lessons Cinderella teaches us. *Huffington Post.* Retrieved from https://www.huffingtonpost.com/audrey-van-petegem/have-courage-and-always-be-kind-and-7-other-lessons-cinderella-teaches-us_b_8710602.html

Appendix A
ProQOL Tool for
Self-Assessment
of PQOL

COMPASSION SATISFACTION AND COMPASSION FATIGUE
(PROQOL) VERSION 5 (2009)

When you [help] people, you have direct contact with their lives. As you may have found, your compassion for those you [help] can affect you in positive and negative ways. The following are some questions about your experiences, both positive and negative, as a [helper]. Consider each of the following questions about you and your current work situation. Select the number that honestly reflects how frequently you experienced these things in the *past 30 days*.

1 = Never	2 = Rarely	3 = Sometimes	4 = Often	5 = Very often

_____ 1.   I am happy.

_____ 2.   I am preoccupied with more than one person I [help].

_____ 3.   I get satisfaction from being able to [help] people.

_____ 4.   I feel connected to others.

_____ 5.   I jump or am startled by unexpected sounds.

_____ 6.   I feel invigorated after working with those I [help].

_____ 7.   I find it difficult to separate my personal life from my life as a [helper].

_____ 8.   I am not as productive at work because I am losing sleep over the traumatic experiences of a person I [help].

_____ 9.   I think that I might have been affected by the traumatic stress of those I [help].

_____ 10. I feel trapped by my job as a [helper].

_____ 11. Because of my [helping], I have felt "on edge" about various things.

_____ 12. I like my work as a [helper].

_____ 13. I feel depressed because of the traumatic experiences of the people I [help].

_____ 14. I feel as though I am experiencing the trauma of someone I have [helped].

_____ 15. I have beliefs that sustain me.

_____ 16. I am pleased with how I am able to keep up with [helping] techniques and protocols.

_____ 17. I am the person I always wanted to be.

_____ 18. My work makes me feel satisfied.

_____ 19. I feel worn out because of my work as a [helper].

_____ 20. I have happy thoughts and feelings about those I [help] and how I could help them.

_____ 21. I feel overwhelmed because my case [work] load seems endless.

_____ 22. I believe I can make a difference through my work.

_____ 23. I avoid certain activities or situations because they remind me of frightening experiences of the people I [help].

_____ 24. I am proud of what I can do to [help].

_____ 25. As a result of my [helping], I have intrusive, frightening thoughts.

_____ 26. I feel "bogged down" by the system.

_____ 27. I have thoughts that I am a "success" as a [helper].

_____ 28. I can't recall important parts of my work with trauma victims.

_____ 29. I am a very caring person.

_____ 30. I am happy that I chose to do this work.

Based on your responses, place your personal scores in the following. If you have any concerns, you should discuss them with a physical or mental healthcare professional.

Compassion Satisfaction _____

Compassion satisfaction is about the pleasure you derive from being able to do your work well. For example, you may feel like it is a pleasure to help others through your work. You may feel positively about your colleagues or your ability to contribute to the work setting or even the greater good of society. Higher scores on this scale represent a greater satisfaction related to your ability to be an effective caregiver in your job.

The average score is 50 (SD 10; alpha scale reliability .88). About 25% of people score higher than 57 and about 25% of people score below 43. If you are in the higher range, you probably derive a good deal of professional satisfaction from your position. If your scores are below 40, you may either find problems with your job, or there may be some other reason—for example, you might derive your satisfaction from activities other than your job.

Burnout _____

Most people have an intuitive idea of what burnout is. From the research perspective, burnout is one of the elements of compassion fatigue (CF). It is associated with feelings of hopelessness and difficulties in dealing with work or in doing your job effectively. These negative feelings usually have a gradual onset. They can reflect the feeling that your efforts make no difference, or they can be associated with a very high workload or a nonsupportive work environment. Higher scores on this scale mean that you are at a higher risk for burnout.

The average score on the burnout scale is 50 (SD 10; alpha scale reliability .75). About 25% of people score above 57, and about 25% of people score below 43. If your score is below 43, this probably reflects positive feelings about your ability to be effective in your work. If you score above 57 you may wish to think about what at work makes you feel like you are not effective in your position. Your score may reflect your mood; perhaps you were having a "bad day" or are in need of some time off. If the high score persists or if it is reflective of other worries, it may be a cause for concern.

Secondary Traumatic Stress _____

The second component of CF is secondary traumatic stress (STS). It is about your work-related, secondary exposure to extremely or traumatically stressful events. Developing problems due to exposure to others' trauma is somewhat rare but does happen to many people who care for those who have experienced extremely or traumatically stressful events. For example, you may repeatedly hear stories about the traumatic things that happen to other people, commonly called vicarious traumatization. If your work puts you directly in the path of danger, for example, field work in a war or area of civil violence, this is not secondary exposure; your exposure is primary. However, if you are exposed to others' traumatic events as a result of your work, for example, as a therapist or an emergency worker, this is secondary exposure. The symptoms of STS are usually rapid in onset and associated with a particular event. They may include being afraid, having difficulty sleeping, having images of the upsetting event pop into your mind, or avoiding things that remind you of the event.

The average score on this scale is 50 (SD 10; alpha scale reliability .81). About 25% of people score below 43, and about 25% of people score above 57. If your score is above 57, you may want to take some time to think about what at work may be frightening to you or if there is some other reason for the elevated score. While higher scores do not mean that you do have a problem, they are an indication that you may want to examine how you feel about your work and your work environment. You may wish to discuss this with your supervisor, a colleague, or a healthcare professional.

WHAT IS MY SCORE AND WHAT DOES IT MEAN?

In this section, you will score your test so you understand the interpretation for you. To find your score on each section, total the questions listed on the left and then find your score in the table on the right of the section.

Compassion Satisfaction Scale

Copy your rating on each of these questions on to this table and add them up. When you have added them up, you can find your score on the table to the right.

3. ____
6. ____
12. ____
16. ____
18. ____
20. ____
22. ____
24. ____
27. ____
30. ____

Total: ____

The sum of my Compassion Satisfaction questions is	So my score equals	And my Compassion Satisfaction level is
22 or less	43 or less	Low
Between 23 and 41	Around 50	Average
42 or more	57 or more	High

Burnout Scale

On the burnout scale you will need to take an extra step. Starred items are "reverse scored." If you scored the item 1, write a 5 beside it. The reason we ask you to reverse the scores is because scientifically the measure works better when these questions are asked in a positive way though they

*1. ___ = ___
*4. ___ = ___
8. ___
10. ___
*15. ___ = ___
*17. ___ = ___
19. ___
21. ___
26. ___
*29. ___ = ___

Total: ___

The sum of my Burnout questions is	So my score equals	And my Burnout level is
22 or less	43 or less	Low
Between 23 and 41	Around 50	Average
42 or more	57 or more	High

can tell us more about their negative form. For example, question 1, "I am happy," tells us more about the effects of helping when you are not happy, so you reverse the score.

You Wrote	Change to
1	5
2	4
3	3
4	2
5	1

Secondary Traumatic Stress Scale

Just like you did on Compassion Satisfaction, copy your rating on each of these questions on to this table and add them up. When you have added them up, you can find your score on the table to the right.

2. ____
5. ____
7. ____
9. ____
11. ____
13. ____
14. ____
23. ____
25. ____
28. ____

Total: ____

The sum of my Secondary Trauma questions is	So my score equals	And my Secondary Traumatic Stress level is
22 or less	43 or less	Low
Between 23 and 41	Around 50	Average
42 or more	57 or more	High

Appendix B
PPACD Tool for Preparedness and Ability to Care for the Dying

PERCEPTION OF PREPAREDNESS AND ABILITY TO CARE FOR THE DYING (PPACD) R-I SCALE © TODARO-FRANCESCHI

DIRECTIONS: Please circle one best answer for each question	Comments
1. I feel very comfortable listening and talking to patients and their loved ones about death, dying, and bereavement. • *Strongly agree* • *Agree* • *Disagree* • *Strongly disagree*	
2. I rate myself as highly competent in my ability to talk to patients and their loved ones about death, dying, and bereavement. • *Strongly agree* • *Agree* • *Disagree* • *Strongly disagree*	
3. Compared to your colleagues, how would you rate your competency regarding your ability to talk and listen to patients and their loved ones about death and bereavement? • *Much more* • *More* • *A little less* • *Much less*	
4. I rate myself as highly competent in my ability to provide pain and symptom management at the end of life. • *Strongly agree* • *Agree* • *Disagree* • *Strongly disagree*	
5. Compared to your colleagues, how would you rate your competency regarding your ability to provide pain and symptom management at the end of life? • *Much more* • *More* • *A little less* • *Much less*	
6. Generally speaking, do you feel able to provide quality care to the dying and their loved ones? • *Yes* • *No*	

Appendix C
Resources

The following list is a small sample of the materials available on the Internet related to topics covered herein. It is meant to be only a starting point for more information. Please note that some of these resources may fit other categories as well—it is all one!

All of these websites were accessible as we went to press. Since then, they may have changed or may no longer be available.

HEALING COMPASSION FATIGUE

Quality Caring: This website is my own. You can find information and resources related to my work (www.qualitycaring.org).

Professional Quality of Life Elements Theory and Measurement: Provides extensive, free access to research and data regarding compassion satisfaction, compassion fatigue (secondary traumatic stress), and burnout. Includes Beth Stamm's "Professional Quality of Life" (ProQOL) Scale to assess compassion satisfaction, fatigue, and burnout. Additional materials can be accessed at this site, along with an extensive reference list compiled by Beth Stamm and colleagues (www.proqol.org).

Compassion Fatigue Awareness Project: Provides information to promote awareness about compassion fatigue and its effects on carers. Offers educational workshops, suggested reading, self-tests, and other resources.

Sterling Heart: Caring for Caregivers: Identifies resources for healthcare professionals regarding compassion fatigue, burnout, grief/loss, and stress relief through the use of readings, music, self-care tips, and workshops. Also acknowledges the importance of spirituality and provides guidance for deepening spirituality (www.sterlingheart.com/index.html).

© Springer Publishing Company DOI: 10.1891/9780826155214.ap03   **269**

The Headington Institute: Care for Caregivers Worldwide: Specifically targets relief and humanitarian workers. Offers trainings, counseling, and a variety of online resources, including podcasts, self-assessment questionnaires, and workshop outlines (www.headington-institute.org).

Watson Caring Science Institute: Dr. Jean Watson is a distinguished nurse scholar, theorist, and educator. She offers insight into the caring and healing we do as nurses and encouragement to persevere through hardship (www .watsoncaringscience.org).

Companion Arts: This is a nonprofit organization dedicated to providing resources to caregivers and includes links to other influential speakers (www.companionarts.org).

Dr. Elizabeth Barrett: Elizabeth A. M. Barrett is a distinguished nurse scholar, theorist, and practitioner. This site gives an overview of her theory of power as knowing participation in change, along with information on health patterning, power prescriptions, and the Power-Imagery Process codeveloped with imagery pioneer and physician Jerry Epstein (www.drelizabethbarrett.com).

Commonweal: This nonprofit health and research institute aims to create a safer world for all people. More specifically, the Institute for the Study of Health & Illness offers a variety of programs for healthcare professionals to reconnect with compassionate healing work (www.commonweal .org).

ORGANIZATIONS DEDICATED TO HEALING TRAUMA

The Center for Victims of Torture: This international organization is engaged in healing, research, training and advocacy efforts for victims of torture. They have also taken over management of the ProQOL tool and website since founder, Beth Stamm's retirement (www.cvt.org).

Traumatology Institute: Dedicated to alleviating trauma through education, research, and training. This organization offers training and certification in a variety of areas related to trauma, including compassion fatigue, and also courses to become a clinical traumatologist and a compassion fatigue specialist (psychink.com).

Gifts From Within: PTSD Resources for Survivors and Caregivers: DVDs, background information, an extensive collection of webcasts, art, music, poetry (for members), support groups, retreats, conferences, workshops, meditation techniques, and both humorous and inspirational stories (www.giftfromwithin. org/html/What-is-Compassion-Fatigue-Dr-Charles-Figley.html).

The Figley Institute: This institute aims to alleviate the impact of trauma for both professionals and nonprofessionals through trauma training at various education levels. They provide online courses, workshops, and trainings. They also offer certification courses to become a field traumatologist, compassion fatigue educator, and certified traumatologist (www .figleyinstitute.com).

The Sidran Institute: traumatic stress education and advocacy—The philosophy of this institute is to help heal trauma through connection and empowerment. They offer an extensive resource list to promote education and self-help, which includes books, workbooks, textbooks, training manuals, DVDs and videos, and educational tools. They also have ongoing projects nationwide, education programming, and trainings (www.sidran.org).

Traumatic Incident Reduction Association: Traumatic incident reduction therapy is a method used to reduce stress associated with past traumatic experiences. The website offers links to professionals, trainings, and workshops to help cope with and overcome trauma (includes a recovery program specific to compassion fatigue; www.tira.org).

The Green Cross: This traumatology academy offers support and guidance in times of acute crisis or trauma through crisis counseling, ongoing counseling, and referral services. Additionally, this institute contains training programs to become a certified traumatologist or compassion fatigue educator/therapist (greencross.org).

INCIVILITY/BULLYING RESOURCES

The Workplace Bullying Institute: Founded by psychologists Drs. Gary and Ruth Namie, experts on workplace violence, the goal of this organization (the first and to date, only one in the United States focused on workplace bullying and incivility) is to understand and prevent workplace abuse. The website is very extensive and offers a wealth of information about bullying, emphasizing that the victim is not alone and not helpless. Resources include access to research and legislation, a blog, training for individuals, professionals, and employers, coaching and the creation of an action plan for individuals being bullied, speeches, books, audio recordings, and DVDs. Recently a two-book volume on workplace mobbing in the United States was published, edited by Duffy and Yamada—more information on this can be found online (www.workplacebullying.org).

American Nurses Association: The organization offers resource materials for nurses, including information on workplace violence and safety (www.nursingworld.org/practice-policy/work-environment). Specific to nurse incivility and bullying: www.nursingworld.org/practice-policy/work-environment/violence-incivility-bullying

HEALING ADDICTION RESOURCES

Addiction Recovery Resources for the Professional: Includes information on addiction and recovery, self-test, book list and resources list, stories, and support for finding help (www.lapage.com/arr).

Hazelden: This organization specializes in addiction treatment and has a specific program for healthcare professionals. The program includes group therapy, tips for reentry into the workplace, lectures, and peer-to-peer support (www.hazelden.org/web/public/addiction_treatment_health_care_professionals.page).

Unbecoming a Nurse: Bypassing the Hidden Chemical Dependency Trap: This website was developed by nurse Paula Davies Scimeca and is a supplement for her authored book on the subject, to offer help for nurses struggling with substance abuse. The website has a variety of resources including FAQs, interviews, a blog, articles, events, retreats, a self-survey, and a list of other resources (www.unbecominganurse.org).

Peer Advocacy for Impaired Nurses: Founded by Jack Stem, a recovering CRNA, this website offers a wealth of information and resourceful links. He also offers educational workshops, recovery mentoring, and relapse prevention to individual nurses (www.peeradvocacyforimpairednurses.com).

The Addiction Recovery Guide: Extensive guide to help with addiction recovery for anyone suffering with substance abuse/addiction. Includes links to programs nationwide, a message board, alternative therapies, and relapse prevention resources (www.addictionrecoveryguide.org).

ON MINDFULNESS AND SELF-CARE

Mindful: All about being mindful—"living with awareness and compassion." Created by Shambhala Sun Foundation (www.mindful.org).

Mindful Hub: Wellbeing, Right Now: This website is dedicated to encouraging healthcare professionals to practice being mindful and also has specific information regarding compassion fatigue. It offers free worksheets and newsletters, articles, resources, and e-consultation (for a fee); www.mindfulhub.com/category/topics/well-being

Stress Relief Choices: This website addresses stress relief for healthcare professionals and offers tips such as including exercise and healthy eating as well as meditation, deep breathing, and visualization. Coaching, classes, as well as free resources, a newsletter, and recommended reading are also available (www.stress-relief-choices.com/stress-management-for-nurses.html).

American Holistic Nurses Association: The organization focuses on holistic healthcare and emphasizes caring for the carers. Their website offers a lot of useful information on self-care and techniques for stress management, including, yoga, tai chi, dance, art, massage, journaling, energy work, and prayer (www.ahna.org/Resources).

Assertiveness Quiz: This quiz evaluates one's level of assertiveness and offers links to articles regarding conflict resolution and communication, including benefits of assertiveness, daily stress tips, and how to improve relationships (stress.about.com/library/assertiveness_quiz/bl_assertiveness_quiz.htm).

Skills Converged: Training Materials on Productivity, Soft Skills, and Personal Development: This website offers free training resources, games, icebreakers, role-plays, and exercises regarding team building, time management, communication skills, conflict resolution, and emotional intelligence for all ages and groups. My favorite: *The Butterfly Effect*, an exercise that demonstrates how a subtle change can have a lasting and far-reaching impact (www.skillsconverged.com/Home/tabid/229/Default.aspx).

Quality Caring: Drop into my healing garden room for a refresher on being mindfully aware and appreciating your moments (www.qualitycaring.org/healing-garden-room).

MORAL DISTRESS AND HELP WITH ETHICAL DILEMMAS

American Nurses Association: Link to our code of ethics, position statements, and a number of excellent online journal articles related to moral distress and moral courage (www.nursingworld.org/practice-policy/nursing-excellence/ethics).

American Association of Critical-Care Nurses (AACN) Ask Affirm Assess Act: The 4 A's to Rise Above Moral Distress is a wonderful guide to help nurses recognize and address moral distress at the workplace (www.aacn.org/WD/Practice/Docs/4As_to_Rise_Above_Moral_Distress.pdf).

AACN also offers a free Healthy Work Environment Assessment Tool: www.aacn.org/nursing-excellence/healthy-work-environments

ALL ABOUT COMPASSION AND HEALTHY WORK ENVIRONMENTS

Center for Building a Culture of Empathy: Dedicated to building a worldwide community of compassion and empathy. Includes articles, conferences, definitions, expert opinions, historical and scientific information, interviews, and videos (cultureofempathy.com).

Empathy and Healthcare (from the aforementioned website): A collection of articles from the news about empathy and healthcare (www.scoop.it/t/empathy-and-healthcare).

Compassion Lab: This organization is made up of a collection of researchers offering resources to enable the creation of organizations using a compassionate foundation. The website includes teaching materials, presentations, publications, and access to like-minded researchers (www .compassionlab.com).

TED Conferences: A collection of inspirational speeches and talks regarding compassion (www.ted.com/themes/the_charter_for_compassion .html).

Positive Psychology: This website is dedicated to promoting positivity and happiness, in thought and action. There is access to literature, related resources, and an annual conference (www.positivepsychology.net).

The Center for Nonviolent Communication: This international organization is founded on the basis that we are all compassionate, nonviolent beings. Through trainings, video, audio, resources, bookstore, e-forums, connection to others, and more, they encourage embracing a nonviolent ideology to resolve conflict peacefully and effectively (www.cnvc.org).

AACN's Healthy Work Environments Initiative: Promotes healthy work environments through conferences, continuing education, research, and collaboration (www.aacn.org/wd/hwe/content/hwehome.pcms?menu=hwe).

HeartMath: Aims to promote health and well-being through training programs, publications, and "emWave" technology, resulting in outcomes including: employee retention, reduced costs, decreased stress and anxiety, and increased productivity. Contains a section specific to healthcare (www .heartmath.com).

Center for Positive Organizational Scholarship: Dedicated to improving leadership through "positive organizing." The website offers a wide array of substantial resources, including suggestions for beginners, education opportunities, literature, teaching materials, and video (https://positiveorgs .bus.umich.edu).

Project Resilience: This website provides a lot of information related to resilience, which supports those interested in creating a more supportive work environment. They also offer a train-the-trainer program for those interested in working with youth or adults (projectresilience .com/index.htm).

Adventures in Caring: This organization is engaged in teaching "the art and practice of compassion in the service of healing." They offer many materials, resources, and training for both formal and informal carers. One of their more recent programs, developed after the first edition of this text had been published, focuses on preventing and healing burnout "Oxygen for Caregivers." The program can be found on their website (www.adventures incaring.org).

INFORMATION ON BURNOUT

European Institute for Intervention and Research on Burnout: This website includes information, self-test, news, coping techniques, trainings, and seminars (www.burnout-institute.org/index_en.php).

Headington Institute: Provides a description of burnout, ways to protect yourself against burnout, and various self-tests (www.headington-institute .org).

Psychology Today: This website offers a number of informational and self-help articles on burnout (www.psychologytoday.com/us/basics/ burnout).

END-OF-LIFE CARE (AND EDUCATION)

American Association of Colleges in Nursing ELNEC: End-of-Life Nursing Education Consortium (ELNEC) program information is available through their website along with a frequently updated list of ELNEC program offerings. There is also a link to web resources related to end-of-life care (www.aacnnursing.org/ELNEC).

City of Hope Pain and Palliative Care Resource Center: Their website offers a database of reference materials regarding end-of-life care, along with an extensive web-based listing of other Internet websites (prc.coh.org).

Hospice and Palliative Nurses Association: This organization is dedicated to promoting excellence in hospice and palliative nursing care. The website offers information on education and resources for nurses (www.hpna.org).

National Hospice and Palliative Care Organization (NHPCO): Dedicated to improving the quality of care at the end of life through hospice and palliative care efforts. A wealth of materials is available (www.nhpco.org/ templates/1/homepage.cfm).

National Hospice Foundation: A partner organization of NHPCO, their website offers additional information on end-of-life care (www.national hospicefoundation.org).

Center to Advance Palliative Care: Offers materials to aid in development of palliative care programs. Palliative care tools, education, resources, and training for healthcare professionals can be accessed through their site (www.capc.org).

Hastings Center: This organization is dedicated to addressing, through research, education, and policy making, ethical issues in health, medicine, and the environment that affect people. A significant part of their work deals with end-of-life care (www.thehastingscenter.org).

ON APPRECIATIVE INQUIRY AND
MEANINGFUL RECOGNITION

Appreciative Inquiry Commons: Dedicated to the study, application, and dissemination of information related to appreciative inquiry. They offer many resources, including access to classic articles and case exemplars (appreciativeinquiry.case.edu).

The Daisy Foundation: This foundation was created in honor of J. Patrick Barnes who suffered and died from an autoimmune disease. The family created this nonprofit organization and brought meaningful recognition in nursing to the forefront with their establishment of the DAISY award for extraordinary nurses, an inspirational recognition program that has been adopted in facilities throughout the world (www .daisyfoundation.org).

Also see prior listings for both the American Nurses Association and the AACN. Through their websites articles on meaningful recognition may be accessed.

WELL-BEING AND HAPPINESS

Mayo Clinic Well-Being Index: A tool invented by Mayo Clinic to measure and focus on professional carer well-being. Housed at MedEd (www.mededwebs.com/well-being-index).

The Science of Well-Being: Yale University's most popular course is available for free online. (www.coursera.org/learn/the-science-of-well-being).

Action For Happiness: This movement is "committed to building a happier and more caring society." The patron of this movement is the Dalai Lama. There is a wealth of inspiring information and resources on their website (www.actionforhappiness.org).

Positive Psychology Program: Their website offers a large array of materials related to many of the topics in this book. In particular, there are many articles and accessible exercises on compassion, self-compassion, and mindfulness (positivepsychologyprogram.com/category/happiness).

TO SEE THINGS YOU NORMALLY DO NOT SEE

The Energy Enigma: My website on the enigma of energy, death and dying, and synchronicity (www.energy-enigma.com).

Journey North: On this website, you can sign up to receive e-news on the migration of various wildlife—monarchs, hummingbirds, whooping cranes, and several other signs of spring news. You can also report your sightings (learner.org/jnorth).

Monarch Watch: For more information on the monarch butterfly and the migration (www.monarchwatch.org).

To follow my work on this subject:

Quality Caring: A website for nurses and other healthcare professionals interested in enhancing quality caring for both the cared for and the carers. Blog, links, and other resources (www.qualitycaring.org).

All of the opinions and information on these websites are theirs, not mine. I have no investment or interest (other than my own website). Readers should make note of individual website policies regarding privacy and membership. Every website differs.

Appendix D
Nurse Leader Resource Kit

The following is meant to be a companion to the book:

Todaro-Franceschi, V. (2019). *Compassion Fatigue and Burnout in Nursing: Enhancing Professional Quality of Life, 2nd Edition.* New York, NY: Springer Publishing.

Suggestions are made related to each part of the book to help guide leaders and educators to enhance staff work-life environment and quality of patient care. Use creativity; some of these activities can be continuous quality improvement (CQI) activities, too!

PART I: PROFESSIONAL QUALITY OF LIFE

1. The Good, Bad, and Ugly of Professional Quality of Life
2. Transforming Both Health and Care in Healthcare

Goal

To begin a discourse with staff (or students) about the meaning of professional quality of life and how it relates to quality caring.

The following can be done during 15 to 30 minutes of a staff meeting or class.

Provide the following basic information (you might want to use poster board):

- *Compassion contentment*: Feeling heartful—happy or joyful about the work one does

  Compassion fatigue: Feeling heart heavy—cosuffering with others—feeling emotionally and physically drained or like "I just cannot do this right now"

  Burnout: Feeling empty-hearted—apathetic, dragging, no energy, exhausted, cynical, "nothing I do matters" and "I just do not care." Feeling ROBOTIC

Questions for Reflection

- Why did you choose nursing (or a caring profession)?
- What does it mean to be a nurse, a carer?
- What does it mean to be healthy?
- What is the nature of healing?
- What does it mean to care for another?
- Do we need to *care* to contribute to health and healing?

Actions

Invite participants to share their thoughts and feelings about their own professional quality of life. Ask them to consider what contributes to how they feel at work. If they do not wish to share their thoughts publicly, you can offer a paper and pencil. Ask them to anonymously jot down their thoughts and feelings. Have someone collect the papers, and then, if you have time, as a group you can identify themes. The goal of this exercise is to identify feelings related to the good, the bad, and the ugly of professional quality of life.

Chart for Themes and Contributing Factors

Break up into small groups to identify and discuss what purposeful actions can be taken to replicate the good and minimize the bad. You can make another chart as in the preceding for actions.

Heartful	Heart heavy	Empty-hearted

(continued)

(*continued*)

Heartful	Heart heavy	Empty-hearted

Butterfly Effect Exercise

During a meeting or class take 30 minutes to do the butterfly effect exercise. It is posted around the Internet and has been used in many organizations for team building.

The exercise will have everyone laughing while learning the butterfly power of even the smallest subtle actions and that everything is connected to everything else. If you have a group larger than 15, break up into smaller groups of 8 to 10. After doing the exercise, discuss what happened, making note of how it changed the workings of the whole collectively. When I use this exercise with a group of individuals, I like to use a small, lightweight butterfly (flitter) beanie.

See *Skills Converged* (2011) for a free one-page download guide for the exercise: www.skillsconverged.com/FreeTrainingMaterials/tabid/258/article Type/ArticleView/articleId/855/The-Butterfly-Effect.aspx or for a slightly different and more in-depth variation at the Center for Quality Improvement (previously known as the National Quality Center) (2006) click on: national qualitycenter.org/files/nqc-game-guide-chapters/07-butterfly-effect-game

PART II: UNITY, PURPOSE, AND THE GOOD: AN ETHIC OF CARING

3. Compassion and Contentment: Being Heartful and Happy at Work
4. Values and Excellences in Nursing
5. The *ART* of Reaffirming Purpose: A Healing Model for Carers

Goal

To underscore how our connectedness and compassion provokes purposeful action, which in turn renews our sense of purpose as carers.

Each of the following exercises can be done in 30 minutes. The American Nurses Association (ANA, 2015) *Code of Ethics for Nurses* can help to guide this discussion. See the ANA website to view the code (www.nursingworld.org/practice-policy/nursing-excellence/ethics/code-of-ethics-for-nurses). You can have an introductory discussion about an ethic of care and the values/excellences in nursing or jump right into the exercises (see the following).

Questions for Reflection

- What is an ethic of care?
- What are our professional values and how do they relate to individual and collective professional quality of life?
- How do they contribute to our contentment (or feeling heartful) at work?

Actions

Provoking empathy thoughts is a great way to enhance awareness of ways to go about being more compassionate. During a staff meeting, show the 4-minute Cleveland Clinic (2013) video on empathy (www.youtube.com/watch?v=cDDWvj_q-o8) and then ask staff what came to mind while watching it. You might want to make a poster board to display on the unit as an "empathy" reminder. . .

One-Minute Mindfulness Exercise: STOP

If your facility has an outdoor area, and it is a nice day, it would be ideal to go outside. If not, you can do this in any area as long as there is space for everyone to stand. Have everyone Stop whatever they are doing and stand with their feet on the ground. Ask them to close their eyes, and focus attention on their connection to the floor/ground. Take a few deep breaths focusing on the in and out movement of air or you can take a few moments to Turn Toward yourself, acknowledging thoughts, emotions, or sensations. If there is anything negative, push it away from you on an exhalation. If it is positive, breathe it in. Then, open your eyes and Observe your surroundings slowly, and really notice them, seeing what you normally wouldn't see. Seek out something pleasant to focus on and be grateful for (there is always something to be grateful for). Proceed to explore how you are feeling right now in this moment and try to remain centered in it for a few more. . .

ART for Joy and Contentment

Take 15 minutes of a meeting (or class) to introduce the *ART*© model (Todaro-Franceschi, 2008, 2013, 2015). Break up into small focus groups to discuss each of the steps. Have one person take notes on common themes to share with the larger group. Future talks can entail focusing on *ART* for the bad, ugly, and uglier; for this first discussion the focus should be on the things that bring joy and/or make us feel good about our work (*ART* and life in general). Participants should be encouraged to also jot down notes on their individual reflections.

A—Acknowledging how one is feeling. Ask:

- Have you felt joyful or happy at work? When? What contributed to feeling that way? You can even expand on this if there is time by encouraging them to reflect upon what brings joy to their lives in general.

R—Recognizing choices and choosing purposeful actions to take. Think about how to replicate that happy feeling. Ask:

- What actions can be taken to enhance the joy in work and life? List them.

T—Turning toward self and other.[1] Encourage them to share thoughts and feelings with others in and out of work. After identifying what brings joy to the workplace, the goal is to turn toward those things mindfully, and get everyone to work together to replicate that joy. The same holds true for life in general.

PART III: THE BAD: COMPASSION FATIGUE AND MORAL DISTRESS

    6. Compassion Fatigue: A Heavy Heart Hurts
    7. Moral Distress: I Know What I Ought to Do!

Goal

To identify what compassion fatigue and moral distress feel like, if participants have ever experienced either/or both, and what can be done to heal from it.

Actions

Take 15 minutes to discuss compassion fatigue. Have someone read the narrative on John Doe to the group or alternatively, if you have Internet access you can have staff view *Vestiges*, a 5-minute digital story, at www.qualitycaring .org (Todaro-Franceschi, 2011, 2012, 2013). Then you can break up into small focus groups to discuss it or alternatively, ask staff if they want to share their own experiences of feeling heavy hearted.

ART for Compassion Fatigue

Apply the *ART* model (Todaro-Franceschi, 2008, 2013, 2015). *A*cknowledging feelings: Have participants jot down how they felt while watching the story. Ask them to complete the Secondary Traumatic Stress (Compassion Fatigue) part of Beth Stamm's ProQOL tool (Appendix A). Have any participants had similar experiences with feeling heavy hearted? Acknowledge them.

*R*ecognizing choices and actions to take: What did participants who experienced compassion fatigue do to overcome it? Were they successful in overcoming compassion fatigue? Brainstorm other actions that might be taken to help one another in instances where one is suffering with compassion fatigue.

Chart it!

Actions That Contributed to CF	Actions That Lessened CF	Other Possible Actions to Heal

CF, compassion fatigue.

*T*urn toward self and other: Encourage staff (or students) to seek out things that renew their spirit, things that bring them joy.

Based on the information arising from these exercises, the next step is formalizing and activating a plan to help staff who are compassion fatigued and/or avert it in future. Does the unit have a room for quiet reflection? Does your facility have a "Code Lavender" for individuals who need it? Is there something in place so staff can cover for one another when emotionally overwhelmed?

Feeling Free to Be Moral (An *ART* Exercise for Leaders)

You might be aware of ethical dilemmas in your work environment. Are they usually resolved in ways that *prevent* rather than create moral distress among staff? Do you, and does your staff, feel free to be moral? Apply the *ART* model (Todaro-Franceschi, 2008, 2013, 2015). *Acknowledge* whether or not there is a problem. If not, why not? List the reasons. *Recognize choices and purposefully take action*: have you, or can you, facilitate the creation of a safe space for them to enter where they will feel supported and can speak up? *Turn toward self and other*: reflect upon ways you can empower staff; enlist the support of other nurse leaders who might be facing similar issues.

PART IV: THE UGLY, UGLIER, AND UGLIEST: BURNOUT AND WORKPLACE VIOLENCE

8. Burnout: Feeling Empty-Hearted and Disheartened
9. Bullying and Incivility in Nursing: An Oxymoron

Goal

To discuss and address the ugly and uglier aspects of professional quality of life in healthcare.

Have a general discussion about the ugly (burnout) and uglier (bullying and incivility) aspects of professional quality of life. Because burnout can contribute to incivility and bullying, the first question you need to ask your staff (or students) is the one I offered at the beginning of the book. Do they look forward to going to work (or class)? If the answer is no, then they need to explore why that is the case.

Questions for Reflection

- Are you working with people who do nothing but complain and who seem cynical, complaisant, and perhaps callous? Are you one of those people?
- Do you work with patients who are suffering and no longer feel any anguish on their behalf?
- Do you walk into a room with loved ones surrounding the bed of one of your acutely ill patients and shut a switch or block any exchange of feelings with your methodical actions to provide care?

Actions

Encourage participants to make an effort while they are working to be more mindfully aware of the things that they dislike or things that they *used* to dislike and no longer notice. When burnout occurs, we tend to see and react less to things because apathy sets in. They need to recapture those negative feelings related to the things that used to bother them. Have them complete the burnout part of the questionnaire in Stamm's ProQOL survey (in Appendix A). Ask them to identify if they are manifesting any of the negative behaviors, feelings, and physical ailments related to burnout.

ART for Burnout

Apply the *ART* Model (Todaro-Franceschi, 2008, 2013, 2015). *Acknowledge* the feelings and manifestations because they hold the key not only to healing but also to evading compassion fatigue and burnout in the future. It might be helpful to give staff (or students) the following chart to complete for their own enlightenment.

Why I Do Not Want to Go to Work	Why I Want to Go to Work

What seem to be the most outstanding things on the list? What is the deal breaker... is it relational, workload, a lack of resources, the physical environment, or perhaps even the patient population they are working with? It could be anything—identify and acknowledge it. Once it is identified, participants will be ready to proceed to the next step, *Recognizing choices and taking purposeful action*. Everyone can explore together, as a whole, or in focused group sessions, how to facilitate whatever changes are needed to enable everyone to reaffirm purpose in the workplace. Poster board will be helpful here, too.

- What changes do they think can be made in practice or the work environment? What choices do they have that might make things better for each of them and their patients? List them. Now, how you can make them happen?

Self-Care Focus

If you are aware of or think that staff (or students) are suffering from burnout, self-care needs to be an additional focus. Your concern and willingness to show it will go a long way toward helping staff who are suffering from burnout to heal. Ask participants to reflect upon whether they might be suffering from physical or mental health issues as a consequence of their work. Stress the need to make choices that will help them to regain well-being. Then they need to take action—whether it is to seek medical, mental health, or employee assistance, begin an exercise or nutrition program, and so on. Stress that if anyone is feeling depressed or self-medicating with food, alcohol, pills, or some other form of drug, they need to seek appropriate help for it. Emphasize that as knowing participants there are always choices they can make (please see Appendix C, Resources).

Since burnout develops over time and there are usually a lot of things contributing to it, healing from it will not happen overnight. It is important to be kind and patient. Stress that with burnout, it is important to recognize that even though they do have many choices, some may not be able to stay in the work environment that they are currently in and be happy or healthy. Some things can be fixed and some cannot. It is not a failure to *acknowledge* it is time to move on—it is a choice—and it may be the best one for some people. In order to heal from burnout once it has been identified, one must make a real effort to be mindfully aware of how he or she is acting and how others are acting in the workplace. To undo the harm of long-standing toxicity, one needs to *Turn toward* (themselves and other), and be mindfully aware that this is a process of relearning ourselves by noting patterns of negativity and replacing those patterns with attentive listening and presencing for both ourselves and others.

ART Exercise: Have You Been Bullied or Are You a Bully?

This can be done in 30 minutes during a meeting or class time. Ask staff (or students) to pair up and then reflect upon the following (keeping notes). The goal is to apply the *ART* model (Todaro-Franceschi, 2008, 2013, 2015) in order to acknowledge and increase awareness of relational factors in their workplace that may be hindering professional quality of life; not to point any fingers at anyone.

- Was there ever an instance or situation where they felt unsupported and/or bullied by someone at work and if so, what behaviors made them feel badly? They should not allude to any information that would identify anyone specifically.
- Was there ever an instance or situation where they were uncivil to another person at work? If so, what behaviors did they portray that they would change now, having thought about it?

Exercise: The Old Eating the Young and the Young Eating the Old

If you have a small group (no more than 10) you can use a poster board. If larger, break up into groups for small focused discussions and have one person in each group take notes. Ask participants to think about and *acknowledge* their feelings related to coworker relationships (or if teaching, alternatively classmates or faculty), taking specifically into account how the more experienced nurses are treating the newer nurses and vice versa.

- What specific behaviors (on the part of experienced nurses toward new nurses and then conversely, on the part of new nurses toward experienced nurses) have been witnessed or experienced that contribute to feeling badly at work?
- What behaviors have you witnessed or experienced by nurses that contribute to feeling supported?

PART V: FACING DEATH

10. Being Prepared to Care for the Dying
11. Collective Trauma and Healing in Healthcare: Aching, Breaking Hearts

Goal

To prepare staff (or students) to care for those with serious illness/those who are dying and provide needed support to do it well.

Questions for Reflection

- How often does dying and death occur on the unit? How many patients are seriously or critically ill?
- Do the majority of patients have advance directives? If not, what mechanisms are in place on the unit to encourage discussion about how your patients want to live until they die? Remember advance directives are really about quality of living, not dying.

ART for Facing Death (or Caring for the Dying Patient)

Apply the *ART* model (Todaro-Franceschi, 2008, 2013, 2015). Have staff complete the PPACD assessment tool (Appendix B) (*A*cknowledgment of feelings). If there are a number of staff who share specific needs, for example, feeling unprepared to communicate with the dying and their families, or pain and symptom management, you can seek out End-of-Life Nursing Education Consortium (ELNEC) trainers in your facility who may be able to come and offer content-specific sessions for staff on the unit. If there are none, consider who might want to go for ELNEC training and come back to share their lessons with the rest of the staff (please see Appendix C, Resources, for more information). There are always courses being held in a number of locales. There should be a budget you can tap into for continuing education (*Recognizing choices and taking action*).

If your staff (or students) are working in an area where serious illness, dying, and death often occur, it is helpful to view the nature of that work as a collective traumatic experience. Does the facility you work in offer debriefing or support for staff? Are there support groups for patients and their families?

Practice an Occasional Collective OUCH

When things seem particularly stressful, for instance, when there have been emergencies with patients or when a death has occurred on the unit, you can hold an impromptu gathering for a few minutes to share a collective "OUCH" together. During the gathering, you could offer a prayer, or say a few words on making meaning from an experience with patients who are suffering and their loved ones. Connecting with one another to know we are all in it together (including leaders!) and making meaning benefit all of us engaged in healthcare practice (*Turning toward self and other*).

PART VI: BEATING THE ODDS

12. Changing the Mindset in Nursing Education
13. Cultivating Collective Mindful Awareness in Nursing: A Leadership Agenda
14. Imagining and Actualizing the Power of Nursing

Goal

To emphasize the importance of nursing, nurses, and self-compassion; the importance of mindful practice and compassionate caring.

Most of the following exercises can be found in the book in more detail (in the final chapters) and can be done in a brief period of time.

Making Time to See Things You Normally Do Not See

Have that occasional collective "OUCH" session and make it a time where people can get to know how others feel. Being able to say OUCH collectively means that you have to see, and encourage others to see, things you might not normally see (or that you have not been acknowledging)—becoming more mindfully aware. It also means that you have to go to places you normally avoid, and perhaps even the places that scare you.

Appreciating Moments Exercise

Share, or if you are a nurse leader, have your frontline nurses share, stories of their *caring moments* (Watson, 1999). Offering opportunities to share these moments not only shows recognition of their value, it also serves as teaching moments for other staff who may be distancing themselves for whatever reason. Whenever and wherever you can, build opportunities for storytelling of caring moments into the work environment. Build in time to make known the unknown about each other. Focus on the positive aspects of the environment and try to build upon them.

Hear Me, Hear You Exercise

Choose a partner. For 5 minutes one person talks—sharing some important experience in his or her life. To also work on the development of compassion skills, you can ask the person to share a loss of some kind—it does not have to be the death of a loved one; it can be any loss. During the 5 minutes one person is speaking, the other person must do nothing but listen. Those who are listening are not allowed to speak at all. At the end of the 5 minutes, have them switch places; the person being listened to becomes the listener and the other person gets to share a meaningful experience or loss. After the second 5 minutes is up, go around the room and have everyone share how they felt when they were listened to, and alternatively, how they felt when they listened. If there is not enough time to go around the room, have everyone reflect upon and later write down the following:

> I felt . . . when I was listened to.
> I felt . . . when I listened.

- Post their responses anonymously in the nursing lounge or on the course board. Have a discussion about them at your next meeting (or class).

Caution: Some folks have a *really* hard time with this exercise.

"I See Me and I See You" Exercise

This exercise, which I have arbitrarily named, is an adaption from Melodie Chenevert's (1988) shared gold mine of assertiveness training techniques. In a staff meeting (or a class), have everyone jot down one personal thing about themselves (e.g., I like to garden, and I love butterflies!), one good thing they like about themselves, and then one good thing they like about the person sitting on their left. Afterward, have each person in turn, going around the room, share how they felt when asked to do this and what they wrote about themselves and their colleague.

Having your staff or students do this exercise helps everyone get to know and appreciate one another.

Enhancing Self-Compassion

The following exercise entails becoming your own friend. The original exercise was developed by Kristin Neff (n.d.), who is an expert on self-compassion, and some variation of it is being used in many organizations. The following is a shortened version. More details on this and other exercises can be accessed at self-compassion.org/category/exercises.

Take a pen and paper to jot down your thoughts for each of the following:

- Think about a friend or loved one who has a rough day or experience.
- How would you (or did you) support that friend?
- Now think about yourself having the same rough day or experience.
- What do you do for yourself?

Most will probably *Acknowledge* that you do not treat yourself as well as you do others.

Recognize what choices you have and take purposeful action to become your own friend.

Turn toward yourself the same way you are compassionate toward others!

Teaching Compassion

Have a WOW! session with your staff if you can make the time. The TED talk *The Power of Empathy* by Helen Riess (2013) at TEDxMiddlebury gives some great rationale for everyone to cultivate human-to-human connection (www.youtube.com/watch?v=baHrcC8B4WM). Alternatively, try to find time to view it yourself, and then think about ways you might incorporate it into a staff meeting—even a piece of it would spur enhanced awareness of the importance and power of connectedness.

Mini CQI on Compassion

The following can be suggested to staff (or students) as something they can try during one of their shifts. Share the results in a staff meeting (and/or publishing it as a poster for everyone to see). Instruct each staff member (or student) to take two or three 5-minute periods during the course of a shift and simply observe one person during each period of time. While observing the person they should make note of the things that come to mind about the person and consider: What might be that person's story? What might the person they are observing be thinking or feeling? Finally ask them if, having done this exercise to observe others, it might prompt a change in their approach to care. There should not be any identifying information—the person should remain anonymous.

Have a *Wit* Moment, a *Patch Adams* Moment, or a *Tuesdays With Morrie* Moment

Check out YouTube for clips from these and other motion pictures that poignantly capture what it means to feel compassion (and what it can do when one tries to flick the shutoff switch). Show one or two short clips at a staff meeting and have a focused group discussion on key points (or, alternatively, ask participants to jot down their feelings about the clip and reflect upon them later).

Do a CQI Activity. . . on Compassion Contentment or Bringing JOY to the Workplace!

How about brainstorming with other leaders to do a systemwide CQI, which focuses primarily on compassion for the cared for *and* the carers, a CQI that explores the issues that feed into productivity, recruitment, and retention of the carers, as well as quality and safety of care for the patients—you know, the *whole*, everything together. Things that might be explored would evolve around compassion contentment for everyone, and in this way you could spruce up the quality of care rendered *and* quality of professional life at the same time. Imagine it and actualize it!

NOTE

1. The use of "self and other" is not a typo, it is a statement, based on a philosophic view that there are no other(s); all is one, and everything is inextricably connected (Todaro-Franceschi, 1999).

REFERENCES

American Nurses Association. (2015). *Code of ethics for nurses*. Retrieved from https://www.nursingworld.org/practice-policy/nursing-excellence/ethics/code-of-ethics-for-nurses

Center for Quality Improvement (previously known as the National Quality Center). (2006). *Butterfly effect game.* Retrieved from http://nationalqualitycenter.org/files/nqc-game-guide-chapters/07-butterfly-effect-game

Chenevert, M. (1988). *STAT: Special techniques in assertiveness training for women in the health professions.* St. Louis, MO: C.V. Mosby.

Cleveland Clinic. (2013). *Empathy: The human connection to patient care.* Retrieved from https://www.youtube.com/watch?v=cDDWvj_q-o8

Neff, K. (n.d.). *How would you treat a friend? Self-compassion exercise.* Retrieved from http://self-compassion.org/category/exercises

Riess, H. (2013). *The power of empathy: Helen Riess at TEDxMiddlebury.* Retrieved from http://www.youtube.com/watch?v=baHrcC8B4WM

Skills Converged. (2011). *The butterfly effect exercise.* Retrieved from http://www.skillsconverged.com/FreeTrainingMaterials/tabid/258/articleType/ArticleView/articleId/855/The-Butterfly-Effect.aspx

Todaro-Franceschi, V. (1999). *The enigma of energy: Where science and religion converge.* New York, NY: Crossroad.

Todaro-Franceschi, V. (2008). Preventing compassion fatigue and reaffirming purpose in nursing. *Proceedings on the 3rd European Federation of Critical Care Nursing Congress and 27th Aniarti Conference, Influencing Critical Care Nursing in Europe*, Florence, Italy (October).

Todaro-Franceschi, V. (2011). *Vestiges.* Retrieved from www.qualitycaring.org

Todaro-Franceschi, V. (2012). *Quality caring.* Retrieved from www.qualitycaring.org

Todaro-Franceschi, V. (2013). *Compassion fatigue and burnout in nursing: Enhancing professional quality of life.* New York, NY: Springer Publishing.

Todaro-Franceschi, V. (2015). The ART of maintaining the "care" in healthcare. *Nursing Management, 46*(6), 53–55. doi:10.1097/01.numa.0000465407.76450.ab

Watson, J. (1999). *Postmodern nursing and beyond.* Edinburgh, UK: Churchill.

Index

AACN. *See* American Association
of Colleges of Nursing and/
or American Association of
Critical-Care Nurses
AACN's Healthy Work Environments
Initiative, 274
*Acknowledging, Recognizing, and
Turning (ART). See ART*© model
Action For Happiness movement, 276
actuality
and *energeia*, 39, 48
and *eudaimonia*, 40, 48
Addiction Recovery Guide, 272
Addiction Recovery Resources for the
Professional, 272
Adventures in Caring, 274
advocacy, 110–111, 257
aesthetic knowledge, 104
alcohol abuse, 92
Alcoholics Anonymous program, 93
alternative-to-discipline (ATD)
programs, 92
altruism, 53–54, 76
American Association of Colleges of
Nursing (AACN), 180, 208,
217, 219
American Association of Critical-Care
Nurses (AACN), 273
4 A's to Rise Above Moral Distress
Model [ask, affirm, assess, and
act], 117, 273

American Holistic Nurses Association,
272–273
American Nurses Association, 271
apathy
and abusive power, 159–161
demoralization, 195
appreciative inquiry, 234–235, 276
ars moriendi (art of dying), 178
ART© model
acknowledgment of our feelings,
68–69, 239–240
applying for burnout, 139–142
applying for compassion fatigue,
93–96
applying for disconnection and
distancing, 64
applying for joy and contentment,
77–78, 282–283
applying for moral distress, 114–117
applying for posttraumatic stress
disorder, 201–202
applying in preparation to care for
the dying, 185–188
assertiveness training techniques,
241
butterfly memorial garden, 243–244
human-to-human connection, 64
listening exercise, 240–241
meaning making, 244
mindful awareness, 67–68
moral distress, 114–117

ART© model (*cont.*)
  nurseculture (see *nurseculture*)
  reaffirming purpose, 65–66
  recognition of choices, 70–75
  shift time overlap, 242–243
  substance use disorder, 91
  total quality management, 241–242
  turning outward toward self and
    other, 75–77
  workplace violence, 164–166
assertiveness
  advocacy skills, 216
  and training techniques, 108, 241
Assertiveness Quiz, 273
associate degree (AD), 109
authenticity, 54–55
autotelic self, 41

Bachelor of Science in Nursing (BSN),
  64, 109, 148, 175, 208
Barrett's theory of power as knowing
  participation in change, 113
bodhichitta, 43
Bohm's dialogue method, 116
brightly burning, 142
Buddhist practice, 67
Buffalo Creek collective trauma,
  194–196
bullying and incivility
  ANA Code of Ethics, 152
  ANA position statement, 152–153
  ANA professional issue panels, 152
  antagonistic environment, 150
  apathy and abusive power,
    159–161
  baby boomer nurses, 149
  culture of unsafety, 153–161
  economic impact, 152
  forms of violence, 149–151
  harm done, 151–153
  in healthcare work environments,
    152
  hierarchical/vertical violence, 150
  horizontal/lateral violence, 150
  new nurse, 148–149
  nursing education, 210–211

  nursing professional quality of life,
    147–148
  resources, 271
  silent voices and witnesses, 162–164
  toxic work environments, 152
  victims and recipients of, 152
  work dissatisfaction, 151
burnin, 142
burnout
  A Burnt-Out Case, Graham Greene,
    123–124
  anger, 131
  ART model, 139–142, 287
  clinical exemplar (Where Was the
    Nurse?), 132–136
  vs. compassion fatigue, 131
  complaisance, 138–139
  consequences, 137–138
  cumulative frustration, 127
  cynicism, 130
  definition, 124
  devaluing caring aspects, 128–129
  dimensions, 130
  disenchantment in action, 125, 126
  dispassionate care, 6, 136
  emotional and physical exhaustion, 5
  emotional exhaustion, 124
  failed survival strategies, 131
  heart empty, 5, 6, 125, 132
  heartless work, 5
  inequitable distribution of rewards
    and respect, 127
  job stress, 124
  male–female disparities, 126–127
  MOLST vs. POLST, 126
  nurses as "full partners," 126
  nursing education, 127–128
  phases, 129–132
  "physician's order," 126
  signs and symptoms, 89–90, 132
  technical skills and lab values, 127
burnout prevention
  brightly burning, 142
  butterfly power, 86
  energy transformation, 132
  nursing education, 127–128

Burnout Scale (ProQOL), 265, 266
butterfly (and butterflies). *See also*
    butterfly effect
  effect, 20, 273, 281
  and energy transformation, 243
  migratory pattern, 20–21
  Monarch, 20, 21
  9/11 memorial garden, 243
  power, 22, 85–88
  Terezin, children, 202
  why, 243
butterfly effect
  "butterfly power," 22
  dispassionate care, 21
  exercise, 281
  medication administering, 21

caring, 60
  compassionate (*see* compassionate
    caring)
  moments, 23, 64–65, 176, 240,
    289–290
  transcultural, 22
  transpersonal, 22
  unitary, 25
  wholeness, 16
caring for the dying. *See also* death
    denying; death education; end-
    of-life care
  applying *ART*, 185–188
  "Changing the Face of Death," 175
  code 99, 172–173
  critical care nurses, 175
  death denying and, 178–182
  importance of, 178–182
  medical necessity vs. futility, 182
  preparation for, 184–185
  teaching about, 173–178
Carper's patterns of knowing, 104
Center for Building a Culture of
    Empathy, 273
Center for Nonviolent
    Communication, 274
Center for Positive Organizational
    Scholarship, 274
Center for Victims of Torture, 270

Center to Advance Palliative Care, 275
"Changing the Face of Death," 175, 252
chaos theory, 20, 22
Chodron, 8, 43, 238, 254
CISD. *See* critical incident stress
    debriefing
City of Hope (COH) Pain and
    Palliative Care Resource
    Center, 275
civility
  interventions, 232
  and professional behavior, 216
  RBC model, 232
clinical nurse leader (CNL), 128,
    216–218, 231
clinical nurse specialist (CNS), 105,
    128, 217
CNL. *See* clinical nurse leader
CNS. *See* clinical nurse specialist
code of ethics, 52–53
collective compassion fatigue, 10
collective healing, 199–201
collective mindful awareness
  appreciative inquiry, 233–234
  ART model, 238–244
  compassion lessons, 219–221
  consciousness transformation, 228
  Magnet model, 234–237
  nursing theory, 235–237
  positive work culture, 232–233
  RBC model, 231–232
  spiritual component, 228
  staff development, 229–231
  transformational leadership,
    229–231
  workplace engagement (*see*
    workplace environment)
collective trauma. *See also*
    posttraumatic stress disorder
  acts of terror and natural disasters,
    192, 193
  ART model, 201–202
  Buffalo Creek disaster, 194–196
  collective healing, 199–201
  critical incident stress debriefing,
    192–193

collective trauma (*cont.*)
  healing, 199–202
  logotherapy, 199
  loss of communality, 194–196
  meaning making, 198–199
  9/11, 193–194
  religious faith, 198
Commonweal, 270
communal, 36
Companion Arts, 270
compassion. *See also* compassionate
    caring
  and Aristotle, 36
  bodhichitta, 43
  and Cassell, 36–37
  and Chodron, 43
  and Dalai Lama, 42
  definition, 36
  and Dossey, 36
  and Frost, 37, 38, 229, 230
  lessons, 219–220, 252
  and Nussbaum, 42
  provokes purposeful action, 37–38,
    238
  values and excellences (or valuing),
    60–61
  virtue, 53
compassion contentment. *See also*
    happiness
  ART model, 77–78
  CQI activity, 241–242
  exemplar (Nurse Katie), 16
  exemplar (Rubies and Gems), 34–36
  heartful work, 5
compassion fatigue
  ART model, 93–96, 283–284
  vs. burnout, 5
  collective, 10
  cosuffering, 89
  critical incidents, 9
  death overload, 7
  definition, 84
  exemplar (*Vestiges: The Story of John
    Doe*), 6–8
  heavy heart, 5

  leadership positions, 11
  negative feelings, 4
  prevention, 93
  signs and symptoms, 89–90
  substance use disorder, 91–93
  suffering, 85
  traumatic stressors, 85–88
  work conditions, 10
Compassion Fatigue Awareness
    Project, 269
Compassion Lab, 274
Compassion Satisfaction Scale, 265,
    266
compassionate caring, 60–61. *See also*
    compassion; nursing and
    compassionate caring
  Antieau's *Ruby's Imagine*, 33–34
  cognitive requirements, 42
  communal, 36
  devaluing, 128–129
  loving-kindness, 42–43
  Magnet® hospital program, 45–46
  open heart, 42–43
  pity, 36
  productivity, 44–45
  purposeful action, 37–38
  RBC model and, 258
  vulnerability, 84
  work satisfaction, 43–44
Competencies And Recommendations
    for Educating undergraduate
    nursing Students (CARES), 219
complaisance, 138–139
consciousness transformation, 228
contentment
  actuality and potentiality, 39
  autotelic self, 41
  awareness and appreciation, 39
  bodhichitta, 43
  creativity, 40
  eudaimonia, 40
  flow, 42
  optimal experiences, 41
  peak experiences, 41
  phenomenon of second wind, 40–41

professional quality of life, 38–39
quality of care, 38
self-actualization, 39
transformational skills, 41–42
continuous quality improvement
(CQI), 105, 241–242
creativity, 40
critical care, 7, 17, 34, 111, 183, 184
critical incident stress debriefing
(CISD), 192–193
cronyism, 150–151
Csikszentmihalyi, 41–42
culture of unsafety, 162–163
cynicism, 130

Daisy Foundation, 276
death denying
cancer patients, 180
coffee drinking, 178
end-of-life care, 180–181
healthy aging, 19, 173
kids die too, 172
Kübler-Ross, 179, 181
living–dying process, 181–182
mandatory death education, 181
medically futile treatment, 180,
182–184
Medicare fee-for-service decedents,
180
slow codes, 172
and weekend exercise, 178
death education
"Changing the Face of Death"
elective class, 175
clinical experiences, 175–178
critical care nurses' perceptions of
preparedness, 175
death overload, 88–89
difference between palliative care
and end-of-life, 174
emotional exhaustion, 177–178
end-of-life care, 174, 175, 177, 178,
184, 186
hospice and palliative care settings,
174, 176–177

importance of, 184–185
Jeanne Quint Benoliel's work, 178
student engagement, 175–176
demoralization, 195
depersonalization, 128–129
disenchantment in action, 125, 127
dispassionate authoritarian
management, 230–231
dispassionate care, 21
do not resuscitate (DNR), 16, 177, 216
doctor of nursing practice (DNP)
program, 128
doctor's orders, 55–57
accountability, 57
questioning, 57–60
dying patients, caring for
death experiences, 172–173
last day memories, 172

eating disturbances, 91
economic impact bullying/incivility,
152
Education in Palliative and End-of-
Life Care (EPEC) project, 180
ELNEC. See End-of-Life Nursing
Education Consortium
EMS, 175, 192
emergency department (ED), 65, 73,
88, 139, 175, 176, 184
"emotional contagion," 84
empathy, 60
Empathy and Healthcare, 273
empirical knowledge, 104
employee assistance program (EAP), 92
end-of-life care, 218–219, 275. See also
death denying; death education
death education, 174, 181, 184
death overload, 88–89
initiatives, 180
Jeanne Quint Benoliel's work, 178
teaching, 69
wholeness of caring work, 16
End-of-Life Nursing Education
Consortium (ELNEC), 180,
217, 275

energy
  actuality and potentiality, 39
  all is one, 41
  Aristotle on, 39
  butterflies and, 20–22
  energy transformation, 18–19
  happiness, contentment and, 39–40
  health and healing, 19–20
  ideas of, 17–19
  James' "The Energies of Man," 40
  purposeful change, 18, 70, 243
  self-actualization and, 39–42
  synchronicity and, 70, 276
Energy Enigma website, 276
ethic of care, 18–19
ethical knowledge, 104
ethics
  bioethics, 209
  code of, 52–53, 102, 152
  nursing, 214
European Institute for Intervention
    and Research on Burnout, 275
exemplary nurse, 54, 231

facing death. See also death denying;
    death education
  and appreciating life, 177
  opportunity, 179
  preparedness for, 184–185
Figley Institute, 270–271
flow
  being hurtful, 132
  connecting with self and other, 93
  optimal experiences, 41
  synchronicity and, 71

Gallup public opinion poll, 110
"gendered labor," 103
good work environment, 233. See also
    healthy work environment
Green Cross, 271

happiness, 237–238. See also
    compassion contentment;
    contentment)

employee happiness, 44, 232–233,
    242
eudaimonia, 40
joy, 77, 237–238
well-being and, 276
Hastings Center, 275
Hazelden organization, 272
Headington Institute, 270, 275
healing addiction resources, 272
health and healing, 17, 19–20
healthy work environment, 45, 47,
    113, 244, 273, 274
HeartMath, 274
hidden curriculum, nursing
    education, 209–210
hierarchical/vertical violence, 150
horizontal/lateral violence, 150
Hospice and Palliative Nurses
    Association, 275
hospice care, 176, 177, 179, 183, 275
hospitalonian captivity, 102
human caring, 55. See also
    compassionate caring

ICU. See intensive care unit
"illusory self," 77
institutional disincentives, 102
instrumental care, 23
intensive care unit (ICU), 11, 17, 34,
    72, 73, 85, 100, 112, 179, 180
intimidating and disruptive
    behaviors, 152

JEWELS program, 163
Journey North website, 276
joy. See happiness

leadership
  compassionate and, 93
  Magnet model and, 45, 46
  nurse leaders, 38, 40, 44, 216–218,
    242
  and quality of care, 11, 38
  sentinel events, 233
  toxic, 229–231

toxin handlers, 229–231
Leininger, M., 22, 23
licensed practical nurse (LPN)
    shortages, 44
life-limiting illnesses, 85
listening exercise, 240–241
logotherapy, 199
loss of communality, 194–196

Magnet® hospital program, 45–46
Magnet model, 234–235
Maslach Burnout Inventory (MBI),
    130
Maslow's idea of self-actualization, 39,
    40, 55
Mayo Clinic Well-Being Index, 276
MBSR. *See* mindfulness-based stress
    reduction
Me Too movement, 163
meaning and purpose of our work, 20,
    28, 93, 220–221, 238
meaningful coincidences, 70–71. *See
    also* synchronicity
Medical Orders for Life-Sustaining
    Treatment (MOLST), 126
medically futile care
    burnout risk, 183
    Callahan's argument, 175
    compassion fatigue risk, 183
    evidence-based practice, 175
    moral distress, 183
    Patient Self-Determination Act,
        183
    qualitatively futile treatment, 175
    quantitatively futile treatment, 175
mindful awareness (mindfulness),
    67–68. *See also ART*© model
    finding joy, 237
    nurseculture and, 215
    in nursing, 67–68
    reaffirming purpose and, 219
    teaching, 222
mindfulness-based stress reduction
    (MBSR), 222
mobbing, 150

MOLST. *See* Medical Orders for Life-
    Sustaining Treatment
Monarch butterfly. *See* butterfly
Monarch Watch, 277
moral distress
    ART model, 114–117, 284
    assertiveness, 108–109
    cause of anguish, 111–112
    choice, 105
    clinical nurse specialists, 105
    continuous quality improvement
        project, 105
    definition, 100
    feeling powerless, 113
    "gendered labor," 103
    hospitalization experience, 99–100
    hospitalonian captivity, 102
    indication, 101
    institutional disincentives, 102
    manifestations, 101
    moral courage, 113
    moral environment, 102–103
    moral residue, 109
    noncredible knowers, 103
    nursing education, 101, 106–107
    opposing internal and external
        factors, 100
    patterns of knowing, 103–104
    power, 106
    self-sacrificing nurse, 112–113
    "whistle-blowers," 110
moral mute, 151

Narcotics Anonymous program, 93
narrative storytelling, 68
National Hospice and Palliative Care
    Organization (NHPCO), 275
National Hospice Foundation, 275
neonatal intensive care unit (NICU),
    172, 173
New York State Nurse Practice Act, 57
NICU. *See* neonatal intensive care unit
Nightingale, 19, 26–28, 136
noncredible knowers, 103
notions of good, 22

nurseculture, 23, 218, 224, 241
  ART model and, 223–224
  assertiveness and advocacy skills, 216
  character building, 215
  CNL role and, 216–218
  compassion lessons
    cheating, 220
    imagery exercise, 220
    Levine's poignant story, 221
    Nussbaum's practical strategies,
      219–220
    self-compassion, 222
    storytelling, 220
  end-of-life and palliative care,
    218–219
  lifelong commitment to service,
    215–216
  mindful awareness, 215
  nursing theory, 216 (*see also* nursing
    and compassionate caring)
nurse practitioner (NP), 105, 128, 153
nursing and compassionate caring.
    See also nursing theory
  Benner's work, 25–26
  "call to care," 16–17
  end-of-life care, 16
  expressive care, 23
  health and healing, 17, 19–20
  ICU setting, 17
  instrumental care, 23
  Leininger's theory of transcultural
    caring work, 22–23
  Newman's health as expanding
    consciousness theory, 25
  Nightingale's symbolic
    representation, 26–27
  nurseculture, 23
  Parse's humanbecoming theory,
    24–25
  Relationship-Based Care (RBC
    model), 25
  Rogers' science of unitary human
    beings, 24
  Smith's unitary caring, 25
  Watson's theory of human caring,
    22–24

nursing education
  apprenticeships, 212
  ART model, 223–224
  Benner's *From Novice to Expert*,
    213–215
  bioethics, 209–210
  burnout, 127–128
  Carnegie Foundation report, 212
  cost and profession, 214–215
  emotional component, caring
    practices, 214
  expert practitioner, 213–214
  fundamental elements, 212–213
  healthcare sectors, 208
  hidden curriculum, 209–210
  incivility, 210–211
  IOM reports, 211
  nurse needs and care, 211–212
  nursing ethics, 214
  oxygen mask importance, 211
  RWJF Initiative, 207–208
  self-care strategies, 214
nursing ethics, 214
nursing theory, 216. *See also* nursing
    and compassionate caring

one-minute mindfulness exercise, 282
optimal experience, 41–42
organizational change management,
    234–235
Overeaters Anonymous program, 93
oxygen mask, 54, 211

palliative care, 174, 218–219
Parse's humanbecoming theory, 24–25
Patient Self-Determination Act, 183
peak experience, 41
pediatric
  emergency room, 14, 172
  intensive care unit (PICU), 172
  trauma, 192
Peer Advocacy for Impaired Nurses, 272
Perception of Preparedness and
    Ability to Care for the Dying
    (PPACD) R-I scale, 267–268
personal knowledge, 104

Physician Orders for Life-Sustaining
    Treatment (POLST), 126
PICU. *See* pediatric intensive care unit
pity, 36
POLST. *See* Physician Orders for
    Life-Sustaining Treatment
Positive Psychology Program, 274,
    276
positive workplace culture
    characteristics, 232–233
    good work environment, 233
posttraumatic stress disorder (PTSD),
    84
    ART model, 201–202
    and collective trauma, 193–194
    and compassion fatigue, 197
    contributing factors, 196
    in healthcare, 195
    and loss of communality, 194–196
    natural disasters, 196
    9/11, 193–194
    potentiality, 39
    symptoms of, 196–197
    terrorism, 192
    veterans of war, 196
power
    and advanced practice nurses,
        96–97, 253
    advocacy, 213
    Barrett's theory of power, 113
    choice and, 96–101
    clinical skill competency, 252
    compassion education, 252
    compassion fatigue and burnout,
        253
    equitable compassionate care,
        254–255
    imagination, 251–252
    nurse as natural warriors, 254
    nurses as primary transformers,
        16–17
    reaffirming purpose, 257
    Remen's nature of healing, 250
    "Speak Up" initiative, 255–257
    tipping points and choices, 258–260
    and voice, 102

PPACD scale. *See* Perception of
    Preparedness and Ability to
    Care for the Dying Scale
preparedness to face death
    ART model, 185–188, 288
    death denying, 178–182
    end-of-life care education, 184
    moral distress and, 180
    why it's important, 184–185
presence, 54–55
primary trauma, 88
Professional Quality of Life Elements
    Theory and Measurement, 269
Professional Quality of Life Scale
    (PROQOL), 263–266, 269
Project Resilience, 274
PROQOL scale. *See* Professional
    Quality of Life Scale
psychic entropy, 41
Psychology Today, 275

quality care, 40, 43, 45, 46, 214
quality caring, 46–47
Quality Caring website, 269, 273, 277
quality and safety, 20, 26, 38, 52, 233,
    242, 292

reaffirm(ing) purpose
    in nursing and healing, 65–66
Relationship-Based Care (RBC)
    model, 25, 231–232, 258
resilience programs, 237–238
Robert Wood Johnson Foundation
    (RWJF) Initiative, 207–208
Rogers' science of unitary human
    beings, 24
root cause analysis, 38
Ruby's Imagine book, 33–34

Science of Happiness, 237. *See also*
    happiness
Science of Well-Being, 276
secondary trauma, 87
secondary traumatic stress (STS), 84
Secondary Traumatic Stress Scale, 265,
    266

self-actualization, 39
  Maslow, 39, 40, 55
self-care, 142, 202, 214, 272–273,
        286–287. *See also* oxygen mask
self-compassion, 291
self-sacrificing nurse, 112–113
senior leadership, 232
sense of oneness, 20, 194
sense of one's own salience, 215, 223
Sidran Institute, 271
silent voices and silent witnesses, 162
  culture of unsafety, 162–163
  JEWELS program, 163
  Me Too movement, 163
  "MeTooinHealthcare" movement,
      164
  silence breakers, 164
  "Speak Up" initiative, 255–257
  Time's Up movement, 164
Stress Relief Choices website, 272
STS. *See* secondary traumatic stress
substance use disorder (SUD), 91–93
suffering
  bearing witness to, 94, 150, 187, 254
  bodhichitta, 43
  bullying and, 151
  burnout and, 131, 132, 286
  collective, 195, 202
  compassion and, 4, 5, 7, 36
  compassion fatigue and, 101, 126
  death overload, 88
  facing death, 187
  finding or making meaning, 198,
      199
  moral distress, 17, 101
  from trauma, 193, 201, 202
synchronicity, 70, 71

theory of human caring (theory of
      transpersonal caring), 22
therapeutic caring presence, 54–55
therapeutic use of self, 64, 129
Time's Up movement, 164
total quality management (TQM),
      241–242

toxic leader, 229
toxic leadership
  exemplar, 230–231
  kinds of, 229
  toxic leader, 229
toxin handlers, 229–231
transcultural caring theory, 22
transformational leadership
  goal for, 229
  good leader, 229, 235
  "handler" of toxicity, 229–230
transpersonal caring theory (theory of
      human caring), 22
trauma (and traumatic stressors)
  collective (*see* collective trauma)
  dying and death, 88–89
  exposure to, 85, 265
  moral distress, 100
  negative subtle influences, 86–87
  primary trauma, 85, 88
  prolonged exposure, 85
  secondary trauma, 87
  technologizing/dehumanizing
      suffering, 86
Traumatic Incident Reduction
      Association, 271
Traumatology Institute, 270

unconditional bodhichitta, 43
unitary caring, 25

values and excellences
  altruism, 53–54
  ANA Code of Ethics, 52–53
  compassion, 53, 60–61
  "doctor's orders," 55–57
  questioning "orders," 57–60
  therapeutic caring presence, 54–55
voice. *See also* assertiveness; power
  complaisance and, 138
  moral courage, 112
  of the nurse, 56, 59, 138, 235
  silent, 162
  vibrant, 24
  of women, 108